T0177643

Sport, Exercise and Performance Psychology

Sport, Exercise and Performance Psychology

Research Directions to Advance the Field

EDSON FILHO AND ITAY BASEVITCH

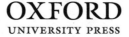

OXFORD

UNIVERSITY PRESS

OXFORD
UNIVERSITY PRESS

Oxford University Press is a department of the University of Oxford. It furthers
the University's objective of excellence in research, scholarship, and education
by publishing worldwide. Oxford is a registered trade mark of Oxford University
Press in the UK and certain other countries.

Published in the United States of America by Oxford University Press
198 Madison Avenue, New York, NY 10016, United States of America.

© Oxford University Press 2021

Library of Congress Cataloging-in-Publication Data
Names: Filho, Edson, editor. | Basevitch, Itay, editor.
Title: Sport, exercise and performance psychology :
research directions to advance the field / Edson Filho, Itay Basevitch.
Other titles: Sport, exercise and performance psychology
(Oxford University Press)
Description: New York, NY : Oxford University Press, 2021. |
Includes bibliographical references and index.
Identifiers: LCCN 2021023962 (print) | LCCN 2021023963 (ebook) |
ISBN 9780197512494 (hardback) | ISBN 9780197512517 (epub) |
ISBN 9780197512524 (online)
Subjects: LCSH: Sports—Psychological aspects—Research. |
Exercise—Psychological aspects—Research | Sports—Physiological
aspects—Research. | Self-efficacy. | Sports sciences.
Classification: LCC GV706.4 .S657 2021 (print) |
LCC GV706.4 (ebook) | DDC 796.01—dc23
LC record available at https://lccn.loc.gov/2021023962
LC ebook record available at https://lccn.loc.gov/2021023963

DOI: 10.1093/oso/9780197512494.001.0001

Printed by Marquis, Canada

Contents

SECTION 2   HEALTH AND WELL-BEING

SECTION 3 CULTURAL AND PROFESSIONAL ISSUES

Foreword

Edson Filho and Itay Basevitch

125 Novel Research Questions to Guide Future Research
in Sport, Exercise and Performance Psychology

Editors' Positionality

Know thyself.

—Oracle of Delphi

In Ancient Greece, thousands of people would visit the Temple of Delphi
to ask questions about their future. A large scripture at the entrance of the
temple reminded the visitors that before seeking knowledge about their
future, they should be attuned to their present, inside world. In editing
this book, we asked experts from around the world, each with a unique
background and theoretical and methodological outlook, to propose
questions that can propel the field of sport, exercise, and performance psychology into the future. We consider ourselves "global citizens" and holistic
researchers, and as such, we believe that multiple theoretical stances and
empirical methods are needed to study the manifold topics that exist in
our field.

The idea for this book originated over a decade ago, when we were both
graduate students, during a drive back to campus from our weekly Monday
night soccer game. At the time we were both reviewing literature for our
dissertations in search for "gaps." On the return trip to campus, we talked
about the difficulty of finding a meaningful research idea to inform our
dissertations, and the challenges with navigating vast amounts of literature without knowing the key essential readings—that is, "Where do you
start when your literature search returns hundreds of articles of both classic
and contemporary literature?" As the conversation progressed over the 25-
minute drive, we discussed how most book chapters and peer-reviewed

manuscripts conclude with a short section (usually one or two paragraphs) discussing avenues for future research; we connected the dots and this was a Eureka moment for us! We decided that night that one day we would edit a book together focusing on (a) open research questions that address the unknown in the field and (b) key readings for a given subfield or topic within the field of sport, exercise, and performance psychology. We were inspired by the writings of some of the best philosophers of all time, and we wanted to put forth a resource that could help students and seasoned researchers to identify some of the key questions that must be addressed to move our field forward. In essence, we envisioned the book to be a database of the most important questions to address—one of the main sources for researchers across the world and at various points in their career, updated every few years in accordance with theoretical, methodological, practical, and of course technological advancements in the field.

Philosophical Positionality

The Socratic Method: A Book About Questions

> True knowledge exists in knowing that you know nothing.
> —Socrates

Socrates, the father of Western Philosophy, never ceased asking questions. We believe scholars need this curiosity and intellectual humility to advance the knowledge base across domains. To this day, the so-called Socratic Method is a fundamental pillar of scientific research and evidence-based practice (e.g., Overholser, 2018; Stenning et al., 2016). Research projects are based on questions that, when addressed properly, might provide us with answers and, most certainly, generate more questions. Likewise, practitioners informed by an evidence-based practice philosophy must ask their clients key questions (e.g., needs assessment or a performance profile) to design an effective and personalized intervention plan (Rousseau & Gunia, 2016). Put plainly, this book is primarily inspired by the Socratic Method. Each chapter starts with a brief overview of "what we know" followed by five open research questions about "what we know that we don't know" that should be addressed to move our field forward.

In Quest for Enlightenment: Theoretical, Methodological, and Applied Questions to Shed Light Into "What We Know That We Don't Know"

Dare to know!

—Immanuel Kant

The rationalist Descartes taught us to use our reasoning to "doubt everything" ("The Omnibus Dubitandum"; see Broughton, 2003), and the empiricist Francis Bacon once said that "by far the best proof is experience." Thanks to Immanuel Kant, who unified Descartes's rationalism and Bacon's empiricism, there is consensus that "enlightenment" comes from both reasoning and empirical data collection and analysis (Stumpf, 2003). Accordingly, we have asked the authors to propose theoretical, empirical, and applied questions. Throughout this book you will find questions labeled "theoretical," "methodological," or "applied," as well as "hybrid" questions (e.g., theoretical-applied). Essentially, these questions reflect three main types of knowledge, namely descriptive (what), explanatory (why), and procedural (how). Altogether, this book reveals 125 research questions on important unknowns in the field of sport, exercise, and performance psychology.

Popperian Falsifiability and Kuhn's Scientific Paradigm Shift: A Book With Hopes to Challenge the Status Quo

In so far as a scientific statement speaks about reality, it must be falsifiable: and in so far as it is not falsifiable, it does not speak about reality.

—Karl Popper

Karl Popper's and Thomas Kuhn's philosophical ideas are also an inspiration for this book (see Kuhn, 2012; Popper, 2005). As Popper noted, science can only progress if scholars try to falsify rather than verify their own models and ideas. It was based on this so-called "Popperian falsifiability principle" that we asked authors to propose questions beyond their own publication records and research agendas. We also asked the authors to summarize in a table the five key readings in each topical area (for a total of 125 suggested key readings) and to include not only their papers but also publications by other scholars and reflecting other schools of thought. As you read through this book, we ask you not to merely accept the ideas presented and the questions proposed, but rather to critically counterpoint each one so that you can generate your own set of questions to inform future research in the field. To this point, Kuhn has warned us that "the answers you get depend on the questions you ask" and that real scientific progress can only happen if we are willing to challenge our most engrained paradigms. In this spirit, we invite you to dive into this book, which is intended to stimulate research and encourage scholarly debate on novel theoretical, methodological, and applied paradigms in the field.

What to Expect From This Book

Each chapter starts with a brief summary of the "State of the Art" literature and includes a table with five must-read papers for that specific area. The five questions that must be addressed to move the field forward are then presented. In total, this volume presents 125 questions and 125 key readings to help guide scholars of all levels to address novel theoretical, methodological, and applied research in the field. Overall, we hope that you read each page bearing in mind the importance of asking more questions, "daring to know!," "doubting everything," trying to falsify rather than verify your ideas, and having the ambition to conduct novel and potentially paradigm-shifting research in sport, exercise, and performance psychology.

References

Broughton, J. (2003). *Descartes's method of doubt*. Princeton University Press.

Kuhn, T. S. (2012). *The structure of scientific revolutions*. University of Chicago Press.

Overholser, J. C. (2018). Guided discovery: A clinical strategy derived from the Socratic Method. *International Journal of Cognitive Therapy, 11*, 124–139.

Popper, K. (2005). *The logic of scientific discovery*. Routledge.

Rousseau, D. M., & Gunia, B. C. (2016). Evidence-based practice: The psychology of EBP implementation. *Annual Review of Psychology, 67*, 667–692.

Stenning, K., Schmoelz, A., Wren, H., Stouraitis, E., Scaltsas, T., Alexopoulos, K., & Aichhorn, A. (2016). Socratic dialogue as a teaching and research method for co-creativity? *Digital Culture & Education, 8*(2), 154–168.

Stumpf, S. E. (2003). *Socrates to Sartre and beyond: A history of philosophy*. McGraw-Hill Education.

Preface

Sport, exercise, and performance psychology researchers and practitioners will be inspired by the information and variety of topics presented in this unique and essential book, edited by Edson Filho and Itay Basevitch. I have known Edson and Itay since they were doctoral students at Florida State University (FSU), where I was the head coach of the women's volleyball team for 26 years and then a faculty member in the Sport Management Department for 15 years.

During my academic tenure at FSU, I had the pleasure of having numerous doctoral students work with me on the design and delivery of a graduate-level coaching certificate. Two of those doctoral students were Edson and Itay. I used to meet with Edson and Itay each week and we would work on designing these courses. We often found ourselves getting sidetracked, and instead of talking about the actual classes, we would end up talking about many of the topics that are in this book. So, while the young doctoral students thought they were learning something in my office, I was constantly fascinated with what they taught me. Usually after our meetings or lunches we would have more questions than answers, but isn't that what higher education is supposed to be about? And maybe that is what inspired them and planted the seed for the idea of this book. It has been nearly a decade since they left FSU and I have enjoyed following their successful careers. I am so proud of them for editing this much-needed book, which will provide professionals in the field with the depth and breadth of knowledge to conduct top-notch research with real-world implications.

I know there will be much more outstanding work from Itay and Edson to come in the future, but for now I invite you to dive into this fascinating book that will most certainly change the landscape of the field in the years to come.

Contributors

Nathalie André, PhD
Associate Professor
Sport Sciences Faculty
University of Poitiers
Poitiers, France

Michel Audiffren, PhD
Full Professor
Sport Sciences
University of Poitiers
Poitiers, France

Joe Baker, PhD
Professor
School of Kinesiology and Health
Science
York University
Toronto, ON, Canada

Vassilis Barkoukis, PhD
Associate Professor
Department of Physical Education and
Sport Science
Aristotle University of Thessaloniki
Thessaloniki, Greece

Itay Basevitch, PhD
Adjunct Professor
Department of Psychology
College of Management Academic
Studies
Rishon, Lezion, Israel

Mark R. Beauchamp, PhD
Professor
School of Kinesiology
The University of British Columbia
Vancouver, BC, Canada

Marika Berchicci, PhD
Associate Professor
Department of Psychological,
Humanistic and Territorial Sciences
University "G. d'Annunzio" Chieti
Chieti, Italy

Maurizio Bertollo, PhD
Professor
Department of Medicine and Aging
Sciences
University G. d'Annunzio of Chieti and
Pescara
Chieti, Italy

Matthieu M. Boisvert, PhD(c)
Department of Kinesiology
University of Windsor
Windsor, ON, Canada

Gavin Breslin, BSc, PhD, FHEA
Senior Lecturer in Psychology
School of Psychology
Ulster University
Coleraine, GB, UK

Joanne Butt, PhD
Professor of Sport Psychology
School of Sport and Exercise Sciences
Liverpool John Moores University
Liverpool, UK

Megan Byrd, PhD
Assistant Professor
Department of Health Sciences and
Kinesiology
Georgia Southern University
Statesboro, GA, USA

Jeffrey G. Caron, PhD
Assistant Professor
School of Kinesiology and Physical
Activity Sciences
Université de Montréal
Montreal, PQ, Canada

**Charlotte Chandler, PhD, MSc,
BSc, FHEA**
Senior Lecturer in Sport and Exercise
Psychology
University of Derby
Derby, GB, UK

Dave Collins, PhD, CPsychol, CSci
Professorial Fellow in Human
Performance Science
Moray House School of Education
and Sport
University of Edinburgh
Edinburgh, GB, UK

Anne E. Cox, PhD
Professor
Kinesiology and Educational
Psychology
Washington State University
Pullman, WA, USA

J. D. DeFreese, PhD
Clinical Assistant Professor
Department of Exercise and Sport
Science
University of North Carolina at
Chapel Hill
Chapel Hill, NC, USA

Brad Donohue, PhD
Distinguished Professor
Department of Psychology
University of Nevada
Las Vegas, NV, USA

Felix Ehrlenspiel, Dr
Department of Sport and Health
Sciences
Technische Universität München
München, Germany

Panteleimon Ekkekakis, PhD
Professor
Department of Kinesiology
Iowa State University
Ames, IA, USA

Robert C. Eklund, PhD
Associate Dean for Faculty
Development and Advancement
College of Education
Florida State University
Tallahassee, FL, USA

Anne-Marie Elbe, PhD
Professor
Department of Sport Psychology
Leipzig University
Leipzig, Germany

Martin Eubank, PhD
Subject Head and Principal Lecturer in
Sport Psychology
School of Sport and Exercise Sciences
Liverpool John Moores University
Liverpool, GB, UK

Deborah L. Feltz, PhD
Distinguished Professor Emerita
Department of Kinesiology
Michigan State University
East Lansing, MI, USA

Edson Filho, PhD
Associate Professor of Sport Psychology
and Counseling
Wheelock College of Education and
Human Development
Boston University
Boston, MA, USA

Selenia di Fronso, PhD
Assistant Professor
Department of Medicine and Aging
Sciences, Behavioral Imaging and
Neural Dynamics (BIND) Center
"G. d'Annunzio" University of
Chieti-Pescara
Chieti, Italy

Cole E. Giffin, Doctoral Student in
Human Kinetics
Student
School of Kinesiology and Life Sciences
Laurentian University
Sudbury, Ontario, Canada

Scott G. Goddard, BPsych(Hons)
(SCU)
PhD Candidate and Causal Academic
Faculty of Health
Southern Cross University
Coffs Harbour, New South Wales,
Australia

Daniel Gould, PhD
Director, Institute for the Study of Youth
Sports and Professor
Department of Kinesiology
Michigan State University
East Lansing, MI, USA

Peter Gröpel, PhD
Professor
Department of Sport Science
University of Vienna
Vienna, Austria

Brandonn S. Harris, PhD, CMPC,
NCC, LAPC
Program Director and Professor of
Sport and Exercise Psychology
Department of Health Sciences and
Kinesiology
Georgia Southern University
Statesboro, GA, USA

Mark E. Hartman, PhD
Assistant Professor
Department of Kinesiology
University of Rhode Island
Kingston, Rhode Island, USA

Katherine E. Hirsch, MHK
PhD Student
Department of Kinesiology
University of Windsor
Windsor, ON, Canada

Patricia C. Jackman, PhD
Lecturer
School of Sport and Exercise Science
University of Lincoln
Lincoln, GB, UK

Moira Lafferty, PhD
Professor
School of Psychology
University of Chester
Chester, GB, UK

Francisco Miguel Leo, PhD
Associate Professor
Department of Didactics of Musical,
Plastic and Corporal Expression
University of Extremadura
Cáceres, ES, Spain

Ronnie Lidor, PhD
Professor and President of the
Academic College at Wingate, Wingate
Institute, Israel
The Motor Behavior Laboratory
The Academic College at Wingate
Netanya, IL

Todd M. Loughead, PhD
Professor
Department of Kinesiology
University of Windsor
Windsor, ON, Canada

Hayley E. Mcewan, PhD
Senior Lecturer
Division of Sport and Exercise
University of the West of Scotland
Lanarkshire, GB, UK

Christopher Mesagno, PhD,
MSESS, BS
Associate Professor
School of Science, Psychology, and Sport
Federation University Australia
Ballarat, Australia

Thierry R. F. Middleton, MSSc, MSc
PhD Candidate
Human Studies and Interdisciplinarity
Program
Laurentian University
Sudbury, ON, Canada

Michael Mignano, MS, MBA
Doctoral Candidate/Instructor Institute
for the Study of Youth Sports
Department of Kinesiology
Michigan State University
East Lansing, MI, USA

Krista J. Munroe-Chandler, PhD
Professor
Department of Kinesiology
The University of Windsor
Windsor, ON, Canada

Shane Murphy, PhD
Professor and Graduate Coordinator
Department of Psychology
Western Connecticut State University
Danbury, CT, USA

Brennan Petersen, PhD Candidate
Department of Human Kinetics
Laurentian University
Sudbury, ON, Canada

Leslie Podlog, BA, MA, PhD
Associate Professor, Sport and Exercise
Psychology
Department of Health and Kinesiology
University of Utah
Salt Lake City, UT, USA

Stefanie Podlog, PhD, MSc,
BSc (Exercise Science), RN
(German), CHW
Professor at the University of St.
Augustine for Health Sciences
College of Health Sciences
St. Augustine, FL, USA

Selen Razon, PhD
Associate Professor
Department of Kinesiology
West Chester University
West Chester, PA, USA

Hugh Richards, MSc, CPsychol
Senior Lecturer
Institute of Sport, Physical Education
and Health Sciences
University of Edinburgh
Edinburgh, GB, UK

Michael Sachs, PhD, CMPC
Professor Emeritus
Department of Kinesiology
Temple University
Philadelphia, PA, USA

Roy David Samuel, PhD
Lecturer
Baruch Ivcher School of Psychology
Interdisciplinary Center (IDC)
Herzliya, Israel

Robert J. Schinke
Doctorate of Education
Professor
Department of Kinesiology and Health
Sciences
Laurentian University
Sudbury, ON, Canada

Matthew J. Schweickle, BA, Psyc
(Hons); BA Comm
PhD Candidate
School of Psychology
University of Wollongong
Wollongong, Australia

Christian Swann, PhD, BSc (Hons)
Associate Professor
Faculty of Health
Southern Cross University
Coffs Harbour, Australia

Gershon Tenenbaum, PhD
Professor
B. Ivcher School of Psychology
Interdisciplinary Center
Herzeliya, Israel

David Tod, PhD
Senior Lecturer
School of Sport and Exercise Science
Liverpool John Moores University
Liverpool, GB, UK

Sarah Ullrich-French, PhD
Professor
Department of Kinesiology and
Educational Psychology
Washington State University
Pullman, WA, USA

Stewart A. Vella, PhD
Senior Lecturer
School of Psychology
University of Wollongong
Wollongong, Australia

Jack C. Watson II, PhD
Dean and Professor
College of Physical Activity and Sport
Sciences
West Virginia University
Morgantown, WV, USA

Robert Weinberg, PhD
Professor
Sport Leadership and Management
Miami University
Oxford, OH, USA

V. Vanessa Wergin, Dr Phil
Postdoctoral Researcher
Chair of Sport Psychology, Department
of Sport and Health Sciences
Technical University of Munich
Munich, Germany

Brad Young, PhD
Professor
School of Human Kinetics
University of Ottawa
Ottawa, ON, Canada

Sigal Ben Zaken, Dr
The Genetic and Molecular Biology
Laboratory, Head
The Genetic and Molecular Biology
Laboratory
The Academic College at Wingate for
Physical Education and Sport Sciences
Wingate Institute, Netanya, Israel

Gal Ziv, PhD
Senior Lecturer
The Academic College at Wingate
Netanya, Israel

SECTION 1
PERFORMANCE AND LEARNING

1

Advancing Research on Efficacy Beliefs

Deborah L. Feltz and Mark R. Beauchamp

Self-efficacy theory has been extensively studied as a cognitive explanation for differences in achievement strivings in sport and physical activity contexts (Beauchamp et al., 2019; Feltz et al., 2008). Since Bandura's seminal publication (1977) on the self-efficacy (SE) construct, there have been over a thousand research articles published on SE and collective efficacy (CE) related to sport and physical activity. Previous reviews have summarized much of this work (e.g., Beauchamp et al., 2019; Feltz et al., 2008; Jackson et al., 2020), but as the field continues to grow, new research questions arise that have the potential to shed light on human behavior across a range of sport and exercise settings.

In this chapter, we pose some of these questions in the hope of stimulating future research. We start with a brief overview of SE theory and CE and provide a summary of key areas of current inquiry within sport and physical activity settings. We then propose and discuss five major research questions that we contend have considerable potential to contribute to the field.

State of the Art

Overview of Self-Efficacy Theory and Collective Efficacy

Bandura's (1977, 1997) theory of SE was developed within the framework of social cognitive theory (SCT), where individuals are posited to use forethought, self-reflection, and self-regulation to influence their own functioning. Within this social cognitive framework, SE, defined as "beliefs in one's capabilities to organize and execute the courses of action required to produce given attainments" (Bandura, 1997, p. 3), addresses the role of

Deborah L. Feltz and Mark R. Beauchamp, *Advancing Research on Efficacy Beliefs* In: *Sport, Exercise and Performance Psychology*. Edited by: Edson Filho and Itay Basevitch, Oxford University Press. © Oxford University Press 2021.
DOI: 10.1093/oso/9780197512494.003.0001

self-referent beliefs as the core agentic factor that determines people's goal-directed behavior. That is, people make conscious efficacy judgments that then influence the challenges they undertake, the effort they expend in the activity, and their perseverance in the face of difficulties. SE judgments can also influence motivation through certain thought patterns and emotional reactions (e.g., pride, shame, happiness, sadness).

Efficacy judgments, in turn, are based on a complex process of self-persuasion that relies on cognitive processing of diverse sources of information (Bandura, 1997). Bandura put these sources into categories of past performance accomplishments, vicarious experiences, verbal persuasion, and physiological/affective states. Performance accomplishments are based on one's own mastery experiences, and thus provide the most dependable source of efficacy information. Vicarious experiences are sources of efficacy information based on gaining information from observing others and comparing one's own capabilities to those observed. Persuasive information includes verbal persuasion, evaluative feedback, expectations by others, self-talk, and imagery. Physiological/affective information includes autonomic arousal that is associated (through perceptual processes) with fear and self-doubt or with being energized and ready for performance, as well as one's level of fitness, fatigue, and pain, such as in strength and endurance contexts (Feltz et al., 2008). Affective states (e.g., mood, anxiety, and depression) are sometimes considered as a separate category of efficacy information that can influence efficacy beliefs (Feltz et al., 2008). Various interventions, based on one or more sources of efficacy information and experiences (e.g., feedback on past performance), can alter SE beliefs (Ashford et al., 2010).

The theory of SE extends to the concept of CE. For instance, whereas SE refers to people's judgments of individual capabilities to perform a given task, CE is defined as a group's judgment of their conjoint capabilities to organize and execute the courses of action required to produce specified levels of collective (e.g., team) performance (Bandura, 1997). Although the concept of CE represents a shift in reference from the self to the collective (e.g., Chan, 1998), it is guided by the same theoretical postulates as SE.

Much of the research on SE and CE within sport and exercise settings has focused on the relationship between efficacy beliefs and achievement-striving behaviors. However, key areas of current research focus on the functional properties of SE, how best to analyze SE and CE, and how efficacy beliefs between individuals (i.e., relational efficacy) influence performance. We provide an overview of this research next and provide key readings in Table 1.1.

Key Areas of Current Research

Functional properties of self-efficacy beliefs in physical activity settings. One of the functional properties of efficacy beliefs that has evolved in physical activity research is the nature of task demands. Early work in the sport domain primarily focused on the effects and predictive utility of efficacy beliefs to perform the various motor behaviors in sport at a given level of difficulty (e.g., diving). Over the ensuing years, however, researchers expanded on the parameters of the original theory to investigate the nature and effects of other forms of efficacy belief. For example, in the exercise domain, a considerable body of research has examined the efficacy beliefs required to engage in effective self-regulation and pursue exercise in the face of multiple demands and obstacles (e.g., Woodgate et al., 2005). Beyond the distinction between task and self-regulatory efficacy beliefs, an array of other forms of efficacy belief have been studied in sport and exercise settings that include coping efficacy, coaching efficacy, and relational efficacy beliefs, to name a few, along with beliefs that groups, people, or teams have in their collective capabilities (for reviews see Beauchamp, 2007; Feltz et al., 2008; Jackson et al., 2020).

Data analysis issues. The current literature on SE and CE includes a number of data analysis considerations. One issue concerns the linearity of the SE and CE relationship to outcome variables. Within SCT, SE is hypothesized to be linearly related to effort, persistence, and performance. This positive, linear relationship has been supported in much of the previous literature on SE in sport and exercise (Feltz et al., 2008). However, Bandura (1997) suggested that there are times when some self-doubt is beneficial for an individual or team to exert optimal effort, particularly in the practice or training phases of a task. The curvilinear relationship between efficacy beliefs and performance has rarely been tested. One study that examined this curvilinear relationship used polynomial regression analyses to show a significant curvilinear, inverted-U relationship with performance in a strength training task (Ede et al., 2017).

A second data analytic issue that has received particular attention within the physical activity domain concerns the way in which CE data are treated when they are derived from individuals nested within groups (e.g., athletes nested within teams). Research on how to measure CE in sport has been summarized by Myers and Feltz (2007), with measures derived from such assessments typically subject to multilevel modeling (MLM). Using this methodology, the relationship between CE and performance has been studied to examine the variability and predictors of CE at both individual and group levels (e.g., Magyar et al., 2004). Although MLM has been used in a number of studies within sport and exercise psychology, how individuals *vary in their perceptions of their team's abilities* and the pattern of those dispersions have not been investigated in published research (Feltz et al., 2008; DeRue et al., 2010). DeRue et al. (2010) described four forms of efficacy dispersion that may exist within teams: (a) shared efficacy (consensus among team members), (b) minority belief (one team member will have either higher or lower perceptions of team efficacy than the rest of the group), (c) bimodal (subgroups will form with different efficacy levels), and (d) fragmented (all members have different team efficacy beliefs).

Relational efficacy. In sport and exercise settings a considerable amount of behavior occurs whereby a person works with or acts to support another to help them achieve their goals. From the perspective of SE theory, a growing body of work has sought to examine the relational efficacy (RE) beliefs that emerge in such settings and their effects on human behavior. Two types of RE have received particular attention. These include the beliefs that one person has in another's capabilities, which is often called other-efficacy (but has also been called proxy efficacy), and relation-inferred self-efficacy (or RISE), which represents a person's appraisals of someone else's efficacy beliefs in them (Lent & Lopez, 2002). Specifically, RISE is a meta-perception in which person A makes an appraisal of person B's confidence in person A.

Research to date has generally found evidence that holding favorable beliefs in a significant other (e.g., an athlete believing in her coach's capabilities, or vice versa) may contribute to the affective states of both the target and holder of those other-efficacy beliefs, as well as relationship quality (see Jackson et al., 2020, for a detailed review). Similarly, believing that a significant other believes in you appears to act as a relational source of SE and support the motivation of the holder of those RISE beliefs (see Jackson et al., 2020).

Table 1.1 Five Key Readings in Efficacy Beliefs in Sport and Physical Activity

Authors	Methodological Design	Key Findings
Beauchamp et al. (2019)	Focus is on SE Review	Critically evaluates empirical evidence related to the theoretical interplay between self-efficacy and other key SCT constructs (e.g., goals, outcome expectations) and physical activity behavior
DeRue et al. (2010)	Focus is on CE Review and theory	Challenges assumption that within-team variability in CE is simply a methodological concern and statistical prerequisite Presents taxonomy that distinguishes four distinct forms of dispersion in CE
Ede et al. (2017)	Focus is on SE Experimental, within-subjects design Participants performed two trial blocks of plank exercise. SE was recorded prior to each trial Performance was used as an indicator of motivational effort	Significant curvilinear relationship between SE and performance on the first trial Significant linear relationship between the two on the second trial Support for the possibility that some self-doubt can be a motivating factor for individuals to exert maximal effort when initially attempting an exercise endurance task
Sparks et al. (2017)	Focus is on RE Cluster randomized controlled trial	Intervention designed to promote relatedness support among teachers resulted in improvements in students' confidence in their teacher (other-efficacy) as well as peer-related RISE beliefs
Williams & Rhodes (2016)	Focus is on SE Conceptual analysis and critique	Presented and reviewed evidence that typical SE measures unintentionally reflect motivation rather than perceived capabilities

CE, collective efficacy; RISE, relation-inferred self-efficacy; SCT, social cognitive theory; SE, self-efficacy.

Questions to Move the Field Forward

1. Theoretical Question: What Directional Paths of SE Work Best to Predict Performance and Behavior in Sport and Physical Activity Contexts?

SCT provides an excellent explanatory framework for understanding the sources of efficacy beliefs and the downstream outcomes associated with those beliefs. However, on the back of a growing and compelling body of research, it may be pertinent to consider extensions/revisions to the original framework, in particular with respect to the causal sequence through which social-cognitive factors shape human behavior. For instance, in much of his writing, Bandura contended that efficacy beliefs constitute "the key factor of human agency" (1997, p. 3) from which subsequent cognitive factors derive. These factors include one's conceived goals, envisioned outcomes, and approaches to socio-structural barriers and obstacles that might impede subsequent behavior. That is, those clusters of social-cognitive factors act as explanatory variables that mediate the effects of SE on behavior.

However, balanced against these theoretical postulates, empirical evidence has accumulated that suggests that when outcome expectations are targeted (and manipulated through intervention), through either monetary incentives or by people being encouraged to envision the consequences of a particular behavior, people's SE beliefs improved (for a review, see Williams & Rhodes, 2016). In short, and contrary to the tenets of SCT, outcome expectations may causally precede efficacy beliefs. In a similar regard, there is compelling evidence that goals may causally precede, and influence, SE beliefs, and so the positioning of goals within the broader SCT framework might require some realignment/repositioning (Beauchamp et al., 2019).

Why is it important to address the question? This question helps researchers understand exactly how different psychological processes emerge and influence behavior and has a major bearing on which psychological factors are prioritized through intervention. *What is the best way to address this question?* A good theory should acknowledge its contradictions (Smaldino, 2019) and be reconfigured if data are inconsistent with the theory's postulates. What this may mean for SCT is the need to (a) better reflect the complexity of relations between key elements of the model and (b) test those postulates using robust experimental methods. In the physical activity domain, the role of socio-structural factors has received relatively scant research attention, but in moving forward it might be prudent to ascertain exactly how complex socio-structural factors (e.g., local health care providers, family income supports and benefits, school systems and educational policy) shape beliefs of human agency, as well as the processes by which agentic thought might differentially overcome barriers to human accomplishment in physical activity pursuits. In the first instance, socio-structural factors might be considered as inputs/antecedents of efficacy beliefs (e.g., a well-resourced school system providing opportunities for sport participation contributing to an adolescent's confidence to be active), whereas in the latter case they might represent a moderator or even a downstream consequence of a person's SE beliefs (e.g., a new immigrant's lack of confidence to speak the local language inhibiting her pursuit of, and access to, local services).

2. Methodological Question: What Measurement, Methodological, and Analytical Tools Can Be Used to Advance Our Understanding of the Dynamic Processes in the Efficacy Belief and Performance Relationship?

There are a number of subquestions within this larger question. In the subsections that follow we address three major issues that relate to ensuring participants' response processes reflect assessments of capability and not motivation, the importance of using analytic methods that allow for examination of nonlinear (efficacy-behavior) relations, and the need to consider the dispersion of efficacy beliefs on sport teams in relation to salient group-related outcomes.

How can assessments ensure that responses reflect a person's perceived capabilities and not motivation? As recent research designed to examine participants' response processes reveals, traditional SE questionnaires may unintentionally tap into conceptions of intention (i.e., an element of motivation) rather than a person's perceived capabilities that they "can" complete the target behavior (Williams & Rhodes, 2016; Williams et al., 2020). *Why is it important to address the question?* Research findings might overestimate explained variance in a targeted behavioral or health outcome due to SE, when the explanatory process might be more motivational in nature. Regardless, improved measurement precision is clearly required to better understand the predictive utility of SE beliefs in physical activity settings. *What is the best way to address this question?* One approach proposed includes the use of brief vignettes, prior to the provision of SE questionnaire items that point out the difference between intentions and perceived capabilities, to ensure that when people are asked about whether they "can" perform a given behavior, perceptions of one's capabilities are actually/appropriately assessed (Rhodes et al., 2016).

What analytical tools can best advance our understanding of nonlinear efficacy-performance relationships? Much of the research on efficacy beliefs and performance in sport and exercise psychology is based on the linear model. However, this assumption could limit the predictive strength of efficacy beliefs on performance or other outcomes in contexts where the relationship may not be linear, such as in practice or training phases (e.g., Ede et al., 2017). *Why is it important to address the question?* Determining what levels of SE and CE are most optimal for performance will help in designing appropriate interventions.

What is the best way to address this question? At a very basic level, this involves collecting repeated measures of SE and the relevant criterion measure (e.g., performance) over time. Furthermore, from a data analytic perspective, as Ede et al. (2017) have done, polynomial regression is one statistical tool to examine the linearity of the efficacy-performance relationship. Experimental designs that manipulate efficacy beliefs should have at least high, moderate, and low efficacy belief conditions. Additionally, cusp catastrophe regression within the cusp catastrophe model has been shown to provide a more nuanced understanding of the relationship between health knowledge (e.g., HIV) and health behavior SE than linear regression (Chen & Chen, 2017). Polynomial regression could also be used within MLM to examine CE within teams (Jansen & Kristof-Brown, 2005). More research is needed using these methods to explore nonlinear characteristics in the efficacy-performance relationship.

What data analytic methods can advance our understanding of *how* different levels of CE within teams contribute to team functioning? An important question that remains to be addressed within sport psychology corresponds to the dispersion of efficacy beliefs within a team (i.e., the inverse of consensus). *Why is it important to address the question?* The variability of athletes' responses within a specific team may have important implications related to the team's functioning, especially at different stages of team development. For instance, dispersion in CE may be positively related to a team's preparatory performance as a result of more structuring, planning, learning, and adapting in the team (DeRue et al., 2010). *What is the best way to address this question?* Using the taxonomy proposed by DeRue et al., MLM can enable researchers to examine a number of variables (e.g., preparatory performance, team viability, cohesion, and dispersion trajectories) in relation to CE beliefs.

3. Theoretical and Applied Question: How Might Teamwork Processes and Structure Foster Improvements in Collective Efficacy?

With a view to ascertain the potential determinants of team performance, several studies within the sport domain have sought to understand the relations between CE, group cohesion, and team performance. A major gap in knowledge corresponds to a broader appraisal of the group dynamics that contribute to CE beliefs in the first instance. Within organizational settings, "teamwork" has been identified as an important behavioral contributor to team effectiveness outcomes, with this relationship mediated by a set of emergent states that include CE and group cohesion (LePine et al., 2008; McEwan & Beauchamp, 2014). Teamwork represents "a dynamic process involving a collaborative effort by team members to effectively carry out the independent and interdependent behaviors that are required to maximize a team's likelihood of achieving its purposes" (McEwan & Beauchamp, 2014, p. 233). Some preliminary evidence exists in support of teamwork being a correlate of CE in sport (McEwan, 2020); however, research has yet to provide causal evidence for a teamwork–CE–team effectiveness effect.

Why is it important to address the question? First, in light of the fact that teamwork represents a set of behavioral processes that exist in the regulation of team performance and the management of team maintenance (McEwan & Beauchamp, 2014), the subcomponents of teamwork (e.g., preparation and execution) provide very clear and tangible targets for intervention and training. Meta-analytic evidence provides strong support for teamwork interventions being able to enhance team effectiveness outcomes outside of sport settings (McEwan et al., 2017), and so an understanding of whether (and the extent to which) teamwork is able to bolster CE beliefs and subsequent team effectiveness outcomes (through experimental intervention-based designs) would appear a viable research question to be pursued within sport.

Another group-related psychological process that is worthy of particular empirical inquiry corresponds to the influence that one teammate might have on the SE and CE of other team members. The effects of a slumping athlete or athlete on a hot streak (CE "contagion") on a team's CE has not been studied. This influence may depend on the status of the impacting athlete (e.g., team captain, starter, nonstarter). Displays of ineffective or inspirational performance could "infect" other teammates' sense of CE.

What are the best ways to address these questions? In terms of understanding the effects of a specific athlete's teamwork behaviors on CE, two approaches would appear particularly worthy of pursuit. First, longitudinal approaches that examine the prospective effects of teamwork behaviors on CE would enable researchers to ascertain exactly which facets of a focal athlete's teamwork might be particularly salient in predicting subsequent confidence among team members in their collective capabilities. In addition, experimental research that systematically targets (through intervention) each of the subcomponents of teamwork would enable researchers to ascertain causality in the extent to which factors such as preparation, execution, and conflict resolution (either by a specific team member or among all team members) causally influence subsequent CE and thereafter team effectiveness outcomes. In addition, researchers should include measures of other-efficacy along with CE when investigating team effectiveness. One way to track such "contagious" influences is through the use of a simulation technique called agent-based modeling (ABM; Oldham & Crooks, 2019). ABM captures emergent phenomena by simulating the behavior of players (i.e., agents) and their interactions, capturing the emergence of structure and patterns of the collective behavior from the bottom up. For example, Oldham and Crooks (2019) provide an example of ABM in a simulation of the hot-streak effect using an agent-based simulation of a basketball game.

4. Methodological Question: How Can We Disentangle the Interrelationships Among Relational Efficacy Beliefs?

A notable contribution to research within the physical activity domain corresponds to examination of the efficacy beliefs that exist within relational settings. Early work by Feltz and colleagues (1999) on coaching efficacy highlighted the importance of coaches having confidence in their coaching capabilities, and the effects of such thought processes on shaping the development and learning of the athletes under their charge. With the contribution of Lent and Lopez's (2002) conceptual model, subsequent research sought to examine the correlates of the two forms of RE described earlier in the chapter, namely other-efficacy and RISE. This corpus of research has generally found these relationship-based efficacy cognitions to be related to important outcomes for both the holder of those cognitions (i.e., actor effects) and the other person in the relationship (i.e., partner effects). Where insights derived from this work are limited is that the research designs used to examine these processes have tended to be correlational (i.e., either cross-sectional or passive prospective analyses over time) or qualitative (based on interviews with coaches and athletes).

Why is it important to address the question? Disentangling the interrelationships among the distinct types of efficacy beliefs that exist within close relationships in physical activity settings has the potential to increase understanding of how to best support the effective functioning of dyads in physical activity settings. For example, if the confidence that a coach has in their athlete's capabilities (i.e., other-efficacy) drives both the coach's commitment to the athlete and the athlete's confidence in themselves, then any intervention might be best served through encouraging coaches to make overt (and clear) their beliefs in their athletes' capabilities. Conversely, if an athlete's RISE beliefs are particularly salient in bolstering the athlete's confidence in themselves, concerted efforts could be made to persuade an athlete that their coach's remarks, body language, and training methods are indicative of the coach's confidence in the athlete. In the former case (i.e., should other-efficacy be a salient predictor), the intervention would involve targeting the coach (encouraging the coach to display confidence in the athlete). However, in the latter case (i.e., should RISE be a salient predictor), the intervention might involve targeting the athlete (helping them to reappraise the coach's interactions as indicative of the coach's confidence in the athlete).

What are the best ways to answer this question? With this in mind, high-quality experimental work that looks to disentangle the relationships among SE, other-efficacy, and RISE in relation to intraindividual and interindividual behavioral processes is clearly needed. Some experimental research has sought to examine the relative contributions of SE and other-efficacy on individual performance in dyadic physical activity tasks (e.g., Dunlop et al., 2011). However, there has been a distinct absence of work that has sought to examine how other-efficacy and RISE beliefs emerge and causally influence behavioral responses (e.g., sport performance), and whether they may operate as viable interpersonal sources of SE beliefs that complement the primary sources of SE articulated by Bandura (1997) within SCT.

Experimental designs can be difficult when trying to control for extraneous variables and still have some ecological validity. One way to understand the predictive strength of other-efficacy and RISE is to use a virtual reality environment with a computer-generated coach, teacher, trainer, or teammate who could be manipulated to be perceived as having differing levels of efficacy beliefs in the participants. Although these would not be real people, there is evidence from media equation theory that people often interact with non-human agents as if they represented reality (Reeves & Nass, 1996).

5. Theoretical and Methodological Question: What Do the Trajectories of Self-Efficacy Beliefs Look Like Across the Life Course in the Context of Sport and/or Physical Activity Settings?

Across the life span, from childhood to adulthood, SE has been identified as one of the most consistent modifiable determinants of physical activity behavior (Bauman et al., 2012). One of the limitations of this research, however, corresponds to the fact that we have very limited insight into the development (and within-person fluctuations) of efficacy beliefs over the life course, or even within/across specific life transitions (e.g., from childhood to late adolescence, from adolescence to early adulthood, and so forth).

In a recent passive prospective study that tracked a large sample of adolescents from the fifth to the seventh grade in the United States, Dishman and colleagues (2017) examined the relationships between participants' self-regulatory efficacy beliefs and physical activity. They found that declines in physical activity (that mirror typical physical activity trajectories among adolescent populations) were buffered to a certain extent among those who had higher efficacy beliefs to overcome barriers. Although this study points to a protective role of SE beliefs over time, the sampled timeframe (2 years) would still be considered short term in nature.

Why is it important to address the question? In the same way that cohort studies in epidemiology track salient lifestyle behaviors over the life course, it would be revealing to track the trajectories of SE beliefs across the life span, and in particular in relation to salient life events in sport (and transition out of sport), as well as in relation to the pursuit of health-enhancing physical activity. If one takes the example of professional athletes, it could be important to see how their efficacy beliefs in sport evolve from childhood to adulthood. Similarly, given established links between SE and health-enhancing physical activity, it would be useful to examine what basic resources (such as fundamental movement skills developed in early childhood) are accrued in early childhood and adolescence that promote downstream SE beliefs and lifelong trajectories that manifest in active lifestyles.

What is the best way to address this question? In light of the fact that SE beliefs represent domain-specific conceptions related to one's perceived capabilities, a life course approach to studying SE beliefs would have considerable potential to examine the "generality" of SE beliefs (Bandura, 1997) across the different physical activity domains that one might sample from childhood to early adulthood and beyond. The study of generality effects has received limited empirical attention in the physical activity domain; however, by sampling, for example, children and adolescents as they attempt each new physical activity in school-based physical education, recreational play, and organized sport, researchers would be well placed to examine how physical competencies and efficacy beliefs accrued in one domain might transfer to each new activity that people sample. Similarly, it would be revealing to ascertain how efficacy beliefs, derived during early adulthood and midlife, contribute to activities pursued during old age.

Conclusion

SE and CE research in sport and physical activity has continued to grow over the four decades since Bandura's (1977) seminal paper, expanding to focus on the functional properties of SE, improved analyses of SE and CE, and how relational efficacy influences performance. To stimulate further research that contributes to the field, we have presented five broad questions that expand on theoretical, methodological, and applied issues, suggesting research approaches that examine the complexities of key theoretical elements, using more robust experimental methods, newer sophisticated analytical tools, virtual technologies, and lifespan research designs.

References

Ashford, S., Edmunds, J., & French, D. P. (2010). What is the best way to change self-efficacy to promote lifestyle and recreational physical activity? A systematic review with meta-analysis. *British Journal of Health Psychology, 15*, 265–288. http://dx.doi.org/10.1348/135910709X461752

Bandura, A. (1977). Self-efficacy: Toward a unifying theory of behavioral change. *Psychological Review, 84*, 191–215.

Bandura, A. (1997). *Self-efficacy. The exercise of control*. W. H. Freeman and Company.

Bauman, A. E., Reis, R. S., Sallis, J. F., Wells, J. C., Loos, R. J., Martin, B. W., & Lancet Physical Activity Series Working Group. (2012). Correlates of physical activity: Why are some people physically active and others not? *Lancet, 380*(9838), 258–271.

Beauchamp, M. R. (2007). Efficacy beliefs within relational and group contexts in sport. In S. Jowett & D. Lavallee (Eds.), *Social psychology in sport* (pp. 181–193). Human Kinetics.

Beauchamp, M. R., Crawford, K. L., & Jackson, B. (2019). Social cognitive theory and physical activity: Mechanisms of behavior change, critique, and legacy. *Psychology of Sport and Exercise, 42*, 110–117.

Chan, D. (1998). Functional relations among constructs in the same content domain at different levels of analysis: A typology of composition models. *Journal of Applied Psychology, 83*, 234–246.

Chen, D-G., & Chen, X. (2017). Cusp catastrophe regression and its application in public health and behavioral research. *International Journal of Environmental Research and Public Health, 14*, 1220. doi:10.3390/ijerph14101220

DeRue, D. S., Hollenbeck, J. R., Ilgen, D. R., & Feltz, D. L. (2010). Efficacy dispersion in teams: Moving beyond agreement and aggregation. *Personnel Psychology, 63*, 1–40.

Dishman, R. K., Dowda, M., McIver, K. L., Saunders, R. P., & Pate, R. R. (2017). Naturally-occurring changes in social-cognitive factors modify change in physical activity during early adolescence. *PLoS ONE, 12*(2), 1–16.

Dunlop, W. L., Beatty, D. J., & Beauchamp, M. R. (2011). Examining the influence of other-efficacy and self-efficacy on personal performance. *Journal of Sport and Exercise Psychology, 33*(4), 586–593.

Ede, A., Sullivan, P. J., & Feltz, D. L. (2017). Self-doubt: Uncertainty as a motivating factor on effort in an exercise endurance task. *Psychology of Sport and Exercise, 28*, 31–36.

Feltz, D. L., Chase, M. A., Moritz, S. E., & Sullivan, P. J. (1999). A conceptual model of coaching efficacy: Preliminary investigation and instrument development. *Journal of Educational Psychology, 91*, 765–776.

Feltz, D. L., Short, S. E., & Sullivan, P. J. (2008). *Self-efficacy in sport*. Human Kinetics.

Jackson, B., Beauchamp, M. R., & Dimmock, J. (2020). Efficacy beliefs in physical activity settings: Contemporary debate and unanswered questions. In G. Tenenbaum & R. C. Eklund (Eds.), *Handbook of sport psychology* (4th ed., pp. 57–80). Wiley & Sons.

Jansen, K. J., & Kristof-Brown, A. L. (2005). Marching to the beat of a different drummer: Examining the impact of pacing congruence. *Organizational Behavior and Human Decision Processes, 97*, 93–105.

Lent, R. W., & Lopez, F. G. (2002). Cognitive ties that bind: A tripartite view of efficacy beliefs in growth-promoting relationships. *Journal of Social and Clinical Psychology, 21*, 256–286.

LePine, J. A., Piccolo, R. F., Jackson, C. L., Mathieu, J. E., & Saul, J. R. (2008). A meta-analysis of teamwork processes: Tests of a multidimensional model and relationships with team effectiveness criteria. *Personnel Psychology, 61*, 273–307.

Magyar, T. M., Feltz, D. L., & Simpson, I. P. (2004). Individual and crew level determinants of collective efficacy in rowing. *Journal of Sport and Exercise Psychology, 26*, 136–153.

McEwan, D. (2020). The effects of perceived teamwork on emergent states and satisfaction with performance among team sport athletes. *Sport, Exercise, and Performance Psychology, 9*(1), 1–15.

McEwan, D., & Beauchamp, M. R. (2014). Teamwork in sport: A theoretical and integrative review. *International Review of Sport and Exercise Psychology, 7*(1), 229–250.

McEwan, D., Ruissen, G. R., Eys, M. A., Zumbo, B. D., & Beauchamp, M. R. (2017). The effectiveness of teamwork training on teamwork behaviors and team performance: A systematic review and meta-analysis of controlled interventions. *PLoS ONE, 12*, e0169604.

Myers, N. D., & Feltz, D. L. (2007). From self-efficacy to collective efficacy in sport: Transitional methodological issues. In G. Tenenbaum & R. C. Eklund (Eds.), *The handbook of sport psychology* (3rd ed., pp. 799–819). Wiley.

Oldham, M., & Crooks, A. T. (2019, April–May). Drafting agent-based modeling into basketball analytics. Paper presented at Spring Simulation Conference, Tuscan, AZ.

Reeves, B., & Nass, C. (1996). *The media equation: How people treat computers, television, and new media like real people and places.* Cambridge University Press.

Rhodes, R. E., Williams, D. M., & Mistry, C. (2016). Using short vignettes to disentangle perceived capability from motivation: A test using walking and resistance training behaviors. *Psychology, Health, and Medicine, 21*, 639–651.

Smaldino, P. E. (2019). Better methods can't make up for mediocre theory. *Nature, 575*, 9.

Sparks, C., Lonsdale, C., Dimmock, J. A., & Jackson, B. (2017). An intervention to improve teachers' interpersonally-involving instructional practices in high school physical education: Implications for student relatedness support and in-class experiences. *Journal of Sport and Exercise Psychology, 39*, 120–133.

Williams, D. M., Dunsiger, S., Emerson, J. A., Dionne, L., Rhodes, R. E., & Beauchamp, M. R. (2020). Are self-efficacy measures confounded with motivation? An experimental test. *Psychology and Health, 35*(6), 685–700.

Williams, D. M., & Rhodes, R. E. (2016). The confounded self-efficacy construct: Conceptual analysis and recommendations for future research. *Health Psychology Review, 10*, 113–128.

Woodgate, J., Brawley, L. R., & Weston, Z. J. (2005). Maintenance cardiac rehabilitation exercise adherence: Effects of task and self-regulatory self-efficacy. *Journal of Applied Social Psychology, 35*, 183–197.

2

Attention

Ronnie Lidor and Gal Ziv

State of the Art

Attention—the ability to focus on a selected stimulus and sustain that focus and shift it at will (Shiel, 2019)—is fundamental for skilled motor performance. The performance of motor skills is linked with paying attention to the task at hand and/or to relevant cues associated with the environment where the individual/team is performing (e.g., Moran, 2010; Schmidt et al., 2019; Wulf, 2007). In this chapter, we focus on two major concepts of attention that have been studied extensively in the literature of sport and exercise psychology: *attentional instructions* (internal and external) and *visual attention*. The chapter is composed of two parts. In the first part, we provide an updated overview of the research findings on the two aforementioned concepts. In the second part, we identify five questions associated with attention and skilled performance that have the potential to advance theory, methodology, and applied interventions in the domain.

Attentional Instructions and Visual Attention

Attentional instructions and visual attention are associated with sporting tasks performed in both stable and dynamic settings (Lidor, 2007). In stable settings, performance occurs in a predictable environment wherein athletes know in advance what they are going to do, such as a floor routine in gymnastics or a free-throw shot in basketball. In these events, performers are mainly required to focus attention on one relevant environmental cue. For example, while standing at the line and preparing themselves for a free-throw shot, the shooter is focusing at one specific cue related to the shooting environment—the front edge of the rim. In dynamic settings, performance occurs in an open environment wherein athletes are required to attend to

Ronnie Lidor and Gal Ziv, *Attention* In: *Sport, Exercise and Performance Psychology.* Edited by: Edson Filho and Itay Basevitch, Oxford University Press. © Oxford University Press 2021. DOI: 10.1093/oso/9780197512494.003.0002 multiple environmental cues and search for the most relevant one, for example, when passing the ball in soccer. Attentional instructions are typically associated with settings that are more stable, while visual attention is more related to dynamic environments. Presumably, in both settings performers should maximize their ability to attend to the most relevant cues to achieve a high level of proficiency.

Internal/External Focus of Attention

In a typical study on attentional focus, participants are assigned to one of two conditions—internal instructions (e.g., the body's own movements) or external instructions (e.g., the intended movement effect). Empirical evidence emerging from an extensive line of studies (see Wulf, 2007, 2013) has revealed that participants who were taught how to focus externally outperformed those who were instructed to attend internally.

The advantage of using external instructions has been observed in several motor tasks (e.g., putting in golf, shooting free throws in basketball, balancing), at different skill levels, and in various age groups (Wulf, 2013). In addition, external attention instructions have been shown to impact both immediate *performance* (i.e., in the practice sessions where the instructions were initially introduced to the participants) and *learning* (i.e., a phase that reflects a more permanent change in the capability to perform the learned skill). Finally, both movement effectiveness (e.g., accuracy, consistency, balance) and movement efficiency (e.g., muscular activity, force production, cardiovascular responses) have been shown to improve with the use of external focusing attention guidance (for a review, see Wulf, 2013).

Two main possible explanations for the superiority of external focus of attention have been proposed by researchers. According to the *constrained action hypothesis* (see Wulf, 2007, 2013), attention instructions induce a conscious type of control, causing performers to constrain their motor system by interfering with the automatic processes. External attention instructions promote a more automatic mode of control, by utilizing unconscious, fast, and reflexive control processes.

The second explanation for the superiority of external attention instructions is found in an expansion of the constrained action hypothesis. According to Wulf and Lewthwaite (2010), references to one's body parts or movements (i.e., internal focus of attention) facilitate access to the neural representation of the self, resulting in self-evaluative and self-regulatory processing. Conditions that trigger neural activation of the self-system result in what Wulf and Lewthwaite (2010) call "micro-choking" episodes, and when these episodes occur performance is hampered.

The expansion of the constrained action hypothesis is one of the pillars of the *OPTIMAL* (Optimizing Performance through Intrinsic Motivation and Attention for Learning) theory proposed by Wulf and Lewthwaite (2016). According to this theory, (a) providing instructions for external focus of attention, (b) increasing learners' sense of autonomy in learning, and (c) providing enhanced expectancies all facilitate motor skill acquisition.

Visual Attention

Athletes are usually required to search visually for relevant information in the sporting environment. However, the ability of humans to visually process a scene is limited. Therefore, how do athletes find objects in the environment or perceive stimuli? Wolfe and Horowitz (2017) proposed five factors that guide our visual attention: (a) top-down guidance—individuals purposefully search for desired targets; (b) bottom-up salience—the shift in visual attention toward salient environmental features, even if one is not purposefully looking for them; (c) scene meaning—guiding attention toward locations in which one is likely to find certain targets; (d) previous history of search—in which targets that were searched for previously may attract more attention in a subsequent search; and (e) relative value of the targets and distractors—in which being rewarded for finding certain targets in previous searches will make them more prominent in a subsequent search.

Understanding how athletes guide their searches can increase knowledge on how they perceive their sporting environments and why they display specific search patterns of behavior. For example, athletes might fail to perceive targets in these environments that are salient to us as an audience. If the visual search was guided to a certain area (based on a combination of the aforementioned five factors affecting the search), it can be understood why another area in the visual field was disregarded—even though searching that area might have led to a better result. Indeed, the relationship between gaze and performance is of major importance in sport (for a review, see Brams et al., 2019).

Three theories on the relationships between gaze and performance have been proposed (see Gegenfurtner et al., 2011). According to these theories, certain gaze features may characterize expert performers. The *information reduction hypothesis* posits that experts are better than novices at attending to relevant areas of interest in their visual field and disregarding areas that are irrelevant to the task at hand (Haider & Frensch, 1999). Based on this hypothesis, experts make more fixations of longer durations to relevant areas and fewer fixations of longer durations to distracting areas.

The *long-term working memory theory* purports that experts have more context-related information stored in their long-term memory that can be rapidly retrieved than novices (Ericsson & Kintsch, 1995). Therefore, when experts need to perform a motor task or make a decision, they can quickly compare the current environmental information with that stored from previous experiences. According to this theory, experts can retrieve relevant information from fewer fixations of shorter durations compared to novices. This theory may seem to contradict the *information reduction hypothesis*; however, a number of studies suggest that these two theories may complement one another (see Brams et al., 2019).

The *holistic model of image perception* suggests that visual scanning starts with a brief glimpse, followed by intentional fixations to relevant areas based on the information received during that glimpse (Kundel et al., 2007). Compared to novices, experts can extract more information during the first glimpse and are then able to more quickly fixate on the relevant areas (Gegenfurtner et al., 2011). Therefore, eye-tracking data of experts should show shorter times until the first fixation toward a relevant area in the visual field.

A recent systematic review examined the relationships between gaze behavior and expertise in sport and in other domains (Brams et al., 2019). In this review, support was provided for the *long-term working memory theory*, which claims that experts in sport have shorter fixation durations during the performance of perceptual-cognitive tasks, respective to their less expert counterparts. In addition, strong support was provided for the *information-reduction hypothesis*, which states that compared to nonexperts, experts make more fixations of longer duration on relevant areas of interest. It is worth noting that an insufficient number of studies have examined the *holistic model of image perception* in the sport domain, and therefore no conclusion can be drawn regarding the importance of this model in sport. Five key readings concerning attention (i.e., attentional instructions and visual attention) and skilled motor performance are presented in Table 2.1.

Table 2.1 Five Key Readings in Attention and Skilled Motor Performance

Authors	Methodological Design	Key Findings
Brams et al. (2019)	Systematic review of visual search and expert performance[1]	Thirty-six studies examining gaze behavior and expert perceptual-cognitive skills in sports were found. Strong support for the information-reduction hypothesis. Experts make more fixations and dwell longer on relevant AOIs. Experts are also better at ignoring irrelevant AOIs.
Park et al. (2015)	Narrative review/ conceptual article on mobile EEG and sport performance[3]	This review discusses frequency- and time-domain analysis of EEG in sport. The review suggests that mobile EEG technology offers opportunities to study sport in ecologically valid settings. Certain brain waves and certain EEG potentials known to be related to attentional processes can therefore supplement our behavioral/ performance measures to provide more robust applied learning strategies.
Toner & Moran (2015)	Literature review and position statement[3]	The review draws on empirical evidence and theory to elucidate the role of bodily awareness in facilitating continuous improvement at the elite level of sport. Based on the reviewed evidence, the authors sketched a number of theoretical and practical implications of the theory of "somaesthetics" for research on expertise in sport.
Vater et al. (2020)	Systematic review on the role of peripheral vision in sport[1]	Twenty-nine studies examined the role of peripheral vision in sports: basketball (2), soccer (9), squash (2), table tennis (1), volleyball (4), baseball (1), cricket (1), combat sports (5), other (4). Three main gaze strategies for perception were discussed: foveal spot, gaze anchor, and visual pivot.
Wulf (2013)	Narrative review of attentional focus effects[2]	A review of the effects of external and internal focus on motor performance. Generally, external focus of attention is more beneficial to motor performance and learning than internal focus of attention.

[1] Related mainly to visual attention. [2] Related mainly to attentional instructions. [3] Related to both visual attention and attentional instructions.

AOI = area of interest; EEG, electroencephalography.

Questions to Move the Field Forward

We identify five questions associated with attentional instructions and visual attention that may advance theory, methodology, and applied interventions, as follows.

1. Applied Question: Can Internal Focus of Attention Be Preferable at Times to an External One?

Based on her review of studies examining the effectiveness of attentional instructions, Wulf (2013) concluded that an external focus of attention applies to all types of tasks and all skill levels, and facilitates both movement effectiveness and movement efficiency. However, a number of researchers have questioned the breadth of the external attentional focus effect (e.g., Montero et al., 2019; Toner & Moran, 2015; Ziv & Lidor, 2015). According to these researchers, an internal focus of attention may be more useful when certain motor tasks are performed, or when the learners who are involved in the learning process are novices.

Montero and colleagues (2019) investigated the difficulty of eliminating confounds in experiments examining the effectiveness of external and internal instructions. One such confound is whether internal focus and external focus are equally natural to participants. For example, in targeting tasks (e.g., dart throwing, free-throw shooting in basketball), an external focus may be more natural than an internal focus, as athletes are required to focus on the target to perform well. This difference alone can lead to superior performance under external focus conditions. Montero and colleagues (2019) also argued that an internal focus of attention can facilitate performance in certain motor skills. Among these skills are those that are defined in terms of attaining an internal focus (e.g., dance, meditation, yoga), skills that may benefit from conscious control (e.g., putting in golf), and skills that are enjoyable to practice. Importantly, Montero and colleagues (2019) did not doubt that sometimes consequence-centered (external) attention leads to a superior outcome compared with body-centered (internal) attention. However, they questioned the breadth of this guidance.

In one study, the relationships between attentional instructions, accuracy of golf putting, and gaze behavior in learners who had not played golf prior to their participation in the study were examined (Ziv & Lidor, 2015). It was found that participants in both the internal and the external attentional instruction groups achieved a higher level of proficiency than those in the control group (i.e., attentional instructions were not provided). However, there were no differences in the performance of participants between the internal and the external attention groups. The authors of this study suggested that a possible explanation for these findings is related to the fact that different types of information can be termed as either internal or external. For example, in golf putting an internal focus of attention can be directed to the arms, the wrists, or the swing of the arms. Similarly, an external focus of attention can be directed to the club, the ball, the hole, or an imaginary line on which the golf ball should roll. In the current study, the external focus of attention was placed on the head of the golf club. However, it is possible that in golf putting the external focus should be directed elsewhere. Therefore, additional empirical evidence on the specific focus of attention is needed for (a) a given learned/performed task and (b) the specific learning stage of the learners.

2. Applied and Theoretical Question: What Is the Role of Peripheral Vision When the Performer Is Attending to the Task/Environment, and How Does Peripheral Vision Influence Attention?

Most studies on visual attention examine foveal (constituting the area of maximum visual acuity and color discrimination) attention by using eye-tracking technology. However, attention can be overt (i.e., directed to the gaze location) or covert (i.e., directed to a location different than the location of gaze). Unfortunately, eye-tracking technology can only inform us *where* one is looking but cannot provide information on *what* an athlete is attending to, which is our main interest.

The role of peripheral vision in sport was discussed in a recent review of 29 studies (Vater et al., 2020). In this review, three definitions of possible gaze strategies were put forward: first, a foveal spot—overt attention, where information is processed via the fovea; second, a gaze anchor—where gaze is directed to one point that is located between several relevant areas, from which information can be covertly gathered using peripheral vision; and lastly, a visual pivot—where a fixation is located at a strategic point between several areas of interest, and gaze can frequently be directed to each of these areas for foveal perception and then return to the central location. Each of these strategies may be beneficial for tasks within a sport or between sports. For a closed, self-paced motor task, for example, a foveal spot and overt attention to the fovea are mostly advised. However, in dynamic situations where there are several areas of interest, it is perhaps more useful to use a gaze anchor and gather information from the peripheral vision.

The literature suggests that peripheral vision plays an important role in our ability to visually search for or visually attend to relevant stimuli (for a review, see Rosenholtz, 2016). Peripheral vision is especially important when there is more than one location on which to fixate or when there is a need to detect motion. A recent review discussed several studies that examined the role of peripheral vision in sport, among them two in basketball, four in volleyball, one in baseball, and nine in soccer (Vater et al., 2020). However, those studies mostly measured natural gaze behavior. While this approach increases external validity, it reduces internal validity and the ability to clearly identify when attention is directed to the peripheral vision.

While methodologies that emphasize external or ecological validity are important in sport and coaching sciences, perhaps it is time to design studies in which internal validity is emphasized. This can be achieved by (a) constraining the head and recording eye movements in front of a computer screen or (b) occluding the foveal field of view or the peripheral field of view to require the participants to use the information from one field or the other (see, e.g., Ryu et al., 2015). Such strategies will improve our understanding of the interplay between foveal and peripheral vision in various motor tasks, as previously suggest by Vater et al. (2020).

3. Applied and Theoretical Question: What Are the Mechanisms That Contribute to Visual Attention in a Number of Individuals Performing Together to Achieve a Shared Goal?

The vast majority of studies on visual attention or gaze behavior in sport have been conducted on the individual athlete. However, in team sports most of the tasks require team coordination. For example, when two basketball players find themselves trying to score a basket against two opposing players, their behavior should be coordinated. To accomplish this, their gaze behavior should be coordinated as well. This is true for the attacking players as well as the defending players. If only one player on the team shows "optimal" gaze behavior and the other player does not, the team may not achieve its goal.

It is important, therefore, to measure gaze behavior of teams rather than only of individual athletes. By synchronizing the recordings of eye movements of two or more expert players, researchers should be able to show how team visual attention leads to expert team performance. It may then be possible to teach "optimal" team visual attention to less expert players, or to novices, and thus improve team performance. Understanding shared gaze behavior can complement the literature on team cognition, coordination, and shared cognition in sport (see Cooke et al., 2013; Gray et al., 2017; McNeese et al., 2016).

We suggest that researchers start with examining the gaze behavior of a team of two participants (i.e., dyads) in relevant sports. For example, an examination of the synchronized gaze behavior of two players in doubles tennis or in two-on-two basketball game scenarios can lead to important findings for the required shared gaze behavior of the two players. After characterizing the gaze behavior of the team, researchers could then examine whether this shared gaze behavior is trainable. Finally, researchers can attempt to increase the size of the team and measure gaze behaviors of three or more players. We believe that this line of research is feasible, as modern eye-tracking technology is now relatively inexpensive and allows for relatively easy synchronization between a number of systems.

4. Theoretical Question: What Are the Neural Correlates of Attentional and Visual Processes in Sport?

In most studies on attention in sport, researchers measure performance variables (e.g., accuracy and consistency), which are sometimes augmented by physiological measures (e.g., heart rate and electromyography). While data have been accumulated on the contribution of attentional strategies to the enhancement of sport performance, the underlying brain mechanisms have been much less researched. More specifically, it would be beneficial to find the neural correlates to different attentional and visual search strategies that are related to improved performance. Once we understand the underlying brain mechanisms, such findings could improve our ability to recommend certain learning strategies that are more robust. Indeed, it can sometimes be difficult to show causation using performance variables only, especially when direct measurements of attention are unavailable. For example, using electroencephalography (EEG) may help researchers show changes in certain brain waves that represent less or more attentive/alert states that accompany behavioral and performance measures (for a review on the relationship between such neurophysiological signals and alertness/mental workload/drowsiness, see Borghini et al., 2014).

In studies in which participants use different types of attentional focus, or when they are required to fixate their gaze at a certain location for a certain duration prior to movement execution, EEG measures can show (a) that one's attention is indeed elevated and/or (b) that the attentional instructions are related to specific brain activity. For example, Mann and colleagues (2011) showed how one specific gaze measure, the Quiet Eye—the final fixation on a specific location before the onset of a critical movement execution (Vickers, 2016)—is related to a specific brain potential, the Bereitschaftspotential, which represents a preparatory period before task execution. Indeed, longer Quiet Eye durations characterize experts (Mann et al., 2007) and the finding by Mann et al. (2011) suggests that behavioral characterization is represented by a specific brain potential.

Research paradigms that include such neurophysiological measures are feasible in sport science, since mobile EEG technology is now available and is relatively inexpensive (for a review of the mobile EEG capabilities for sport performance, see Park, Fairweather, and Donaldson, 2015). For example, Bertollo et al. (2016) used EEG recordings to explore the neural correlates of processing efficiency and performance states in 10 elite shooters. They found that different neural dynamics are associated with either optimal/automatic performance or optimal/controlled performance. Such findings can lead to the development of cognitive and neuro-feedback strategies to improve performance. EEG recordings can also be used when examining team shared cognition (e.g., Filho et al., 2016) and can complement the usage of gaze recordings of multiple participants striving for a shared goal. Finally, from an ecological validity perspective, the availability of mobile eye trackers and mobile EEG systems can enable researchers to understand attentional processes and expert performance in conditions that mimic real-life situations. In addition, the use of virtual reality can allow researchers to mimic real-life situations while still maintaining control over the research environment.

5. Applied and Methodological Question: What Do We Actually Know About the Ecological Validity of the Attentional Instructions/Visual Attention Field Training?

The primary goal of any instructional program is to facilitate long-term learning (Soderstrom & Bjork, 2015). More specifically, instructions should create relatively enduring changes in the comprehension, understanding, and skills that will provide support for long-term retention and transfer. Both attentional instructions and visual attention strategies were mainly studied with short-term retention intervals. Although the attentional studies allowed the researchers to argue that attentional practice enhanced both performance and learning of motor tasks (e.g., Wulf, 2013), studies on long-term retention (e.g., months, years) are still needed. While we acknowledge the difficulties of running such longitudinal studies, we believe that efforts should be made to conduct them. In addition, we have relatively little knowledge on training in the field. For example, how do coaches, instructors, and sport psychology consultants plan short- and long-term attentional training? Do we know if they do this as part of their practice sessions where the sport skills are learned/performed, or as part of the consultation/psychological sessions that complement the practice sessions?

Answers to the aforementioned questions will strengthen the ecological validity of attentional training in both stable and dynamic sport environments. Additional studies—field studies, evaluative studies, and case studies—should be performed to obtain evidence-based information on the applicability effect of attentional instructions and visual attention practice.

Conclusion

This chapter discussed the relationship between two aspects of attention (i.e., focus of attention and visual attention) and performance. After presenting the main theories related to both aspects of attention, five questions that could move the field forward were discussed. A few of these questions are applied in nature and the others are more theoretical. We suggest that researchers increase the use of current technology (e.g., modern eye trackers, mobile EEG systems) that can help understand how attention is related to expert performance—both in theory and in practice. Specifically, we propose that research should be expanded on (a) foveal and parafoveal vision and their relationships with performance, (b) gaze behavior and attention of teams who have a shared goal rather than individuals within teams, and (c) understanding the neural activity that supports both individual and team performance. By doing so, we should also be able to explore the applicability of learning strategies that are based on attentional processes, and therefore provide evidence-based practical instructions to practitioners who work with athletes with the goal of improving performance.

References

Bertollo, M., di Fronso, S., Filho, E., Conforto, S., Schmid, M., Bortoli, L., Comani, S., & Robazza, C. (2016). Proficient brain for optimal performance: The MAP model perspective. *PeerJ, 4,* e2082.

Borghini, G., Astolfi, L., Vecchiato, G., Mattia, D., & Babiloni, F. (2014). Measuring neurophysiological signals in aircraft pilots and car drivers for the assessment of mental workload, fatigue and drowsiness. *Neuroscience & Biobehavioral Reviews, 44,* 58–75.

Brams, S., Ziv, G., Levin, O., Spitz, J., Wagemans, J., Williams, A. M., & Helsen, W. F. (2019). The relationship between gaze behavior, expertise, and performance: A systematic review. *Psychological Bulletin, 145,* 980–1027.

Cooke, N. J., Gorman, J. C., Myers, C. W., & Duran, J. L. (2013). Interactive team cognition. *Cognitive Science, 37,* 255–285.

Ericsson, K. A., & Kintsch, W. (1995). Long-term working memory. *Psychological Review, 102,* 211–245.

Filho, E., Bertollo, M., Tamburro, G., Schinaia, L., Chatel-Goldman, J., Di Fronso, S., Robazza, C., & Comani, S. (2016). Hyperbrain features of team mental models within a juggling paradigm: A proof of concept. *PeerJ, 4,* e2457.

Gegenfurtner, A., Lehtinen, E., & Säljö, R. (2011). Expertise differences in the comprehension of visualizations: A meta-analysis of eye-tracking research in professional domains. *Educational Psychology Review, 23,* 523–552.

Gray, R., Cooke, N. J., McNeese, N. J., & McNabb, J. (2017). Investigating team coordination in baseball using a novel joint decision making paradigm. *Frontiers in Psychology, 8,* 907.

Haider, H., & Frensch, P. A. (1999). Eye movement during skill acquisition: More evidence for the information-reduction hypothesis. *Journal of Experimental Psychology: Learning, Memory, and Cognition, 25,* 172–190.

Kundel, H. L., Nodine, C. F., Conant, E. F., & Weinstein, S. P. (2007). Holistic component of image perception in mammogram interpretation: Gaze-tracking study. *Radiology, 242,* 396–402.

Lidor, R. (2007). Preparatory routines in self-paced events: Do they benefit the skilled athletes? Can they help the beginners? In G. Tenenbaum & R. C. Eklund (Eds.), *Handbook of sport psychology* (3rd ed., pp. 445–465). Wiley.

Mann, D. T., Coombes, S. A., Mousseau, M. B., & Janelle, C. M. (2011). Quiet eye and the Bereitschaftspotential: Visuomotor mechanisms of expert motor performance. *Cognitive Processing, 12,* 223–234.

Mann, D. T., Williams, A. M., Ward, P., & Janelle, C. M. (2007). Perceptual-cognitive expertise in sport: A meta-analysis. *Journal of Sport and Exercise Psychology*, *29*, 457–478.

McNeese, N., Cooke, N. J., Fedele, M., & Gray, R. (2016). Perspectives on team cognition and team sports. In M. Raab, P. Wylleman, R. Seiler, A-M. Elbe, & A. Hatzigeorgiadis (Eds.), *Sport and exercise psychology research* (pp. 123–141). Academic Press.

Montero, B. G., Toner, J., & Moran, A. P. (2019). Questioning the breadth of the attentional focus effect. In M. L. Cappuccio (Ed.), *Handbook of embodied cognition and sport psychology* (pp. 199–221). MIT Press.

Moran, A. (2010). Concentration/attention. In S. J. Hanrahan & M. B. Andersen (Eds.), *Routledge handbook of applied sport psychology* (pp. 500–509). Routledge.

Park, J. L., Fairweather, M. M., & Donaldson, D. I. (2015). Making the case for mobile cognition: EEG and sports performance. *Neuroscience & Biobehavioral Reviews*, *52*, 117–130.

Rosenholtz, R. (2016). Capabilities and limitations of peripheral vision. *Annual Review of Vision Science*, *2*, 437–457.

Ryu, D., Abernethy, B., Mann, D. L., & Poolton, J. M. (2015). The contributions of central and peripheral vision to expertise in basketball: How blur helps to provide a clearer picture. *Journal of Experimental Psychology: Human Perception and Performance*, *41*, 167–185.

Schmidt, R. A., Lee, T. D., Winstein, C. J., Wulf, G., & Zelaznik, H. N. (2019). *Motor control and learning – A behavioral emphasis* (6th ed.). Human Kinetics.

Shiel, W. C. (2019). Attention. Retrieved from MedTerms medical dictionary. https://www.medicinenet.com/medterms-medical-dictionary/article.htm

Soderstrom, N. C., & Bjork, R. A. (2015). Learning versus performance: An integrative review. *Perspectives on Psychological Science*, *10*, 176–199.

Toner, J., & Moran, A. (2015). Enhancing performance proficiency at the expert level: Considering the role of somaesthetic awareness. *Psychology of Sport and Exercise*, *16*, 110–117.

Vater, C., Williams, A. M., & Hossner, E.-J. (2020). What do we see out of the corner of our eye? The role of visual pivots and gaze anchors in sport. *International Review of Sport and Exercise Psychology*, *13*, 81–103.

Vickers, J. N. (2016). Origins and current issues in Quiet Eye research. *Current Issues in Sport Science*, *1*.

Wolfe, J. M., & Horowitz, T. S. (2017). Five factors that guide attention in visual search. *Nature Human Behaviour*, *1*, 1–8.

Wulf, G. (2007). *Attention and motor skill learning*. Human Kinetics.

Wulf, G. (2013). Attentional focus and motor learning: A review of 15 years. *International Review of Sport and Exercise Psychology*, *6*, 77–104.

Wulf, G., & Lewthwaite, R. (2010). Effortless motor learning? An external focus of attention enhances movement effectiveness and efficiency. In B. Bruya (Ed.), *Effortless attention: A new perspective in the cognitive science of attention and action* (pp. 75–101). MIT Press.

Wulf, G., & Lewthwaite, R. (2016). Optimizing performance through intrinsic motivation and attention for learning: The OPTIMAL theory of motor learning. *Psychonomic Bulletin & Review*, *23*, 1382–1414.

Ziv, G., & Lidor, R. (2015). Focusing attention instructions, accuracy, and quiet eye in a self- paced task – An exploratory study. *International Journal of Sport and Exercise Psychology*, *13*, 104–120.

3

Choking Under Pressure

*Christopher Mesagno, Felix Ehrlenspiel,
V. Vanessa Wergin, and Peter Gröpel*

The pressure of competition helps develop athletes who can focus their attention well, performing better than normal in big moments. Often, however, competitive pressure leads athletes to perform worse than normal (e.g., as displayed in practice), which is known as choking under pressure (i.e., choking). In this chapter, we first provide a brief, contemporary summary of the choking literature, which mainly includes choking in individuals but also incorporates team choking (i.e., collective team collapse). We then offer unknown questions for future researchers.

State of the Art

Researchers who experimentally examine choking have advanced the literature exponentially since Baumeister's (1984) seminal work, which investigated the effects of personality, and anxiety, on choking. Six main areas discussed within choking research include definitions of, personality characteristics predicting, models of, neurophysiological correlates of, interventions of, and "team" choking. The "key readings" in Table 3.1 (ordered alphabetically) are choking-specific papers meeting the following criteria: (a) an "influential" choking paper, (b) robust study design, and (c) related to existing choking models or "theory-matched" choking interventions. Ultimately, we chose one article that supports the self-focus, distraction, and self-presentation models of choking, and one theory-matched choking intervention article that relates to either the self-focus or distraction model. Since Baumeister's work initiated this research, it is an assumed key reading and was excluded. We have also excluded literature (or systematic) reviews because we include them in the choking summaries later.

Christopher Mesagno, Felix Ehrlenspiel, V. Vanessa Wergin, and Peter Gröpel, *Choking Under Pressure* In: *Sport, Exercise and Performance Psychology*. Edited by: Edson Filho and Itay Basevitch, Oxford University Press. © Oxford University Press 2021. DOI: 10.1093/oso/9780197512494.003.0003

Choking Definitions Debate

Recent literature has provided conjecture about how much of a magnitude of performance decrement equates to choking. Initially, Baumeister (1984) defined choking as "performance decrements under pressure circumstances" (p. 610), which implies that "any" performance decrease constitutes choking. Other researchers (e.g., Hill et al., 2009; Mesagno & Hill, 2013), however, have questioned whether choking should be reserved for large performance decreases because differences in thought patterns may exist between small (i.e., underperformance) and substantial (i.e., choking) performance decrements. Mesagno and Hill (2013) initiated a within-journal issue debate (see *International Journal of Sport Psychology [IJSP]*, 2013 issue) arguing for clarity of the choking definition and more investigations dedicated to a magnitude of performance decrease under pressure to determine if cognitive processing differences between "underperformance" and choking exist. Jackson (2013) agreed that the underperformance and choking dichotomy could be investigated through hypothesis testing, and other researchers (in the *IJSP* special issue) agreed that examining the underperformance and choking dichotomy could advance choking research. Nevertheless, Mesagno and Hill suggested choking is defined as "an acute and considerable decrease in skill execution and performance when self-expected standards are normally achievable, which is the result of increased anxiety under perceived pressure" (p. 273). Mesagno and Hill acknowledged this as an underdeveloped definition suggesting that researchers investigate the dichotomy further to agree on a magnitude for decreased performance. Although no agreed-upon choking definition exists, we (the authors of this chapter), in independent recent publications, have needed to justify the selected choking definition to reviewers. This may signify a paradigm shift in reporting definitions and links to research findings, which was less monitored prior to the Mesagno and Hill choking definition debate.

Personality Characteristics of Choking

Researchers have continued to investigate the link between personality and choking, which may include trait anxiety, self-consciousness, dispositional reinvestment, fear of negative evaluation and failure, coping, self-confidence, and narcissism. With the exception of self-confidence and narcissism, these personality characteristics have a positive correlation with choking.

Self-confidence and narcissism are negatively linked to choking; as self-confidence or narcissism increases, choking decreases.

Generally, researchers investigate the predictive nature of these personality characteristics, whereby participants complete a self-report questionnaire prior to an experiment. During the experiment, participants perform a sporting task under low and high pressure and then the trait is analyzed using correlational or regression analyses on the low- and high-pressure performance (and anxiety) scores. Researchers have also combined three personality characteristics (i.e., trait anxiety, self-consciousness, and coping) in an attempt to identify and help choking-susceptible (i.e., more prone to experience decreases in performance under pressure) athletes improve performance (Mesagno et al., 2008). For in-depth discussions of personality characteristics and choking, the reader is referred to Mesagno et al. (2015).

Choking Models

Researchers who investigate explanatory theories of choking would agree that a heightened anxiety is essential for an experience to be labeled choking (e.g., Baumeister, 1984; Mesagno et al., 2015). Explanations, to date, focus on attentional changes that occur as a consequence of the anxiety increase, or antecedents that predispose someone to become more anxiety stricken. Most research support is focused on the attention-based consequences of heightened state anxiety through the self-focus and distraction models of choking (Mesagno & Beckmann, 2017). Self-focus explanations (e.g., explicit monitoring hypothesis or reinvestment theory) indicate that, as anxiety increases, explicit attention is allocated to task execution (see Masters & Maxwell, 2008, for a review on reinvestment theory). That is, attention shifts from task-relevant information to internal monitoring of skill-based knowledge in order to consciously control movement, which decreases smooth, coordinated actions, usually processed intuitively. Distraction-based explanations indicate that as anxiety increases, the combined effects of worry and explicit self-instruction exceed a threshold of attentional capacity, which diminishes high-level performance. Ultimately, anxiety shifts attention toward threat-based and task-irrelevant stimuli, reducing available attention to process task-relevant cues and decreasing performance.

Recently, researchers have proposed theoretical descriptions about the antecedents of increased state anxiety via self-presentation. The central premise of the self-presentation model (Mesagno et al., 2011, 2012), which has limited support to date, is that certain personality characteristics predispose athletes to being more choking susceptible. When these characteristics are associated with choking-susceptibility, athletes are predisposed to higher cognitive state anxiety and self-presentation concerns. Self-presentation is the process by which people attempt to monitor and control how they are perceived and evaluated by others (Schlenker, 1980). People engage in self-presentation behaviors to help create a public identity. Given that athletes likely have a strong (or exclusive) athletic identity, self-presentation concerns and behaviors may emerge because athletes want to create a positive public image to other athletes and supporters to confirm their own beliefs about themselves. To deal with the cognitive anxiety increases, attentional shifts occur to control public image and avoid relational devaluation, which exacerbate performance decrements. The reader is referred to other reviews (e.g., Christensen et al., 2015; Roberts et al., 2019) for recent discussions about choking models and theoretical debates.

Neurophysiological Correlates of Choking

Although the choking theories are considered cognitive and specifically propose attentional mechanisms, they also imply neurophysiological underpinnings (i.e., brain areas and functions). Choking theories have been examined mainly employing electroencephalography (EEG) equipment to assess cortical activity and communication.

Self-focus theories imply greater activity of the left, "analytic" hemisphere, especially in the temporal lobe, where verbal-analytic processing originates. Such ideas resonate in findings that expert performers show a comparably relaxed and refined cortical state, especially in the left temporal region (Del Percio et al., 2011), and that explicit motor learning (but not control) is associated with strong neural communication (called coherence) between the verbal-analytic regions of the temporal lobe and central motor areas (Gallicchio et al., 2017). Furthermore, improved performance under pressure is accompanied by reduced connectivity between motor and nonmotor areas (Rietschel et al., 2011), whereas an elevated coherence between verbal-analytic areas and motor planning is found in "chokers" (Lo et al., 2019). Finally, performing under pressure appears to increase an error-specific EEG signal, the error-related negativity, which is an indicator of enhanced error monitoring (Masaki et al., 2017). Taken together, these studies provide general evidence for neurophysiological underpinnings of self-focus theories.

Distraction theories, however, imply less interference with motor processes from verbal-analytic areas but rather problems with executive control. The prefrontal cortex (PFC) is associated with executive functions (Banich, 2009), and it is thought that frontal influences on motor activity are necessary to protect performance from interference. Using brain imaging methods, Lee and Grafton (2015) showed that activity in the right anterior cingulate cortex and the medial PFC is indeed related to enhanced performance in a visuomotor coordination task. Moreover, elevated coherence between the dorsolateral PFC and motor areas protected against performance failure under pressure, again highlighting the role of executive functions (Lee & Grafton, 2015). We were unable to identify neurophysiological choking reviews; thus, we encourage readers to review the articles discussed in this section.

Choking Intervention

To ameliorate choking, sport psychologists have developed "theory-matched" choking interventions (see Gröpel & Mesagno, 2019, for a review). *Distraction-based* interventions aim to prevent internal or external distractions and promote task-relevant attention. These interventions often include a preperformance routine (PPR), which is a set of cognitive and behavioral elements that an athlete systematically engages in prior to performance execution (Cotterill, 2010). Researchers have found that effective PPRs are individualized and typically consist of (but are not limited to) a combination of relaxation, mental imagery, cue words, external focus, and temporal consistency (Mesagno & Mullane-Grant, 2010). *Self-focus-based* interventions are used to minimize the conscious, step-by-step control of skill execution, often applying distal methods or ad hoc interventions. Distal methods include implicit (or analogy) learning (i.e., biomechanical metaphors; hitting a table tennis forehand as if drawing a triangle) to reduce the likelihood of "reinvestment" occurring (Masters & Maxwell, 2008). The most effective ad hoc interventions are dual task and left-hand dynamic handgrip interventions. When performing a dual task, athletes focus attention toward the dual task rather than skill execution, which facilitates the smooth skill execution and minimizes reinvestment. Alternatively, athletes may use a dynamic handgrip and squeeze a soft ball in their left hand prior to skill execution (Beckmann et al., 2013), which leads to a state of cortical relaxation and prevents overcontrol (Cross-Villasana et al., 2015). Finally, *acclimatization* interventions focus on reducing the anxiety that leads to distraction or self-focus. These interventions may include (but are not limited to) practice under mild anxiety conditions, such as when being videotaped or watched by an audience, with the goal to familiarize participants with pressure (Oudejans & Pijpers, 2010).

Collective Team Choking

While choking in individual athletes is well investigated, research into team choking is still in its infancy. A competitive situation where a team's perfor- mance suddenly breaks down is called a collective collapse (Apitzsch, 2009a, 2009b) or collective sport team collapse (Wergin et al., 2018). Collective team collapse can be defined as "a sudden, collective, and extreme underper- formance of a team within a competition, which is triggered by a critical sit- uation that interferes with the team's interplay, a loss of control of the game, and ultimately the inability of the team to regain their previous performance level within the game" (Wergin et al., 2018, p. 5).

Existing evidence indicates a cascade of causes rather than single triggers of team collapse (Apitzsch, 2009a, 2009b; Wergin et al., 2018, 2019). Wergin and colleagues' model distinguishes antecedents (e.g., increased pressure, over- confidence, lack of attentional focus) and critical events on the court or field (e.g., team errors accumulating, collapse of a key player) that make the collapse more likely. These critical events change the affective, cognitive, and behavioral state of players and the team, which exacerbates the collapse and prohibits the team from returning to their initial level of "normal" performance.

Affective changes or outcomes maintaining the collapse include (but are not limited to) increased anxiety, anger, and frustration, as well as negative emotional contagion. On a cognitive level, insecurity, a lack of accountability, and a shift from goal to prevention orientation (i.e., trying to play safe rather than attempting to score) play a role in collective team collapse. Behavioral changes include (but are not limited to) decreased performance contagion, limited communication, cautious or hectic play, or blaming teammates for failure. Social factors arising from the interaction of players (e.g., limited communication, lack of accountability, blaming each other for failure) are important in evocation and maintenance of a team collapse. The perceived importance of these social factors indicates that team collapse is more than the sum of individual athletes choking concurrently (Wergin et al., 2018).

Table 3.1 Five Key Readings in Choking Research

Authors	Methodological Design	Key Findings
Beckmann et al. (2013)	Multistudy experimental design using three different sports under low and high pressure to determine if left-hand dynamic handgrip (theory-matched intervention to self-focus model) could prevent choking.	Left-hand dynamic handgrip optimized performance under pressure (and minimized choking) in the three studies compared to a control group.
Beilock & Carr (2001)	Multistudy experimental design to test the self-focus model with novice and experts' generic and episodic knowledge generation (Experiments 1–2) and using arithmetic or sensorimotor tasks with dual-task and self-consciousness training (Experiments 3–4).	Choking occurred in the sensorimotor task and dual-task training, but not in the arithmetic task or self-consciousness training. Step-by-step control of procedural knowledge harms experts' performance under pressure, supporting self-focus models of choking.
Mesagno et al. (2012)	Single-study experimental design with "preselection" into an experimental stage. Preselection involved 138 athletes completing questionnaires to select 34 athletes, categorized as either low or high in fear of negative evaluation, to perform basketball shots under low and high pressure.	The group with high (but not low) fear of negative evaluation experienced choking, with cognitive anxiety partially mediating the fear-performance relationship. This adds support to the self-presentation model of choking.
Mesagno & Mullane-Grant (2010)	Single-study experimental design with five separate PPR groups (theory-matched intervention to distraction model) performing football kicks under low and high pressure.	PPR groups improved performance under pressure compared to a control group.
Oudejans et al. (2011)	Robust qualitative methodology using retrospective verbal reports and concept mapping of expert athletes to determine common attentional focus under pressure. Statements were clustered (in common choking themes) and rated on the frequency of occurrence and how important statements were for choking.	Expert athletes commonly attended to worries (statements concerning distracting thoughts and worries), with minimal thoughts about movement execution, under pressure, favoring distraction models of choking.

PPR, preperformance routine.

Questions to Move the Field Forward

Our major research questions, which are in order of the topics discussed previously—interventions of, neurophysiology of, and team choking—could advance the "unknown" in choking. We have also included another nonexistent choking topic: mental health of "chokers."

1. Applied Question: How Do We Target Choking Interventions to Specific Sports?

The benefits of choking interventions have been evidenced for various sport skills, but substantial variations in their effectiveness exist, possibly because they are not sport specific. A targeted intervention seems appropriate to help performers deal with the particular demands of a sport task. For example, researchers have begun speculating that externally and self-paced skills can fail because of different attentional mechanisms (Roberts et al., 2019). Externally paced skills (e.g., baseball batting) demand rapid reaction to a moving stimulus, whereas self-paced skills (e.g., golf putt) allow the performer to decide when to initiate action. Experts of externally paced skills use nonverbal cues to anticipate and prepare for action, and thus misplaced attentional resources due to distraction (rather than self-focus) can harm anticipation and performance. The challenge of self-paced skills is the opportunity for distracting thoughts to occur prior to execution, which allows for both distraction and self-focus choking mechanisms to emerge. Consequently, future researchers may test the benefits of targeting distraction-based interventions to externally paced skills, and both distraction- and self-focus-based interventions for self-paced skills, especially when used in combination.

2. Applied Question: How Do We Tailor Choking Interventions to Specific Personalities?

Targeted interventions can be further tailored and individualized according to the personality characteristics relevant to choking. A tailored approach using personality characteristics would provide interventions based on an individual's score on those traits. If, for example, trait anxiety and self-consciousness were high, the individual would presumably benefit from acclimatization training and specific elements (e.g., external focus, left-hand dynamic handgrip) within a PPR to adapt to enhanced pressure and prevent conscious control, respectively. The tailored approach seems important as targeted interventions alone may not be equally appropriate for everyone. A tailored intervention might produce more visible benefits, which may strengthen the individual's willingness to apply the intervention. Methodologically, tailored intervention studies could test how independent interventions interact with specific personality characteristics, initially using hypothesis testing with single personality characteristics together with pre- and postintervention designs. In addition, single-case (or perhaps mixed-methods) designs with "chronic chokers" (i.e., athletes who perform poorly under pressure frequently and consistently) may provide valuable details on how interventions work for different personalities. Researchers could also better predict choking susceptibility using more personality variables than the three applied previously (Mesagno et al., 2008). If we can integrate multiple personality characteristics to better identify the choking-susceptible athlete, researchers could more accurately predict choking and then also prevent it using tailored interventions.

3. Theoretical and Applied Question: How Do Neurophysiological Processes Relate to Cognitive Processes Underlying Choking?

To advance choking theory and also theory-matched interventions, we need to identify the neurophysiological link between cognitive processes and choking. Christensen et al. (2015) suggested that there is a dearth of direct evidence of either self-focus or distraction-based choking because most studies rely on assessing and interpreting performance outcomes rather than directly examining underlying motor or cognitive processes. This extends to a neurophysiology explanation of choking. To date, there is no evidence that the enhanced communication between verbal-analytical areas in the temporal cortex and central motor areas of the brain (indicating self-monitoring) leads to skill breakdown or step-by-step control of execution. Furthermore, there is no direct connection between reduced involvement of the PFC (indicating distraction) and "distracted" cognitive processing (e.g., via a reduced quiet eye). To provide such evidence, the integrated assessment of neurophysiology (via EEG), visual attention (via eye tracking), movement execution (via motion sensors or capture), and performance is needed. Showing and understanding these connections is paramount for at least three reasons.

First, providing links between neurophysiology and cognitive processes might allow a reconciliation of the self-focus and distraction models of choking. Such a reconciliation has been attempted (e.g., Mesagno et al., 2015; Nieuwenhuys & Oudejans, 2012), but the current neurophysiological evidence indicates that the two explanations are not just "overlapping" (Mesagno et al., 2015). For example, Lo et al. (2019) found not only elevated coherence between motor planning and verbal-analytic areas ("self-monitoring") but also increased high-alpha in the occipital area, indicating impaired visual processing ("distraction"). Thus, distraction and self-focus are separate processes that could occur in parallel, within a single choking experience. Second, understanding the neurophysiology and cognitive processing links better will allow more accurate evaluation of choking interventions, which may create more precise tailoring to conditions and people. For example, given that the propensity for reinvestment is related to interindividual differences in coherence between verbal and motor areas, dynamic handgrip might be tailored for individuals with high reinvestment tendencies (Hoskens et al., 2020). Third, understanding neurophysiological underpinnings and linkages will facilitate the design of neurophysiological interventions. Such interventions could involve distinct technological tools (e.g., EEG neurofeedback; transcranial direct current stimulation) and the easy-to-use, "off the shelf" mobile recording devices already available. This "stimulation" might enhance activity of the PFC to augment executive control or inhibit communication between verbal and motor areas and improve performance (under pressure).

4. Applied Question: Which Social or Team-Related Factors Should Be Addressed When Designing Team Choking Prevention and Intervention Strategies?

Given the causes and processes of team choking discussed earlier, further research investigating the relationship between causes of team choking is needed. In particular, social or team-related factors should be of interest because they are a major element of evocation of a team collapse (Wergin et al., 2018) and thus could provide future approaches for preventions and interventions.

One approach to identify team factors may be to expand the process model of collective sport team collapse (Wergin et al., 2018, 2019). While the occurrence of critical, uncontrollable events happening on the field (e.g., wrong referee decision, opponent scoring) may not be influenceable, but may adversely affect the game, future prevention and intervention strategies should focus on antecedents, and facilitating factors, underlying the team collapse. For example, poor preparation, physical exhaustion of players, or young and inexperienced players are antecedents, which can be addressed by coaches prior to a game. Psychological antecedents (e.g., team overconfidence, high respect for the opponent, or lack of self-confidence) or facilitating factors (e.g., emotional contagion among team members, lack of accountability, or immobility) could be addressed by providing sport psychology education to the players and team throughout the season.

Moreover, a better understanding of the interrelatedness of affective, cognitive, and behavioral factors causing and maintaining team collapse is needed. Affective, cognitive, and behavioral connections may be explored by conducting qualitative focus groups with sport teams and coaching staff on team collapses. Methodologically, organizing such focus groups shortly after (i.e., within a week) a collective team collapse would allow for sufficient memory recall. Furthermore, providing video recordings, and maybe using the "think aloud" technique (Eccles & Arsal, 2017) while players are watching the video footage, may support athletes and coaches in recalling the event more accurately. Further ideas may include (but are not limited to) the use of a continuous assessment of emotion and/or thoughts while watching the video. During the focus group, social or team-related affective, cognitive, and behavioral factors along with identifying key factors that evoke the team collapse could be explored. The type of sport, as well as individual experiences of the team in the past, should be considered. The most salient social causes of team collapse (e.g., negative emotional contagion or blaming each other for failure) could then be addressed in the development of team-based interventions.

5.   Applied and Methodological Question: Is There a Connection Between Choking and Mental Health Issues?

Many sport psychology associations (e.g., International Society for Sport Psychology—Schinke et al., 2018; European Federation of Sport Psychology [FEPSAC]—Moesch et al., 2018) and international committees (e.g., International Olympic Committee—Reardon et al. 2019) have recently provided guidelines for improving mental health for high-performance athletes. Because choking is connected to elite sport and athlete identity, and being a successful athlete may be important theoretically (e.g., self-presentation model of choking; Mesagno et al., 2011, 2012), elite athletes who experience choking may either be predisposed to mental health problems or experience mental health issues following a "choke." This is exacerbated with "chronic chokers," who "choke" repeatedly and may be devastated and embarrassed after the incident. Although not the main purpose, Hill and colleagues (e.g., 2011, 2019) provided qualitative evidence that suicidal ideation (Hill et al., 2011) or risky behavior (e.g., drunk driving; Hill et al., 2019) may be a destructive consequence of chronic choking, but only for certain athletes (which also needs further examination). Thus, correlational, qualitative, experimental, case study, and/or longitudinal designs, with the sole purpose of determining the mental health effect of choking, could be used in future research.

Conclusion

In summary, researchers who investigate (individual) choking have increased our understanding since Baumeister's (1984) first investigations. Researchers who examine team choking, however, have only begun to explore the characteristics and antecedents associated with a team's catastrophic decline in performance during a competition. There is still much to be learned about models of team choking, which are largely grounded in qualitative exploration and need substantiation through rigorous experimental designs. The "unknown" suggestions we have provided should give aspiring sport psychology researchers our view on where the choking literature should develop and also provide insight into what questions could be investigated based on current choking literature.

References

Apitzsch, E. (2009a). A case study of a collapsing handball team. In S. Jern & J. Näslund (Eds.), *Dynamics within and outside the lab* (pp. 35–52). LiU-Tryck.

Apitzsch, E. (2009b). Coaches' and elite team players perception and experiencing of collective collapse. *Athletic Insight, 1*(2), 57–74.

Banich, M. T. (2009). Executive function: The search for an integrated account. *Current Directions in Psychological Science, 18,* 89–94. doi:10.1111/j.1467-8721.2009.01615.x

Baumeister, R. F. (1984). Choking under pressure: Self-consciousness and paradoxical effects of incentives on skillful performance. *Journal of Personality and Social Psychology, 46,* 610–620.

Beckmann, J., Gröpel, P., & Ehrenspiel, F. (2013). Preventing motor skill failure through hemisphere-specific priming: Cases from choking under pressure. *Journal of Experimental Psychology: General, 142,* 679–691. doi:10.1037/a0029852

Beilock, S. L., & Carr, T. H. (2001). On the fragility of skilled performance: What governs choking under pressure. *Journal of Experimental Psychology, 130,* 701–725. doi.org/10.1037/0096-3445.130.4.701

Christensen, W., Sutton, J., & McIlwain, D. (2015). Putting pressure on theories of choking: Towards an expanded perspective on breakdown in skilled performance. *Phenomenology and the Cognitive Sciences, 14,* 253–293.

Cotterill, S. (2010). Pre-performance routines in sport: Current understanding and future directions. *International Review of Sport and Exercise Psychology, 3,* 132–153. doi:10.1080/1750984X.2010.488269

Cross-Villasana, F., Gröpel, P., Doppelmayr, M., & Beckmann, J. (2015). Unilateral left-hand contractions produce widespread depression of cortical activity after their execution. *PLoS ONE, 10*(12), e0145867. doi:10.1371/journal.pone.0145867

Del Percio, C., Iacoboni, M., Lizio, R., Marzano, N., Infarinato, F., Vecchio, F., . . . Babiloni, C. (2011). Functional coupling of parietal alpha rhythms is enhanced in athletes before visuomotor performance: A coherence electroencephalographic study. *Neuroscience, 175,* 198–211.

Eccles, D. W., & Arsal, G. (2017). The think aloud protocol? What is it and how do I use it? *Qualitative Research in Sport, Exercise and Health, 9,* 513–541.

Gallicchio, G., Cooke, A., & Ring, C. (2017). Practice makes efficient: Cortical alpha oscillations are associated with improved golf putting performance. *Sport, Exercise, and Performance Psychology, 6,* 89–102. doi:10.1037/spy0000077

Gröpel, P., & Mesagno, C. (2019). Choking interventions in sports: A systematic review. *International Review of Sport and Exercise Psychology, 12,* 176–201. doi:10.1080/1750984X.2017.1408134

Hill, D. M., Cheesbrough, M., Gorczynski, P., & Matthews, N. (2019). The consequences of choking in sport: A constructive or destructive experience? *Sport Psychologist, 33,* 12–22.

Hill, D. M., Hanton, S., Fleming, S., & Matthews, N. (2009). A re-examination of choking in sport. *European Journal of Sport Science, 9,* 203–212.

Hill, D. M., Hanton, S., Matthews, N., & Fleming, S. (2011). Alleviation of choking under pressure in elite golf: An action research study. *Sport Psychologist, 25,* 465–488.

Hoskens, M. C., Bellomo, E., Uiga, L., Cooke, A., & Masters, R. S. (2020). The effect of unilateral hand contractions on psychophysiological activity during motor performance: Evidence of verbal-analytical engagement. *Psychology of Sport and Exercise, 48,* 101668. doi:10.1016/j.psychsport.2020.101668

Jackson, R. C. (2013). Babies and bathwater: Commentary on Mesagno and Hill's proposed re-definition of "choking." *International Journal of Sport Psychology, 44,* 281–284.

Lee, T. G., & Grafton, S. T. (2015). Out of control: Diminished prefrontal activity coincides with impaired motor performance due to choking under pressure. *NeuroImage, 105,* 145–155.

Lo, L. C., Hatfield, B. D., Wu, C. T., Chang, C. C., & Hung, T. M. (2019). Elevated state anxiety alters cerebral cortical dynamics and degrades precision cognitive-motor performance. *Sport, Exercise, and Performance Psychology, 8,* 21–37.

Masaki, H., Maruo, Y., Meyer, A., & Hajcak, G. (2017). Neural correlates of choking under pressure: Athletes high in sports anxiety monitor errors more when performance is being evaluated. *Developmental Neuropsychology, 42,* 104–112. doi:10.1080/87565641.2016.1274314

Masters, R. S. W., & Maxwell, J. (2008). The theory of reinvestment. *International Review of Sport and Exercise Psychology, 1,* 160–184.

Mesagno, C., & Beckmann, J. (2017). Choking under pressure: Theoretical models and interventions. *Current Opinions in Psychology, 16,* 170–175.

Mesagno, C., Geukes, K., & Larkin, P. (2015). Choking under pressure: A review of current debates, literature, and interventions. In S. Mellalieu & S. Hanton (Eds.), *Contemporary advances in sport psychology: A review* (pp. 148–174). Routledge.

Mesagno, C., Harvey, J. T., & Janelle, C. M. (2011). Self-presentational origins of choking: Evidence from separate pressure manipulations. *Journal of Sport & Exercise Psychology, 33,* 441–459.

Mesagno, C., Harvey, J. T., & Janelle, C. M. (2012). Choking under pressure: The role of fear of negative evaluation. *Psychology of Sport and Exercise, 13,* 60–68.

Mesagno, C., & Hill, D. M. (2013). Definition of choking in sport: Re-conceptualization and debate. *International Journal of Sport Psychology-Performance Under Pressure, 44,* 267–277.

Mesagno, C., Marchant, D., & Morris, T. (2008). Using a pre-performance routine to alleviate choking under pressure in "choking-susceptible" athletes. *Sport Psychologist, 22,* 439–457. doi:10.1123/tsp.22.4.439

Mesagno, C., & Mullane-Grant, T. (2010). A comparison of different pre-performance routines as possible choking interventions. *Journal of Applied Sport Psychology, 22,* 343–360. doi:10.1080/10413200.2010.491780

Moesch, K., Kenttä, G., Kleinart, J., Quignon-Fleuret, C., Cecil, S., & Bertollo, M. (2018). FEPSAC position statement: Mental health disorders in elite athletes and models of service provision. *Psychology of Sport & Exercise, 38,* 61–71. https://doi.org/10.1016/j.psychsport.2018.05.013

Nieuwenhuys, A., & Oudejans, R. R. D. (2012). Anxiety and perceptual-motor performance: Toward an integrated model of concepts, mechanisms, and processes. *Psychological Research, 76,* 747–759. doi:10.1007/s00426-011-0384-x

Oudejans, R. R. D., Kuijpers, W., Kooijman, C. C., & Bakker, F. C. (2011). Thoughts and attention of athletes under pressure: Skill-focus or performance worries? *Anxiety, Stress & Coping, 24,* 59–73.

Oudejans, R. R., & Pijpers, J. R. (2010). Training with mild anxiety may prevent choking under higher levels of anxiety. *Psychology of Sport and Exercise, 11,* 44–50. doi:10.1016/j.psychsport.2009.05.002

Reardon, C. L., Hainline, B., Miller Aron, C., Baron, D., Baum, A. L., Bindra, A., . . . Engebretsen, L. (2019). Mental health in elite athletes: International Olympic Committee consensus statement (2019). *British Journal of Sports Medicine, 53*, 667–699. doi:10.1136/bjsports-2019-100715

Rietschel, J. C., Goodman, R. N., King, B. R., Lo, L. C., Contreras-Vidal, J. L., & Hatfield, B. D. (2011). Cerebral cortical dynamics and the quality of motor behavior during social evaluative challenge. *Psychophysiology, 48*, 479–487.

Roberts, L. J., Jackson, M. S., & Grundy, I. H. (2019). Choking under pressure: Illuminating the role of distraction and self-focus. *International Review of Sport and Exercise Psychology, 12*, 49–69. doi:10.1080/1750984X.2017.1374432

Schinke, R. J., Stambulova, N. B., Si, G., & Moore, Z. (2018). International Society of Sport Psychology position statement: Athletes' mental health, performance, and development. *International Journal of Sport and Exercise Psychology, 16*, 622–639. https://doi.org/10.1080/1612197X.2017.1295557

Schlenker, B. R. (1980). *Impression management: The self-concept, social identity, and interpersonal relations.* Brooks/Cole.

Wergin, V. V., Mallett, C. J., Mesagno, C., Zimanyi, Z., & Beckmann, J. (2019). When you watch your team fall apart – Coaches' and sport psychologists' perceptions on causes of collective sport team collapse. *Frontiers in Psychology, 10*, 1331. doi:10.3389/fpsyg.2019.01331

Wergin, V. V., Zimanyi, Z., Mesagno, C., & Beckmann, J. (2018). When suddenly nothing works anymore within a team: Causes of collective sport team collapse. *Frontiers in Psychology, 9*, 2115. doi:10.3389/fpsyg.2018.02115

4

Flow and Clutch States

Christian Swann, Scott G. Goddard, Patricia C. Jackman,
Matthew J. Schweickle, and Stewart A. Vella

The Society for Sport, Exercise, and Performance Psychology defines performance psychology as "the study and application of psychological principles of human performance to help people consistently perform in the upper range of their capabilities and more thoroughly enjoy the performance process" (American Psychological Association, Division 47, 2019, p. 9). Episodes of optimal functioning—or optimal experiences—typically involve exceptional performance as well as highly positive subjective experiences (e.g., Csikszentmihalyi, 2002), and are therefore integral to the study and application of sport, exercise, and performance psychology. Such episodes are relatively brief yet typically represent the most enjoyable and memorable times that an individual can have in sport, exercise, or performance contexts, including personal bests, important achievements and successes, and harmonious experiences (e.g., when everything just "flows"; Csikszentmihalyi et al., 2017). In turn, optimal experiences have lasting benefits such as satisfaction, pride, and intrinsic motivation to engage in the activity again (Csikszentmihalyi, 2002) and are highly important in sport, exercise, and performance psychology.

The primary construct in the field of optimal experience, based on the most developed body of literature, is flow (Csikszentmihalyi, 2002). Despite its appeal, and 45 years of research, flow is generally considered to be rare and elusive (Csikszentmihalyi, 2002; Csikszentmihalyi et al., 2017). Indeed, it has been suggested that research in this field "is plagued by a variety of conceptual and methodological problems" (Moran & Toner, 2017, p. 193), and that flow research is approaching a "crisis point" and potential paradigm shift (see Swann et al., 2018, for a review). Against this backdrop, a new perspective outlined recently, the Integrated Model of Flow and Clutch States (Swann et al., 2016, 2017a), has potential to address the existing issues and facilitate

Christian Swann, Scott G. Goddard, Patricia C. Jackman, Matthew J. Schweickle, and Stewart A. Vella, *Flow and Clutch States* In: *Sport, Exercise and Performance Psychology.* Edited by: Edson Filho and Itay Basevitch, Oxford University Press. © Oxford University Press 2021. DOI: 10.1093/oso/9780197512494.003.0004 progress in research and practice. However, the Integrated Model is thus far based on a small number of primarily qualitative studies and needs further testing and refinement. Therefore, it is important and timely to consider the future of research in this field. This chapter reviews the state of the art, before identifying and discussing what we consider to be the five most important questions requiring attention at this point. By doing so, we hope this chapter helps guide scientific progress in this field, to the point that we can meaningfully influence applied practice and better fulfill the promise of this field for sport, exercise, and performance psychology.

State of the Art

Flow

Flow is commonly defined as an intrinsically rewarding and harmonious psychological state that involves concentration and absorption in an activity, with a sense of "everything coming together" or "clicking into place," even in challenging situations (Csikszentmihalyi, 2002). Flow is traditionally conceptualized through Csikszentmihalyi's nine dimensions framework, which involves three conditions (challenge-skill balance, clear goals, unambiguous feedback) and six characteristics (action-awareness merging, sense of control, concentration on the task at hand, loss of self-consciousness, time transformation, and autotelic experience; e.g., Nakamura & Csikszentmihalyi, 2002). In sport, exercise, and performance psychology, this framework is accompanied by measures based explicitly on the nine dimensions (such as the Flow State Scales—Jackson & Eklund, 2002), upon which most of the evidence on flow is based (e.g., Tan & Sin, 2019).

There are a number of reasons as to why flow remains difficult to apply, ranging from definitional to conceptual, measurement, and even philosophical issues. For example, the dimensions of flow are defined in a broad/imprecise manner (Swann et al., 2018); most research has been correlational in nature rather than tapping into the causal mechanisms and explanation of flow (Swann et al., 2018); and there are questions as to whether common measures (e.g., Flow State Scale-2 [FSS-2]; see Jackson & Eklund, 2002) can discriminate between an individual who has experienced flow and someone who has not (Kawabata & Evans, 2016; Moneta, 2021). In turn, we proposed that "given these problems, it is difficult to confidently proceed with the traditional paradigm centered on Csikszentmihalyi's conceptualization of flow as nine dimensions" (Swann et al., 2018, p. 11).

The Integrated Model of Flow and Clutch States

The Integrated Model of Flow and Clutch States was outlined in 2017 (Swann et al., 2017a), based on interviews conducted with athletes within days of an exceptional performance, and through inductive analyses (i.e., rather than deductively "shoe-horning" data into the nine dimensions). As such, this model is based on a recent, detailed, and chronological recall of specific events and experiences, which enabled description of the contexts, processes of occurrence, experience, and outcomes of flow as well as "clutch" states (Figure 4.1).

Clutch performances have commonly been defined as "any performance increment or superior performance that occurs under pressure situations" (Otten, 2009, p. 584). Clutch states are proposed to be the psychological state underlying such performances (Swann et al., 2017b) and are often reported when there is an important outcome on the line (e.g., at the end of a race). Where flow is characterized by effortless attention, positive feedback (e.g., feeling that "everything is going to plan"), and perceptions that the performance is easy or on autopilot, clutch states are characterized by complete and deliberate focus on the task, heightened awareness of the situation and its demands, and intense effort (Swann et al., 2017b). Both states also share overlapping characteristics including absorption and confidence.

The Integrated Model presents clear and testable/falsifiable predictions about the processes through which flow and clutch states occur, as well as the outcomes of each state (see Figure 4.1), which is an improvement on the nine-dimensions framework. Arguably the most important implication of this recent work is that these two distinct psychological states *both* appear to be described by Csikszentmihalyi's nine dimensions (Swann et al., 2018). That is, the nine-dimensions framework conflates flow and "clutch" states. In turn, there are now questions regarding the discriminant validity of measures based on the nine-dimensions framework, such as the FSS-2 (Jackman et al., , 2017; Moneta, 2021).

Interestingly, there are similarities between this work on the Integrated Model and earlier studies by other research groups. In collecting same-day

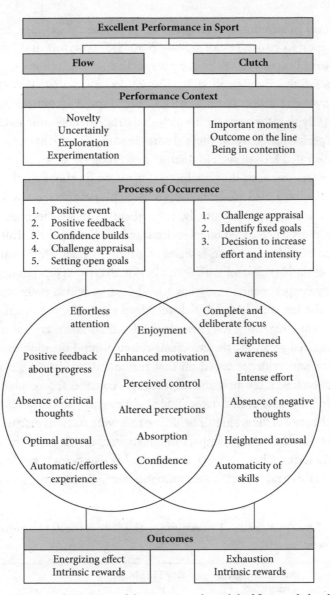

Figure 4.1 The initial iteration of the integrated model of flow and clutch states.

Note: Figure as originally published in Swann, C., Crust, L., Jackman, P.C., Vella, S. A., Allen, M. S., & Keegan, R. (2017). Psychological states underlying excellent performance in sport: Toward an integrated model of flow and clutch states. *Journal of Applied Sport Psychology*, 29, 375–401. doi:10.1080/10413200.2016.1272650

data on flow in adventure recreation, Houge Mackenzie, Hodge, and Boyes (2011) reported two types of flow—"paratelic" (playful) and "telic" (serious)—based on a reversal theory perspective (see Swann et al., 2018, for a critique). Similarly, Bortoli et al., (2012) described a Multi-Action Plan Model involving "Type 1" (automatic) and "Type 2" (controlled) performance in Olympic shooters, which included details of how athletes transition between performance types. These studies lend support for key propositions in the Integrated Model, such as distinct psychological states underlying excellent performance and the possibility of transitioning between those states.

While the Integrated Model holds promise, this new perspective is in need of further testing and, potentially, refinement to make meaningful progress toward evidence-based interventions and applied practice. Thus far, the Integrated Model is based on a series of primarily qualitative studies (e.g., Jackman et al., 2017; Swann et al., 2016, 2017a, 2017b). At this point, only one quantitative/experimental study has tested (and provided preliminary support) for the Integrated Model (Schweickle et al., 2017), but much stronger and more comprehensive tests are required. Additionally, critical investigation is required regarding the criticisms raised around the nine-dimensions framework and evidence based on that framework to date (e.g., using the FSS-2). Therefore, it is timely and important to consider future directions for research on flow and clutch states. Table 4.1 presents five key studies underpinning the state of the art in this field. The following sections discuss what we consider to be the five most impactful questions that will guide the future of this field in terms of how we can move beyond a crisis point to guide scientific progress in this field and ultimately influence applied practice.

Table 4.1 Five Key Readings Underpinning the State of the Art on Flow and Clutch States

Authors	Methodological Design	Key Findings
Bortoli et al. (2012)	Longitudinal evaluation of a 2-year intervention with 15 Olympic shooters	This study reported two types of optimal performance that overlap with flow and clutch states: "Type 1" (automatic) and "Type 2" (controlled) performance. Strategies for transitioning between types of performance were also identified. Although this study was not focused on flow and clutch states specifically, it does lend support for key propositions in the Integrated Model.

Table 4.1 *Continued*

Authors	Methodological Design	Key Findings
Houge Mackenzie et al. (2011)	Interviews with six expert adventure participants; waterproof surveys and recordings via head-mounted video cameras with 10 novice river-surfers	This study provided the first empirical evidence that two distinct psychological states are experienced rather than just flow. Flow and reversal theory were integrated to present evidence of "paratelic" (playful) and "telic" (serious) flow states—descriptions of which are highly similar to those of flow and clutch states in the Integrated Model. Notably, this study employed real-time data collection via head-mounted video cameras and waterproof surveys, enabling the collection of much more recent, detailed, and specific data—similar to event-focused interviews used in later studies.
Jackman et al. (2017)	Longitudinal mixed-method multiple case study with 10 athletes	By collecting interview and questionnaire data about the same performances, this study provided the first empirical evidence that the FSS-2 conflates both flow and clutch states, thereby supporting concerns around discriminant validity. Specifically, this study found that the majority of the 36 items, and all nine of the subscales, in the FSS-2 could represent the experience reported during either flow or clutch states.
Schweickle et al. (2020)	Systematic review of 27 studies on clutch performance	This systematic review found that there is considerable heterogeneity in definitions, conceptualization, and measurement of clutch performance. There are two ways in which clutch performance has primarily been studied: (a) as an ability and (b) as an isolated episode of performance. Stronger evidence exists for clutch performance as an isolated episode. This review provided a series of recommendations to help address issues in the field and guide future research toward refined explanations of clutch performance.
Swann et al. (2017a)	"Event-focused" interviews with 26 athletes, on average 4 days after a specific activity	This study first presented the Integrated Model of Flow and Clutch States, including contexts, processes of occurrence, experience, and outcomes for each state. Psychological skills used to maintain/maximize each state were also reported, whereby dissociative strategies were employed during flow and associative strategies were used during clutch states. Athletes also reported transitioning between states to optimize outcomes.

Note: A broad range of other studies have been highly influential in the development of this field, and to be clear, the studies in this table were identified because they directly address the issues highlighted in this chapter and the specific questions we have posed for future research.

FSS-2, Flow State Scale-2.

Questions to Move the Field Forward

1. Methodological Question: What Is the Best Way to Measure Flow and Clutch States?

Before further testing can take place, new measures of flow and clutch states—consistent with the Integrated Model—are required.[1] With such measures, researchers will be able to test and falsify, support, or refine the Integrated Model. For example, new measures could further assess recent insights such as the processes through which each state is proposed to occur. Furthermore, this step would enable critical examination of the concerns raised over the nine-dimensions framework, accompanying questionnaires, and existing evidence based on those questionnaires (e.g., do measures based on the nine-dimensions framework encompass both flow and clutch states?). As such, the development of measures to test the Integrated Model of Flow and Clutch States is of critical importance to further research.

It is imperative that a critical perspective of the Integrated Model is adopted during the development and validation of new measures. Rather than seeking to provide support for the Integrated Model, the aim should be to try and falsify the model in accordance with Popperian philosophy (see Swann et al., 2018). Measures should be developed based on flow-specific, clutch-specific, and overlapping characteristics. Exploratory factor analysis should first seek to identify the factor structure in a data-driven manner, as opposed to the theory-driven approach used in validation of existing questionnaires such as the FSS-2 (i.e., confirmatory factor analysis based on the nine-dimensions framework; Jackson & Eklund, 2002). Such measures should be able to discriminate between an individual who experienced flow and/or clutch states versus those who did not (i.e., individuals who experienced neither), which is a core critique of the FSS-2 at present (Kawabata & Evans, 2016; Moneta, 2021). The development and validation of these measures is an important next step, before other innovative approaches to measurement may follow in the future (e.g., real-time measures).

---

[1] Note: the dichotomous flow/clutch used in Schweickle et al., (2017) had sound psychometric properties in that study but has not been exposed to rigorous development and validation processes. As such, caution is urged regarding that measure until further testing and validation is conducted.

2. Theoretical Question: What Is the Nature of Clutch Performance?

There are also fundamental questions around clutch states, given that they have only been reported recently. For example, an essential step is to understand whether clutch states are inherent in clutch performance. That is, do clutch states always underlie clutch performances, or could an individual experience clutch states without a clutch performance? Does performance need to be defined objectively (e.g., scoring three points in the last seconds to win a basketball match), or are individuals' subjective appraisals of performance more important (e.g., an individual feeling like they are "giving everything" in terms of effort during a pressure situation)? Such questions are important in understanding the relationship between clutch states and performance, which also has implications for when we may ultimately aim to promote such states or when facilitation of other states (i.e., flow) may be more appropriate. Indeed, similar research is also required to develop better understanding of the relationship between flow and performance.

Inhibiting investigation of these questions, however, are issues surrounding how clutch performance is defined and conceptualized. For example, clutch has been described as "a challenging concept which is inadequately defined in sport" (Seifreid & Papatheodorou, 2010, p. 92). This issue is illustrated in the two primary definitions of clutch performance, which are provided by Otten (2009) and Hibbs (2010). On one hand, Otten (2009) defines clutch performance as "any performance increment . . . under pressure circumstances" (p. 584). On the other hand, Hibbs (2010) defines clutch performance as "succeed[ing] at a competition-related, challenging task during a clutch situation," whereby a clutch situation is when the performance has a significant impact on the outcome of the contest (p. 55). Questions remain, however, over what increment is required to constitute a clutch performance, and further, what the performance should be compared against (e.g., should performance be compared against one's career best or some measure of best performance on that particular day?). It is also unclear as to whether *success* or just *improved performance* is necessary to be a clutch performance, as well as *competition*.

Future research should therefore aim to resolve definitional issues in clutch performance. First, researchers should consider the nature of pressure in clutch performance. For example, clutch states have been found to occur in noncompetitive settings (e.g., exercise; Swann et al., 2019), which suggests that clutch performances may also occur in noncompetitive settings (assuming the performance contains pressure). Second, we know that clutch performance is some form of *positive* performance (i.e., increased or successful performance, either measured objectively or appraised subjectively). As such, researchers should examine the type of indicators athletes use to assess their performance. Specifically, do athletes consider clutch performance based on objective or subjective indicators of performance? Exploration of these questions will illuminate the nature of clutch performance and, consequently, facilitate a robust and conceptually sound investigation of the relationship between clutch states and clutch performance.

3. Theoretical Question: How and Why Do Flow and Clutch States Occur?

A core priority for research in this field is to understand the mechanisms through which flow and clutch states occur. The Integrated Model has promise in that it makes causal predictions about the processes of occurrence for each state (see Figure 4.1). For example, flow is proposed to occur through a positive event, which leads to positive feedback and increased confidence, which in turn results in a challenge appraisal and the setting of open goals—the pursuit of which leads to the experience of flow. Clutch states are proposed to occur through a challenge appraisal, identification of a specific goal (e.g., to birdie the last hole in order to win a golf tournament), and a decision to increase effort and intensity, which results in clutch states (e.g., Swann et al., 2017a, 2017b, 2019). By testing these predictions in the Integrated Model, researchers will be able to support, refine, or falsify the model.

Once new measures are developed and validated, these predictions can be tested experimentally, with the important aim of assessing how to induce flow/clutch states in a laboratory setting. For example, Schweickle et al. (2017) experimentally tested the effects of open versus specific goals on flow and clutch states in a cognitive task and found preliminary support for the Integrated Model; however, flow was reported during significantly lower performance compared to clutch states. Importantly, such experiments will be able to test effects of inducing these states on performance and other hypothesized outcomes such as enjoyment, intrinsic motivation, and well-being. That is, experimental research can address the highly impactful questions: If we can induce a flow or clutch state, will it lead to exceptional performance? What is the relationship between flow/clutch states and performance? This work should also guide research in other performance domains. Flow is suggested to be universal (i.e., experienced across all cultures and activities; Csikszentmihalyi, 2002), which raises the question: Is that the case with clutch states too? And does the Integrated Model apply similarly in other performance domains such as dance and the military? In turn, this knowledge can contribute to the development of a strong, practically useful theory of flow and clutch states in sport, exercise, and performance psychology.

4. Applied Question: Can Individuals Maximize Flow and Clutch States?

Understanding if/how performers and exercisers can manage, prolong, and maximize flow and clutch states is an exciting avenue for future research (Brick et al., 2019). Initial insights have suggested that flow and clutch states can be maximized, for example, by using psychological skills to prolong these states. Athletes have explained that flow can be prolonged through positive distractions (Jackman et al., 2020; Swann et al., 2017a), suggesting that focusing one's attention away from the task can be helpful to avoid the effortful, analytical thoughts that can disrupt flow. The use of distractions to enhance performance or prolong flow is somewhat counterintuitive, however, and requires further research (e.g., in terms of the limits of such distractions for remaining constructive). During clutch states, athletes have reported using motivational self-talk, setting short-term goals, and strategically monitoring their performance/attention to manage and maintain their experience (Jackman et al., 2020; Swann et al., 2017a). Thus, it appears that flow is prolonged by utilizing distractive strategies, while clutch states are managed through active self-regulation (see Brick et al., 2014). The lack of debilitative interpretations of anxiety during flow and clutch states may explain why such cognitive strategies can maintain these states, even though attentional shifts are a primary component in common explanations of choking, such as distraction (e.g., Oudejans et al., 2011) and self-focus (e.g., Beilock & Carr, 2001) theories. Furthermore, athletes have reported transitioning between flow and clutch states during performances to achieve optimal outcomes, through processes of reappraisal and resetting of goals (Swann et al., 2017a).

While these initial insights are interesting and have potential from an applied perspective, several questions exist concerning the management, sustainment, and maximization of flow and clutch states, and especially in terms of what strategies are most effective for each state. One potential line of inquiry is how research on attentional focus and metacognition (e.g., Brick et al., 2014) could be combined with the Integrated Model to build understanding of self-regulation during flow and clutch states (Brick et al., 2019). Such research should initially seek to explore metacognitive processes (e.g., metacognitive feelings, estimations, and judgments) and attentional focus during flow and clutch states (i.e., to determine strategies used, if any), before experimentally testing whether specific strategies are more suitable to prolong, maximize, and manage each state.

Additionally, more research is required on the prospect that individuals can transition between flow and clutch states. Studies are needed to identify the mechanisms of these transitions, whether they can be initiated consciously, and, if so, what strategies are involved. Finally, it is important to examine the mental and physical effects of experiencing flow and clutch states. The Integrated Model proposes that flow is characterized by ease/reduced effort and leaves individuals feeling energized, whereas clutch states involve intense effort and lead to exhaustion (Swann et al., 2017a, 2019). Questions remain, however, as to whether these distinctions in effort are physical and/or mental, and if they are supported by objective data. Researchers could examine psychophysiological demands associated with experiencing flow and clutch states, for example, through heart rate variability, which is a potential physiological marker of flow (e.g., Tozman et al., 2015). Together, these lines of inquiry present promising avenues for future research in terms of whether/how individuals can manipulate these psychological states to optimize performance and experiential outcomes.

5. Applied Question: What Should Flow and Clutch State Interventions Involve?

Understanding how to purposefully induce flow and clutch states remains arguably the most important question for sport and exercise psychologists, representing the "holy grail" for researchers in this field. To reiterate, our role as sport, exercise, and performance psychologists is to apply psychological principles to help individuals "consistently perform in the upper range of their capabilities *and* more thoroughly enjoy the performance process" (American Psychological Association, Division 47, 2019, p. 9). Arguably, promoting optimal experiences of flow and clutch in performers and exercisers concurrently embodies both objectives. Nonetheless, attempts to induce and enhance flow and clutch in sport and exercise have been considered as methodologically flawed and largely unsuccessful (Swann et al., 2012, 2018). As discussed previously, at this point we are unable to provide performers and exercisers with strategies and techniques to reliably experience these optimal states (Swann et al., 2018). Addressing this issue is fundamental in translating optimal experience research into applied settings and, in turn, fulfilling our role as sport, exercise, and performance psychologists. Despite its challenges, we must endeavor to provide practitioners with trainable and effective methods to increase the frequency and intensity of flow and clutch states.

Ideally, researchers, performers/exercisers, and practitioners should be able to create interventions to induce and manage (e.g., prolong/maintain) the occurrence and experience of flow and clutch states (Swann et al., 2018). Interventions should inform performers and exercisers of strategies for inducing and maintaining such states and how/when to use those strategies (e.g., depending on contexts such as the stage or importance of the activity and desired outcomes). Advancing the application of flow and clutch states will require the development of interventions that clearly link the techniques and strategies with a mechanism of change related to flow and clutch. That is, interventions should be developed with clear and logical links between the techniques or strategies employed and proposed mechanisms of action (i.e., processes that influence the occurrence of flow/clutch states), and in doing so, they will have greater potential to be effective (e.g., Connell et al., 2019). Interventions built upon the processes and mechanisms provided by a testable model will either refine the conceptualization or afford genuine strategies for athletes and practitioners to utilize in applied settings.

Conclusion

Optimal experiences and episodes of superior functioning are central to sport, exercise, and performance psychology. Specifically, this chapter reviewed the state of the art of research on flow and clutch states. Despite extensive research, flow states remain rare, elusive, and difficult for researchers or practitioners to induce purposefully—due primarily to a number of conceptual issues in the traditional nine-dimensions framework. We reviewed recent research on the Integrated Model of Flow and Clutch States, which makes several important contributions (including testable/falsifiable hypotheses about the occurrence of each state) and may be able to overcome limitations in the nine-dimensions framework. The Integrated Model is at an early stage of development and requires further testing and refinement. We proposed five key questions that we believe can help guide future research: (a) What is the best way to measure flow and clutch states? (b) What is the nature of clutch performance? (c) How and why do flow and clutch states occur? (d) Can individuals maximize flow and clutch states? and (e) What should flow and clutch state interventions involve? We hope this chapter helps guide scientific progress in this field, with the ultimate aims of meaningfully influencing applied practice and better fulfilling the promise of flow and clutch states in sport, exercise, and performance psychology.

References

American Psychological Association, Division 47. (2019). Defining the practice of sport and performance psychology. https://www.apadivisions.org/division-47/about/resources/defining.pdf

Beilock, S. L., & Carr, T. H. (2001). On the fragility of skilled performance: What governs choking under pressure? *Journal of Experimental Psychology: General, 130*(4), 701–725. https://doi.org/10.1037/0096-3445.130.4.701

Bortoli, L., Bertollo, M., Hanin, Y., & Robazza, C. (2012). Striving for excellence: A multi-action plan intervention model for shooters. *Psychology of Sport and Exercise, 13*(5), 693–701.

Brick, N., Campbell, M., & Swann, C. (2019). Metacognitive processes in the self-regulation of endurance performance. In C. Meijen & S. Marcora (Eds.), *The psychology of endurance performance*. Routledge.

Brick, N., MacIntyre, T., & Campbell, M. (2014). Attentional focus in endurance activity: New paradigms and future directions. *International Review of Sport and Exercise Psychology, 7*(1), 106–134.

Connell, L. E., Carey, R. N., de Bruin, M., Rothman, A. J., Johnston, M., Kelly, M. P., & Michie, S. (2019). Links between behavior change techniques and mechanisms of action: An expert consensus study. *Annals of Behavioral Medicine, 53*, 708–720.

Csikszentmihalyi, M. (2002). *Flow: The psychology of optimal experience* (2nd ed.). Harper & Row.

Csikszentmihalyi, M., Latter, P., & Weinkauff Duranso, C. (2017). *Running flow*. Human Kinetics.

Hibbs, D. (2010). A conceptual analysis of clutch performances in competitive sports. *Journal of the Philosophy of Sport, 37*(1), 47–59.

Houge Mackenzie, S., Hodge, K., & Boyes, M. (2011). Expanding the flow model in adventure activities: A reversal theory perspective. *Journal of Leisure Research, 43*(4), 519–544.

Jackman, P. C., Crust, L., & Swann, C. (2017). Systematically comparing methods used to study flow in sport: A longitudinal multiple-case study. *Psychology of Sport and Exercise, 32,* 113–123.

Jackman, P. C., Crust, L., & Swann, C. (2020). The role of mental toughness in the occurrence of flow and clutch states in sport. *International Journal of Sport Psychology, 51*(1), 1–27.

Jackson, S., & Eklund, R. (2002). Assessing flow in physical activity: The Flow State Scale-2 and Dispositional Flow Scale-2. *Journal of Sport and Exercise Psychology, 24*(2), 133–150.

Kawabata, M., & Evans, R. (2016). How to classify who experienced flow from who did not based on the flow state scale-2 scores: A pilot study of latent class factor analysis. *Sport Psychologist, 30*(3), 267–275.

Moneta, G. B. (2021). On the conceptualization and measurement of flow. In C. Peifer & S. Engeser (Eds.), *Advances in flow research* (2nd ed.). Springer Science.

Moran, A., & Toner, J. (2017). *A critical introduction to sport psychology.* Taylor & Francis.

Nakamura, J., & Csikszentmihalyi, M. (2002). The concept of flow. In C. R. Snyder & S. J. Lopez (Eds.), *Handbook of positive psychology* (pp. 89–105). Oxford University Press.

Otten, M. (2009). Choking vs. clutch performance: A study of sport performance under pressure. *Journal of Sport and Exercise Psychology, 31,* 583–601.

Oudejans, R. R. D., Kuijpers, W., Kooijman, C. C., & Bakker, F. C. (2011). Thoughts and attention of athletes under pressure: Skill-focus or performance worries? *Anxiety, Stress and Coping, 24*(1), 59–73. https://doi.org/10.1080/10615806.2010.481331

Schweickle, M., Groves, S., Vella, S. A., & Swann, C. (2017). The effects of open vs. specific goals on flow and clutch states in a cognitive task. *Psychology of Sport and Exercise, 33,* 45–54.

Schweickle, M., Swann, C., Jackman, P., & Vella, S. (2020). Clutch performance: A systematic review. *International Review of Sport and Exercise Psychology.* https://doi.org/10.1080/1750984X.2020.1771747

Seifreid, C., & Papatheodorou, M. (2010). The concepts of clutch and choking: Recommendations for improving performance under pressure. *Journal of Coaching Education, 3*(1), 91–98.

Swann, C., Crust, L., Jackman, P. C., Vella, S. A., Allen, M. S., & Keegan, R. (2017a). Psychological states underlying excellent performance in sport: Toward an integrated model of flow and clutch states. *Journal of Applied Sport Psychology, 29,* 375–401.

Swann, C., Crust, L., Jackman, P., Vella, S. A., Allen, M. S., & Keegan, R. (2017b). Performing under pressure: Exploring the psychological state underlying clutch performance in sport. *Journal of Sports Sciences, 35*(23), 2272–2280.

Swann, C., Jackman, P. C., Schweickle, M. J., & Vella, S. A. (2019). Optimal experiences in exercise: A qualitative investigation of flow and clutch states. *Psychology of Sport and Exercise, 40,* 87–98.

Swann, C., Keegan, R., Crust, L., & Piggott, D. (2016). Psychological states underlying excellent performance in professional golfers: "Letting it happen" vs. "making it happen." *Psychology of Sport and Exercise, 23,* 101–113.

Swann, C., Keegan, R., Piggott, D., & Crust, L. (2012). A systematic review of the experience, occurrence, and controllability of flow states in elite sport. *Psychology of Sport and Exercise, 13,* 807–819.

Swann, C., Piggott, D., Schweickle, M., & Vella, S. A. (2018). A review of scientific progress in flow in sport and exercise: Normal science, crisis, and a progressive shift. *Journal of Applied Sport Psychology, 30,* 249–271.

Tan, L., & Sin, H. X. (2019). Flow research in music contexts: A systematic literature review. *Musicae Scientiae,* 1029864919877564.

Tozman, T., Magdas, E. S., MacDougall, H. G., & Vollmeyer, R. (2015). Understanding the psychophysiology of flow: A driving simulator experiment to investigate the relationship between flow and heart rate variability. *Computers in Human Behavior, 52,* 408–418.

5

Mental Skills

Dave Collins and Hugh Richards

State of the Art

Sport psychology (SP) is an essentially applied subject that historically has been inextricably linked to concepts of mental skills (MS) and mental skills training (MST). Importantly, however, the view that SP is just concerned with MS is limited, inaccurate, and justifiably criticized (cf. Collins et al., 2011). Such criticism has run parallel to other debates including the role of sport psychologists contrasted with other subdisciplines (particularly clinical and counseling), the services provided (e.g., performance enhancement, individual well-being, or research), and, more recently, the expertise appropriate to address mental health issues of performers (and coaches).

Therefore, our review of what is needed in MS considers not only the "what" of MST but also issues related to the who, how, and why, reflecting the ideas of professional judgment and decision-making (PJDM; Martindale & Collins, 2012, 2013) that underpin effective service provision. Table 5.1 offers our overview of key readings reflecting key issues on MS.

Psychological factors play an important role in performance. This applies equally to skills used "on the performance day," skills to maximize training benefits, and skills to ensure the well-being of the athlete as a person. Additionally, however, other factors critical to performance must be addressed, either directly or indirectly through the sport psychologist working effectively with and through other disciplines. Reflecting this, an effective practitioner will need knowledge and the ability to apply the knowledge in five key areas:

- MST
- Skill acquisition and motor control (cf. Abraham & Collins, 2011a)
- Coaching science (cf. Abraham & Collins, 2011b)

Dave Collins and Hugh Richards, *Mental Skills* In: *Sport, Exercise and Performance Psychology.*
Edited by: Edson Filho and Itay Basevitch, Oxford University Press. © Oxford University Press 2021.
DOI: 10.1093/oso/9780197512494.003.0005

- Organizational behavior for teams and squads (cf. Fletcher & Wagstaff, 2009)
- Mental welfare (cf. Küttal & Larsen, 2019)

Effective SP practice requires the ability to blend and balance knowledge of all of these broad areas, as well as more specialist ones such as talent development, to achieve agreed-upon target outcomes. Thus, for example, psychologists working in sport need to be aware of how a mental health first aid course might be beneficial but might be even more effective when adjusted to meet the social context and culture of sport (cf. Lebrun & Collins, 2017).

The importance of sociocultural factors in delivering effective MS has been previously acknowledged (Vealey, 2007). Accordingly, in this chapter we also highlight specific issues and areas for work that reflect the complexity of sociocultural (e.g., nationality) and sport cultural influences that may coact or compete in determining what works best (cf. Pankhurst, 2014). Additionally, further research is necessary to examine how MS usage—indeed, suitability—may vary between men and women. This issue is relevant in other areas (e.g., talent development; see Curran et al., 2019), which suggests it might be inappropriate to assume that methods developed predominantly on males will apply to females.

But Do We Measure What We NEED to Measure?

Fundamental to any scientific discipline is that it is based on empirical evidence generated through research and the application of systematic method. Few approaches to establishing evidence receive as much credibility as the randomized controlled trial (RCT) because evidence on treatment effects is obtained with minimal bias. Such a design is effective when standardized treatment (e.g., drug dosage by body weight) can be applied. However, this approach is not effective or suitable when the "treatment" is multifactorial/longitudinal/dependent on professional relationships and outcomes are dependent on multiple interacting factors. Thus, there are significant drawbacks in applying RCT approaches to assess the effectiveness of MST. First, principles of RCTs—randomization, comparison to a control group, and double-blind designs—are challenging to achieve in realistic applied settings. Even if these were achieved, an RCT still has potential for biases, which must be minimized or acknowledged (Killin & Della Sala, 2015). Topically, in arguing against over-reliance of RCT evidence informing policy during the COVID-19 pandemic, Greenhalgh (2020) extolls the value of "practice-based evidence" (Ogilvie et al., 2020) to complement limits of traditional RCT-oriented evidence.

If MS were considered only in terms of MST, reducing research focus down to assessing causal linear effects on single/few outcomes, it would be easier to adopt elements of RCTs. For example, Barwood, Thelwell, and Tipton (2008) taught psychological skills (goal setting, arousal regulation, mental imagery, and positive self-talk) to healthy male adults, who showed significantly improved running performance in the heat (8%) compared to pretest, while the control group showed no significant change. An equally robust approach was utilized by Mesagno and Mullane-Grant (2010) to assess relative benefits of preperformance routines (PPRs) to maintain performance under pressure. Those receiving "extensive PPR" showed better performance compared to groups receiving single elements of PPR (such as breathing, cue words, or temporal consistency alone). In both examples, the intervention was standardized and the impact assessed on a single outcome measure. Outside of sport, MST was shown to improve surgical performance of medical residents under stress, using a full RCT design including blinding of evaluators (Anton et al., 2018). Although each high-quality study contributed positively to understanding MST impact, none considered needs assessment, training delivery, provider-participant interactions, or the iterative process of adaptation expected to take place in real applied SP service. Indeed, expert SP practitioners (Henriksen et al., 2019) report that successful interventions with senior performers often have no curricula, focus on the whole person using multiple data sources to assess needs, and are based on "deep, trusting and long term" relationships (p. 79) that include regular contact with/feedback to the client. When features of good practice contrast so strongly with the standardized protocol required for RCT, more appropriate methods are needed to develop a convincing evidence base.

So How COULD We Measure It Better?

Typically, SP interventions comprise multiple components that interact to enhance performance together with other changes influencing more holistic issues for the athlete. Accordingly, such interventions can be construed as complex interventions, notwithstanding that work is often focused on an individual. On this basis, adopting principles from the Medical Research Council guidance on process evaluations could provide a useful approach to building an evidence base that informs practice for developing MS (Moore et al., 2015).

Process evaluations are proposed to complement evidence-based RCT research, emphasizing the importance of context and differential effects of intervention, utilizing qualitative information to assess two dimensions: implementation of interventions and mechanisms of impact. This is completed in tandem with "normal" research that describes the intervention and assesses changes in outcomes. Notably, this approach fits well with the concepts of PJDM (Martindale & Collins, 2012). Process evaluations play a critical role in providing complete evaluation of interventions without which evidence from RCTs cannot be adequately judged. Although stringent publication word limits may work against this, detail on implementation focuses on delivery, training conduct, materials, and resources, which contrasts and complements the detail of experimental protocols typically provided in MS training studies discussed earlier. Additionally, implementation reports on *fidelity* (intervention delivered as intended), *dose* (intensity, frequency, and duration of sessions), and *adaptations* (changes to intervention to fit needs and context) are needed.

Secondly, process evaluation focuses on the mechanism of impact, testing putative pathways such as whether benefits of PPRs may be influenced through changing self-efficacy alone, rather than a specific performance preparation. This focus also considers intervention responses, such as the commitment, adherence, and uptake of MS. Implementation and mechanism of impact are evaluated, along with details about opportunities and barriers in the context to help interpret the effect of treatment and consider generalization. While process evaluations are presented by Moore et al. (2015) in relation to public health research on a much larger scale, the principle can be easily adjusted to support developing robust evidence on MS delivery.

Another approach to guide research on MS interventions is through the organizational training and development literature. Salas et al. (2012) discuss comprehensive training evaluation based on Kirkpatrick's hierarchical four-level model: *reactions, learning, behavior,* and *results.* This model has been criticized for the ordinal structure, purported to suggest that if no learning was assessed, then behavior was not expected to change. However, Salas et al. recommended that thorough training evaluation should focus on all four levels and that this should be conducted with a specific aim with measures linked directly to intended outcomes.

Conclusion: So What Does This Mean?

The potential for evidence from process evaluation or training evaluations to inform effective MS interventions is significant. Such evidence would be superior to that from simple research designs where delivery is reduced to formulaic protocol and effectiveness considered only in relation to limited outcome variables. Professional training requirements could adopt these approaches and the information generated published to inform the professions' evidence base. The practical and ethical issues associated could be effectively addressed. Furthermore, adopting ideas such as premortems and cultures of dialogue and criticism proposed as a partial solution to the "replication crisis" in psychology (Bishop, 2019) would not only benefit professionals completing training but also create stronger and more scientifically rigorous practice.

Table 5.1 Five Key Readings on MS and Related Topics

Authors	Methodological Design	Key Findings
Adler et al. (2015)	RCT in military recruits. Surveys at various points of training	Examination of MST effects. Comparatively small but significant effects of intervention on several indices of training outcome
Behnke et al. (2019)	Psychometric design: five studies using PCA and factorial analysis	Development of an MST-related measurement tool, developed in two languages in parallel
Collins & Kamin (2012)	Desktop study. Literature-based exposition	Three "ages" of a science and how this influences knowledge application. Offers insights on how different aims will influence epistemologies and application
Moore et al. (2015)	Methodology advice	Guidance application of RCTs, stressing the use of process evaluations to offer a richer picture of intervention mechanism and impact
Sharp et al. (2019)	Qualitative study with practitioners and supervisors	Effective use of supervision in applied SP. Examines the ethical challenges experienced in supervised practice

MS, mental skills; MST, mental skills training; PCA, principal component analysis; RCT, randomized controlled trial; SP, sport psychology.

Questions to Move the Field Forward

We now propose five questions that we consider to offer significant opportunity to develop the field. Given that MS is an overwhelmingly applied topic, these questions reflect the critical issues facing sport psychologists to optimize the efficacy and effectiveness of mental skills applications with performers.

1. Methodological Question: Are We Clear on the Link Between Aim and Design in MST?

What
Identifying exact objectives for MS interventions is a key stage in design (Martindale & Collins, 2005), whether these are short-term (e.g., within sessions based on intentions for impact) or long-term outcomes from a program. Current debate exists on optimizing balance across elements such as performance (now or future), well-being, and athletic and/or personal development. Indeed, as SP becomes more accepted, the scope of application is likely to broaden. However, it is important that case conceptualization and subsequent design of MS "packages" be explicitly considered.

Why
Good practice starts with setting mutually agreed-upon targets and includes both outcome and process goals, nested into an overall program (cf. Martindale & Collins, 2007). Interestingly, case conceptualization and planning are increasingly common requirements of professional SP accreditation programs (cf. Tod et al., 2017). Despite this positive development and the increase in published case studies offering underpinning evolution and rationale, the link between aim and design is still comparatively unexplored.

How
In contrast to clinical psychology, where clients contract to a series of sessions to solve a specific problem, SP practitioners commonly form longer term relationships, often as embedded members of support teams. Reflecting this, longer term and longitudinal research is required. The significant change in work timescale necessitates different approaches to evaluating efficacy, moving beyond simplistic consultant evaluation questionnaires.

Evaluation should enable original case conceptualizations and objectives to be assessed against eventual impact together with ongoing refinement and adaptation. Comprehensive triangulation can be achieved by incorporating data-driven needs analyses with case conceptualization, intervention approaches, and consideration of alternative options. Such approaches will also cater to providers' social constructivism in intervention design and deployment. On completion or, more likely in the current climate, when a benchmark is reached, these same measures and planning parameters will inform thorough evaluations against design, ongoing refinement, and endpoint outcomes.

2. Applied Question: How Do We Deliver MST Services?

What

Once case conceptualization has been accurately completed, the optimum "blend" of MST must be designed, incorporating aspects such as timing, sequencing of the skills taught, and how they fit into a nested periodization approach. Recent research (e.g., Collins et al., 2018) has emphasized the importance of periodization, for example, tactical periodization for team sports and emotional periodization in high-risk adventure or action sports. A key point here is that the many forms of sport present a very wide spectrum of challenges and contexts.

Why

SP is no longer a young discipline, yet there is still a significant tendency to draw uncritically on research from the parent discipline of psychology (Collins & Kamin, 2012). Considering the complex demands and particular challenges inherent in performance sport means that practitioners require not just a bespoke set of skills but specific research to underpin them.

How

The overlapping and interacting nature of issues presents significant challenges, for example, how to achieve an optimum blend of MS in a complex social setting with multiple interactions and different personalities with individual needs. An effective solution we believe is to adopt a PJDM approach. This is significantly different from "off-the-peg recipes" disseminated in the pop-psych literature and by social media gurus. Instead, effective SP support is more complicated and time consuming and requires thorough

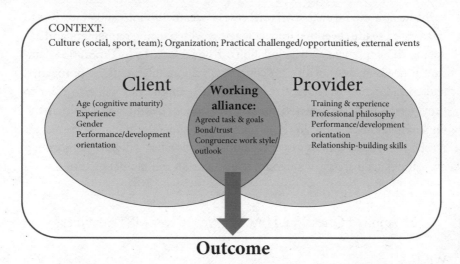

Figure 5.1. Schematic of the key factors affecting intervention impact.

analysis and bespoke intervention. The major issue is how much knowledge and experience are required to deliver this approach.

In the final three questions we discuss the integration of the client, the practitioner, and culture to maximize the effect of MS interventions. As illustrated in Figure 5.1, the effects of MST are all influenced by this interaction and research is required to contribute to a sophisticated understanding to benefit applied practice and SP service. To aid flow, we have collapsed the what-why-how structure within the three interacting factors.

3. Applied Question: What Individual Client Factors Are Relevant in Determining MST Interventions?

Performers differ with respect to many dimensions, which are relevant to effective MS delivery (Table 5.2).

Unlike many other performance domains (e.g., business, military, medicine), sport performers start athletic careers much earlier, often as children and adolescents, and the majority may have retired from competitive performances well before age 40! Consequently, age and cognitive maturity are important factors to include in determining effective design of MST. It is also salient that the sport context usually includes direct and immediate feedback, public performance, and critical evaluation to enhance performance.

Table 5.2 Client Factors Relevant to Effectiveness of MS Development

Age/cognitive maturity	Correlated but not the same. Typically, around puberty, females may show greater cognitive maturity. Performance experience compared to age also varies considerably between sports (e.g., experienced female gymnasts may be quite young), and types of experience (development academy) may influence elements of cognitive maturity.
Gender	Gender differences in response to MS have been identified; however, the evidence is not clear and more specific examination of this issue through research is necessary.
Special populations	Working with athletes with disabilities is one example that may require specific consideration. Athletes with disabilities may have experienced discrimination, have longstanding psychological issues, and/or have experienced specific trauma. In such instances, the importance of quality supervision, awareness of professional boundaries and competencies, and suitable referral systems and networks is particularly high.
	In relation to the pragmatics of MST, careful adaptation is required. For example, imagery and attentional control both typically have strong visual components, so providing explanations and content needs to be reconfigured for use with visually impaired athletes. Peer networks, supervision, and professionals in allied fields (e.g., education) can help to inform work on adaptations.
Injury	Psychosocial and emotional factors associated with injury have been well explored in the literature (e.g., Brewer, 2010). Sport psychologists must demonstrate high levels of rapid adaptability to offer effective service to clients. Timing of service can be critical in such circumstances.
Career stage	Several transitions are relevant to MS interventions such as those between athletic levels, stages of education, independent living, and parenthood. MST can be employed effectively to help address issues, from practical to emotional. There is also a reciprocal relationship in which the transition itself may significantly influence development of the athlete and their MS.
Retirement	Technically a career stage (see previously) but uniquely one in which psychological support may be altered or ceased. Forced retirement is particularly challenging. Many professional sports have player associations that can provide support, information, and resources and in some cases SP provision is maintained for a period, postcareer. Judicious referrals can be critical in assisting athletes and help to compensate if psychological support is not resourced.

MS, mental skills; MST, mental skills training.

Successful sport participation is also predicated upon effective physical and technical training, which require significant levels of motivation to adhere to prolonged training, sleep restriction to enable schedules to be met, and consequent sacrifices in relation to social life. For adolescents specifically, these demands are particularly challenging as detailed by Blakemore (2019), who summarized the most recent evidence identifying the significant neurological transformations that occur for adolescents. Heightened sensitivity to social exclusion from peers, acute self-consciousness, and biochemical adaptations driving changes in sleep patterns (from "lark" to "owl") each present specific issues that sport psychologists must help young athletes carefully navigate.

As one example, the evidence-based emphasis on developing self-regulation to support achievement in high-level sport (Cleary & Zimmeran, 2001; Toering et al., 2009) must at the same time reflect the different brain "architecture" associated with functional differences. Specifically, the limbic (reward) system is well developed and shows little change through adolescence. In contrast, the prefrontal cortex (self-control, planning, and self-awareness) is relatively underdeveloped from the early teenage years onward and continues transforming significantly through to the early 20s (Mills et al., 2014). Social and environmental factors influence this process, which also has significant interindividual variation, requiring sport psychologists to attend especially to needs analysis and monitoring. Such factors might suggest that an early Sunday morning workshop on long-term planning and goalsetting with a group of adolescent athletes would seem particularly ill-conceived scheduling.

4. Applied Question: What Are the Implications of Sport Psychologist Characteristics?

Within counseling and psychotherapy, the importance of the client-professional relationship is well recognized and suggested to have a greater bearing on outcome than theoretical orientation or technique (Horvath & Bedi, 2002). This same issue has also been outlined in relation to SP practice (Petipas et al., 1999). Understanding when and how to flexibly adopt different relationship styles, to best suit both client and context, is what Lazarus (1993) refers to as an "authentic chameleon": a critically important skill to effectively deliver MS interventions. This is not to suggest that psychologists should "play roles," but rather that they focus on making connections to the client that recognize their expectations, needs, and personal characteristics—in other words, an optimum but also broad-ranging application of PJDM in using interpersonal skills.

Forging a working alliance (cf. Figure 5.1) lies at the heart of successful practice, and these principles have been clearly articulated in the fields of counseling and psychotherapy (see, e.g., Taber et al., 2011). An effective working alliance is based on three components: clearly agreed-upon goals, tasks that will help to achieve goals, and a bond between performer and psychologist. Importantly, however, this bond need not necessarily be a "positive" friendship, but rather needs to be effective for the goals agreed upon. For example, while counseling is usually driven by specific problems or concerns, in SP there may be a broader remit on development over a longer period. Consequently, developing an agreed-upon focus requires detailed attention and periodic review as work progresses. In agreeing upon the tasks to achieve such dynamic goals, psychologists must identify the most suitable approaches yet have adaptability to cater to performer preferences and impact. Agreed-upon goals and tasks will create the third component of the alliance: the bond based on trust, respect, and rapport. Notably, how these components are developed will vary according to the performer's age. Simple professional requirements such as explaining how confidentiality works, justifying rationale for the chosen approach, and effective communication skills will all contribute to creating an effective bond.

Reflecting our earlier caveat, being approachable, trustworthy, and effective are much more salient than attempting to be liked. Within a program, psychologists may have to challenge clients, provoke desire to change, and provide honest, critical feedback. Attempting to be friendly and supportive, typically reported by athletes as their preferred style, is *not* the basis for a professional relationship and risks limiting effectiveness and creating potential for dependency, both of which should be avoided.

5. Applied Question: What Cultural Factors Influence Effective Development of MS?

All sport performers train and compete in situations that have a social context. The term *culture* has been used to refer to this social dimension but does not precisely define the scope of the social context. Thus, culture might be used confusingly to describe a social dimension at the largest scale, linked to country, race, and religion, down to the smallest scale, such as a conditioning training group or a coach-athlete dyad. In between these are many other dimensions of culture, for example, types of sports (e.g., individual or team, independent or interactive performance), specific named sports within the same "type" (e.g., Rugby Union or Rugby League; Formula 1 or Rally), outcome focus (development, performance, or recreation), age and gender, team-specific culture, and subgroup of performers (by position/role/training needs). Effective MST requires the sport psychologist to be sensitive to cultural norms at any, and all, of these levels and work hard to suspend their own preconceptions that could limit their ability. There has been significant growth in SP research on team culture generally in the last decade (e.g., Cruickshank et al., 2013). However, research has not focused specifically on showing how MS development can be improved by attending to cultural dimensions. Consequently, while the importance of culture is widely acknowledged at a practical level, evidence is urgently required to underpin professional behavior and training.

Psychology, including SP and, indeed, many research fields, is subject to a broad sampling bias in research that has been referred to by the acronym WEIRD (Western, Educated, Industrialized, Rich, and Democratic; Henrich et al., 2010). In essence, this means that the enormous overreliance on sampling a particular section of society (especially university students) in countries such as the United States and United Kingdom leads to an extremely low generalizability of research to a world population of sport performers. Henrich et al. identify several approaches to try to improve this situation, including systemic (e.g., funding, publication demands) and organizational (e.g., data sharing), that would have significant impact but are hard to achieve. However, they also promote active collaborations between researchers, several approaches to "comparative" studies, and developing relationships with participant pools with different demographics. These latter approaches can be addressed by research groups and individuals and, together with greater publication of SP training experiences suggested earlier in this chapter, could significantly advance research knowledge of MS.

The challenge to sport psychologists to understand and work within a sport or team culture for effective development in MS can appear complex. Research in this area examining and comparing the development of culture in professional sports teams and Olympic sports offers an empirically based model on which SP can begin to analyze and understand the key components of this complex dynamic (Cruickshank et al., 2013, 2014). This relative new contribution must be developed further and of course considered in light of the previous paragraph since the research was primarily based in the United Kingdom. The experience of working with individuals from different world regions, with distinctive cultures, highlights, by contrast, the predominant influence of "Westernized" traditions. The SP literature is typically characterized by a focus on the individual rather than collective and values autonomy, high status, and principles of liberal democracy in groups. Furthermore, the religious and spiritual backdrop to a culture can influence thinking about even basic components of MST, such as attention control or casual attributions. Cultural awareness and sensitivity, at multiple levels, are essential.

Conclusion

As active pracademics (we research it and do it), we hope that our observations are of interest to both sides of the research-practice divide. Indeed, and returning to the point made at the start of this chapter, we hope that we encourage colleagues to erode and eradicate this divide in what is, after all, an applied discipline. In closing, we would stress how useful knowledge from outside a domain, in this case SP, can be, so long as it is critically reviewed and applied. We trust that message has emerged loud and clear!

References

Abraham, A. K., & Collins, D. (2011a). Effective skill development: How should athletes' skills be developed? In D. Collins, A. Button, & H. Richards (Eds.), *Performance psychology: A practitioner's guide* (pp. 207–230). Elsevier.

Abraham, A., & Collins, D. (2011b). Taking the next step: Ways forward for coaching science. *Quest, 63*, 366–384.

Adler, A. B., Bliese, P. D., Williams, J., Csoka, L., Pickering, M. A., Hammermeister, J., Harada, C., Holliday, B., & Ohlson, C. (2015). Mental skills training with basic combat soldiers: A group-randomised trial. *Journal of Applied Psychology, 100*(6), 1752–1764.

Anton, N. E., Beane, J., Yurco, A. M., Howley, L. D., Bean, E., Myers, E. M., & Stefanidis, D. (2018). Mental skills training effectively minimizes operative performance deterioration under stressful conditions: Results of a randomised controlled study. *American Journal of Surgery, 215*, 214–221.

Barwood, M. J., Thelwell, R. C., & Tipton, M. J. (2008). Psychological skills training improves exercise performance in the heat. *Medicine and Science in Sports and Exercise, 40*, 387–396.

Behnke, M., Tomczak, M., Kaczmarek, L. D., Komar, M., & Gracz, J. (2019). The sport mental training questionnaire: Development and validation. *Current Psychology, 38*(2), 504–516. https://doi.org/10.1007/s12144-017-9629-1

Bishop, D. V. M. (2019). The psychology of experimental psychologists: Overcoming cognitive constraints to improve research: The 47th Sir Frederic Bartlett Lecture.

Quarterly Journal of Experimental Psychology, 22, 1–19. https://doi.org/10.1177/1747021819886519

Blakemore, S. J. (2019). Adolescence and mental health. *Lancet, 393*(10185), 2030–2031. doi:10.1016/S0140-6736(19)31013-X. PMID: 31106741.

Brewer, B. (2010). The role of psychological factors in sport injury rehabilitation outcomes. *International Review of Sport and Exercise Psychology, 3*, 40–61. https://doi.org/10.1080/17509840903301207

Clearly, T. J., & Zimmerman, B. J. (2001). Self-regulation differences during athletic practice by experts, non-experts, and novices. *Journal of Applied Sport Psychology, 13*, 185–206. doi.org/10.1080/104132001753149883

Collins, D., Button, A., & Richards, H. (2011). *Performance psychology: A practitioner's guide*. Elsevier.

Collins, D., & Kamin, S. (2012). The performance coach. In S. Murphy (Ed.), *Handbook of sport and performance psychology* (pp. 692–706). Oxford University Press.

Collins, D., Willmott, T., & Collins, L. (2018). Periodisation and self-regulation in action sports: Coping with the emotional load. *Frontiers in Psychology*. https://doi.org/10.3389/fpsyg.2018.01652

Cruickshank, A., Collins, D., & Minten, S. (2013). Culture change in a professional sports team: Shaping environmental contexts and regulating power. *International Journal of Sport Science and Coaching, 8*(2), 319–325. http://dx.doi.org/10–1260/1747-9541.8.2.271

Cruickshank, A., Collins, D., & Minten, S. (2014). Driving and sustaining culture change in Olympic sport performance teams: A first exploration and Grounded Theory. *Journal of Sport & Exercise Psychology, 36*, 107–120.

Curran, O., MacNamara, A., & Passmore, D. (2019). What about the girls? Exploring the gender data gap in talent development. *Frontiers in Sports and Active Living*. ISSN 2624–9367.

Fletcher, D., & Wagstaff, C. (2009). Organizational psychology in elite sport: Its emergence, application, and future. *Psychology of Sport and Exercise, 10*(4), 427–434. https://doi.org/10.1016/j.psychsport.2009.03.009

Henrich, J., Heine, S. J., & Norenzayan, A. (2010). The weirdest people in the world? *Behavioral and Brain Sciences, 33*, 61–83. doi.10.1017/S0140525X0999152X

Henriksen, K., Storm, L. K., Prydol, N., Stambulova, N., & Larsen, C. H. (2019). Successful and less successful interventions with youth and senior athletes: Insights from expert sport psychology practitioners. *Journal of Clinical Sport Psychology, 13*, 72–94.

Horvath, A. O., & Bedi, R. P. (2002). The alliance. In J. C. Norcross (Ed.), *Psychotherapy relationships that work: Therapist contributions and responsiveness to patients* (pp. 37–69). Oxford University Press.

Killin, L., & Della Sala, S. (2015). Seeing through the double blind. *The Psychologist, 28*(4), 288–291.

Küttal, A., & Larsen, C. H. (2019). Risk and protective factors for mental health in elite athletes: A scoping review. *International Review of Sport and Exercise Psychology, 13*(1), 231–265. https://doi.org/10.1080/1750984X.2019.1689574

Lazarus, A. A. (1993). Tailoring the therapeutic relationship, or being an authentic chameleon. *Psychotherapy, 30*, 404–407.

Lebrun, F., & Collins, D. (2017). Is elite sport (really) bad for you? Can we yet answer the question? *Frontiers in Psychology, 8*, 324. doi:10.3389/fpsyg.2017.00324

Martindale, A., & Collins, D. (2005). Professional judgment and decision making: The role of intention for impact. *Sport Psychologist, 19*(3), 303–317.

Martindale, A., & Collins, D. (2007). Enhancing the evaluation of effectiveness with professional judgement and decision making. *Sport Psychologist, 21*, 458–474.

Martindale, A., & Collins, D. (2012). A Professional Judgment and Decision Making Case Study: Reflection-in-Action Research. *The Sport Psychologist (Special Edition), 26*, 500–518.

Martindale, A., & Collins, D. (2013). The development of professional judgment and decision making expertise in applied SP. *Sport Psychologist, 27*, 390–398.

Mesagno, C., & Mullane-Grant, T. (2010). A comparison of different pre-performance routines as possible choking interventions. *Journal of Applied Sport Psychology, 22*, 343–360.

Mills, K. L., Goddings, A-L., Clasen, L. S., Giedd, J. N., & Blakemore, S-J. (2014). The developmental mismatch in structural brain maturation during adolescence. *Developmental Neuroscience, 36*, 147–160.

Moore, G. F., Audrey, S., Barker, M., Bond, L., Bonell, C., Hardeman, W., Moore, L., O'Catain, A., Tinati, T., Wight, D., & Baird, J. (2015). Process evaluation of complex interventions: Medical Research Council guidance. *BMJ, 351*, 350. doi:10.1136/bmj.h1258.

Ogilvie, D., Adams, J., Bauman, A., Gregg, E. W., Panter, J., Siegel, K. R., Warehame, N. J., & White, M. (2020). Using natural experimental studies to guide public health action: Turning the evidence-based medicine paradigm on its head. *Journal of Epidemiology and Community Health, 74*, 203–208. doi:10.1136/jech-2019-213085

Pankhurst, A. (2014). *Exploring stakeholder coherence in an effective talent identification and development environment* (Doctoral dissertation, University of Central Lancashire).

Petipas, A. J., Giges, B., & Danish, S. J. (1999). The sport psychologist-athlete relationship: Implications for training. *Sport Psychologist, 13*(3), 344–357.

Salas, E., Tannenbaum, S. I., Kraiger, K., & Smith-Jentsch, K. A. (2012). The science of training and development in organizations: What matters in practice. *Psychological Science in the Public Interest, 13*(2), 74–101.

Sharp, L-A., Hodge, K., & Danish, S. (2019). "I wouldn't want to operate without it": The ethical challenges faced by experienced Sport Psychology consultants and their engagement with supervision. *Journal of Applied Sport Psychology*. doi:10.1080/10413200.2019.1646838

Taber, B. J., Leibert, T. W., & Agaskar, V. (2011). Relationships among client-therapist personality congruence, working alliance, and therapeutic outcome. *Psychotherapy Theory Research Practice Training, 48*(4), 376–380. doi:10.1037/a0022066

Tod, D. A,, Eubank, M. E., & Hutter, R. I. (2017). Professional development for sport psychology practice. *Current Opinion in Psychology, 16*, 134–137.

Toering, T. T., Elferink-Gemser, M. T., Jordet, G., & Visscher, C. (2009). Self regulation and performance level of elite and non-elite youth soccer players. *Journal of Sports Sciences, 27*(14), 1509–1517. doi:10.1080/02640410903369919

Vealey, R. S. (2007). Mental skills training in sport. In G. Tenenbaum & R. Eklund (Eds.), *Handbook of sport psychology* (3rd ed., pp. 285–309). https://doi.org/10.1002/9781118270011.ch13

6

Mental Toughness

Robert Weinberg and Joanne Butt

Since the upsurge of interest in mental toughness research that was sparked by a seminal paper in 2002 (Jones et al.), researchers have learned a great deal about different aspects of mental toughness. However, despite all this research attention, there are lots of questions and issues that remain unanswered (or are controversial), including the stability of mental toughness, mental versus physical toughness, the relationship between mental toughness and mental health, different types of mental toughness, and the measurement and definition of mental toughness. This chapter will briefly discuss the current state of mental toughness literature, but as the title of the text implies, the focus will be on discussing the unknown and potential areas for future research.

State of the Art

The first section in this chapter will summarize key aspects of mental toughness research where there appears to be general agreement among researchers. This does not mean that all research (or researchers) agree; rather, there is consistency in findings regarding a specific aspect of mental toughness (see Table 6.1).

Psychological Attributes of Mental Toughness

First, an area of research that has been consistent is that mental toughness pertains to a certain set of psychological attributes. In their seminal research, Jones et al. (2002) interviewed elite athletes, used focus groups, and used rating scales to identify the psychological attributes that make up mental toughness. They found 12 different psychological attributes underpinning

Robert Weinberg and Joanne Butt, *Mental Toughness* In: *Sport, Exercise and Performance Psychology*.
Edited by: Edson Filho and Itay Basevitch, Oxford University Press. © Oxford University Press 2021.
DOI: 10.1093/oso/9780197512494.003.0006

mental toughness, but they designated coping with pressure, focused concentration, motivation, and self-belief as the four pillars of mental toughness. Subsequent research has found many other psychological attributes underlying mental toughness, although researchers do not always agree on all the attributes (see Gucciardi, 2017, for a review). The ones that are consistently found in research include focused concentration, self-belief (confidence), coping with pressure, goal-directed motivation (commitment), sense of control, optimism, and resilience (bouncing back from setbacks; see Harmison, 2011).

Genetic Versus Learned Aspects of Mental Toughness

A second area of mental toughness research where there is consensus is that mental toughness has both genetic and learned aspects to it (Harmison, 2011). Specifically, researchers using twin study methodology found that individual differences in mental toughness could be attributed to both genetic and environmental factors (Horsburgh et al., 2009). Specifically, they found individual differences in overall mental toughness to be primarily explained by both genetic and nonshared environmental factors ($r = .52$). Their results also revealed that the correlation coefficients between hereditability and specific aspects of mental toughness (e.g., challenge, commitment) ranged from .36 to .56. These findings led Horsburgh et al. to conclude that mental toughness is similar to just about every other personality trait that has been studied to determine the extent to which genetics or environmental factors determine individual differences.

From a qualitative perspective, research by Connaughton et al. (2008) revealed that mental toughness can be developed in a number of different ways depending on the environment in which an athlete grows up. This can be considered as mental toughness being "caught" as opposed to "taught." Specifically, mental toughness being caught might include natural rivalry with a sibling, "archrival" competitor, overcoming negative critical incidents, creating training simulations, and coach motivational climate. Mental toughness being "taught" has included many of the mental skills to enhance performance and well-being such as anxiety management, focused attention, imagery, goal setting, and self-talk. In addition, researchers have implemented and positively evaluated, both quantitatively and qualitatively, the effectiveness of a mental training program (e.g., Gucciardi et al., 2009a).

Is Mental Toughness Multidimensional or Unidimensional?

A third area of general consensus is that mental toughness is multidimensional in nature and focuses on a collection of values, attitudes, emotions, and cognitions that are hypothesized to enable individuals to behave in such a way as to achieve their goals in the face of obstacles (Hardy et al., 2014). A few examples demonstrate the point of the perceived multidimensionality of mental toughness. Specifically, for Jones et al. (2002), these characteristics are motivation, confidence, attentional focus, and coping. For Gucciardi, Gordon, and Dimmock (2009b), the characteristics include challenge, sport awareness, tough attitudes, and desire for success. Finally, Harmison (2011) conceptualizes mental toughness as a social cognitive personality construct, which by definition is multidimensional. For example, affects, expectancies, and goals are part of the social cognitive approach to mental toughness. In summary, although these characteristics are sometimes similar and sometimes dissimilar, these research studies all view mental toughness as a multidimensional construct.

What Is the Relationship of Mental Toughness to Hardiness and Resilience?

A fourth area of consensus is that mental toughness is more than resilience and hardiness. In fact, hardiness and resilience are seen as part of the larger construct of mental toughness. For example, Clough, Earle, and Sewell (2002) suggested that hardiness, a key concept within the field of health psychology, could be used to help explain mental toughness in sport. Hardiness has been defined as a personality trait that acts as a buffer to influence how an individual copes with stressful life events. Hardiness is thought to comprise the personality components of control, commitment, and challenge, but in terms of mental toughness, Clough et al. (2002) added the component of confidence. Thus, for these authors, hardiness is part of mental toughness, because mental toughness has the added component of confidence. It should be noted that Clough et al. have been criticized for failing to adequately justify the transferring of the health psychology construct of hardiness into a more sport-specific setting (Gucciardi & Gordon, 2009). Researchers understand that one cannot simply take a construct out of mainstream psychology (or health psychology in this specific case) and apply it to a sport-specific setting. Psychometrics need to be conducted to demonstrate the reliability and validity of mainstream psychology constructs being applied to sport.

In terms of the concept of resilience, like hardiness, it is seen as a part of the larger construct of mental toughness. For example, all mentally tough individuals are seen as resilient, but not all resilient individuals are seen as mentally tough. Although both resilience and mental toughness share the ability to bounce back from setbacks, mental toughness also includes an optimistic and confident attitude. The core aspects of resiliency revolve around the concepts of adversity and adaptation, whereas mentally tough individuals see challenges and adversity as an opportunity and not a threat, and have the positive approach to move forward with enhanced performance and well-being. In essence, resiliency is focused on adversity, whereas mental toughness is shown in a variety of situations (positive and negative), not just dealing with adversity and difficult or even horrific events (Weinberg & Gould, 2019)

What Are the Behaviors of Mentally Tough Individuals?

A fifth area of agreement is that the individuals who are considered mentally tough exhibit certain types of behaviors in and around competition. These behaviors do not define a mentally tough individual; rather, they are representative of how a mentally tough individual behaves (Connaughton et al., 2008). For example, Hardy et al. (2014) developed a behavioral scale based on feedback by athletes including behaviors that were thought to be consistently exhibited by mentally tough athletes. The question stem was "an athlete is able to maintain a high level of personal performance in competitive matches," and some example responses included "when the conditions were difficult," "when the match is particularly tight," and "when teammates are struggling." Similarly, Anthony et al. (2018) defined specific behaviors that coaches were trying to teach in developing mental toughness. Examples of behaviors included adapts to changing situations, exhibits positive body language following a personal or team mistake, and displays decisive actions in pressure situations that are effective.

Table 6.1 Five Key Reading in Mental Toughness in Sports

Authors	Methodological Design	Key Findings
Gucciardi (2017)	Narrative review	Different definitions and conceptualizations of mental toughness were discussed before the latest definition, considering previous research was offered.
Hardy et al. (2014)	Test construction	Being mentally tough results in certain behaviors/outcomes opposed to one's psychological attributes.
Horsburgh et al. (2009)	Twin study methodology	Mental toughness has both genetic and environmental influences and thus can sometimes be taught and sometimes be caught.
Jones et al. (2002)	Qualitative interviews	Mental toughness is multidimensional, being composed by a variety of psychological attributes.
Strycharczyk & Clough (2015)	Correlations	Mental toughness encompasses hardiness and resilience, and coaches learn how to build mental toughness.

Questions to Move the Field Forward

While mental toughness research has achieved consistency in some conceptual areas, as noted earlier, there are still some issues surrounding the construct that future research needs to address. In this section of the chapter we will discuss some of these pertinent issues where our knowledge base and understanding are less consistent.

1. Theoretical Question: How Stable Is Mental Toughness?

2. Theoretical Question: Are There Different Types of Mental Toughness?

Two main questions are raised in this section, the first being whether mental toughness is stable or unstable, and the second, which is somewhat connected, being whether there are different types of mental toughness for different situations. To continue to develop the conceptual clarity of mental toughness, it is important to consider whether mental toughness is more of a personality disposition (i.e., trait-like), which tends to be stable over time and situations, or whether it is more unstable (i.e., state-like), and thus changes across different situations. In support of viewing mental toughness as more of a personality disposition, some earlier research studies have suggested that mental toughness consists of various attributes (e.g., confidence, determined, optimistic, handling pressure) that make performers mentally tough in general and across situations (e.g., Connaughton et al., 2008; Gucciardi et al., 2009a; Weinberg et al., 2011). Quantitative studies and the subsequent development of different models of mental toughness have also highlighted specific attributes that are assumed to make performers mentally tough (e.g., 4Cs model; cf. Clough et al., 2002). Within these models it is typically hypothesized that the psychological attributes or personal resources allow individuals to perform effectively across a wide variety of situations, especially when these situations involve coping with pressure or adversity.

Other research studies have found that mental toughness is relatively unstable (i.e., state-like) across (and even within) situations, suggesting that it might be determined by the constraints and requirements of specific situations. That is, some sport-specific research has reported that the requirements of different sports seem to require a different set of mentally tough attributes. Examples of this research can be found in Australian football (Gucciardi et al., 2008), soccer (Thelwell et al., 2005), cricket (Bull et al., 2005), and elite soccer referees (Slack et al., 2014). Moving beyond sport-specific attributes and exploring situational mental toughness, Weinberg et al. (2017) explored tennis players' perceived shifts in mental toughness within and between matches. Findings indicated that athletes' mentally tough behaviors, cognitions, and affect varied across situations and at times many athletes were not able to sustain "being mentally tough." These research findings offer support for the state-like nature of mental toughness, indicating that depending on the situation and athletes' perceptions of the situation, mental toughness can fluctuate. It is recommended that researchers continue to identify the specific situations and athletes' perceptions of situations that elicit behaviors that are (or are not) mentally tough. This research should lead to the development of appropriate interventions that teach coping skills to elicit the most effective cognitions, affects, and behaviors for different situations. For example, gaining an understanding of competitive situations that could potentially evoke fluctuations in mental toughness (i.e., mental weakness) can be integrated into athletes' training environments to help prepare them better for performing in competition and critical moments.

Within the broader issue of stability and situational mental toughness, there is a continued need to explore the different types of mental toughness. In particular, one question that remains is whether different situations require different types of mental toughness rather than being mentally tough in general. As noted earlier, there might be a specific set of attributes necessary for particular sports (e.g., soccer vs. golf), but preliminary research regarding situations within sports (e.g., Weinberg et al., 2017; Bull et al., 2005) would tentatively indicate that certain types of mental toughness are required for certain situations that occur within sport. Being able to identify and assess different types of mental toughness would enable specific mental toughness training programs to be designed to help athletes develop the psychological and physical attributes that are necessary to be successful in their particular sport.

3. Applied Question: Does Mental Toughness Depend on Physical Toughness?

The second issue within mental toughness research that remains uncertain is the role of physical toughness and whether it is an attribute of mental toughness. In some qualitative research, physical toughness (i.e., conditioning, physical fitness) has been reported as being essential for mental toughness to be displayed (e.g., Gucciardi et al., 2009a; Weinberg et al., 2011). That is, physical toughness was not considered an attribute of mental toughness per se, but rather, a necessary platform for individuals to demonstrate the mental attributes such as handling pressure and having strong belief. In an earlier quantitative study that was conducted (Crust & Clough, 2005), results revealed a linkage between mental toughness and physical endurance in which higher levels of mental toughness would "push" individuals to pursue their physical training. Taken together, these findings indicate that there is a connection between mental toughness and physical toughness, although scant research has focused on empirically investigating the relationship.

In a classic model on "toughness," Dienstbier (1991) demonstrated a specific physiological response to stress termed "toughness" or "physiological toughness." In summary, the research highlights the changes in specific biomarkers that are associated with better or poorer performance and also the relationship to positive psychological reactions such as lower anxiety, greater emotional stability, greater adaptability to stress, and enhanced mental/cognitive abilities—many of which are found to be attributes of mental toughness. Taking a psychophysiological approach to further understand mental toughness in the sporting context could be a fruitful line of research, especially when taking into account athletes' perceptions of threat or challenge in response to stressful situations and the mediating role that mental toughness could play. In addition, future research is still needed to explore whether creating pressurized training environments in sport enhance mental toughness. Some research in this area has identified that exposing athletes to certain training demands (e.g., manipulating task, environment) combined with training consequences (e.g., manipulating judgment, forfeit) can increase athletes' perceptions of pressure and cognitive anxiety intensity and directional interpretation (Stoker et al., 2019). However, the role of mental toughness in relation to pressure training and performance needs to be investigated.

4. Theoretical Question: What Is the Relationship Between Mental Toughness, Mental Health, and Physical Health?

The third issue in mental toughness research where questions remain relates to athletes' mental and physical health. In recent years there has been an increased emphasis on the mental health of athletes, and one question being asked is whether mental toughness and mental health are contradictory concepts, especially in elite sport. An editorial by Bauman (2016) brought to light the potentially negative effects that being mentally tough might have on the mental health of elite athletes. Specifically, he argues that the culture of elite sport is one that encourages athletes to be "tough," which in part means not admitting to, reporting, or seeking professional help for mental health issues. Furthermore, there is a stigma that is associated with athletes reporting mental health issues, as they fear that they will be labeled as "mentally weak," or certainly not mentally tough. In response to this editorial, Gucciardi, Hanton, and Fleming (2017) conducted a narrative review to investigate the assertion that mental toughness and mental health are contradictory concepts in elite sport. While no empirical published research investigating the relationship of mental toughness to mental health in elite athletes was found, they did find some studies linking mental toughness and mental health in nonelite sport performers as well as performers in other contexts. For example, several studies with adolescent and adult athletes (e.g., Gucciardi & Jones, 2012) and military personnel (Arthur et al., 2015) have found mental toughness to be positively related to positive affect and enhanced performance, while negatively related to burnout, depression, stress, and anxiety. Therefore, based on some limited research with adolescent athletes, students, and military personnel, an argument can be made that mental toughness appears to represent a positive indicator of mental health, and that it in fact helps to facilitate positive mental health. Future research is needed to determine the relationship between mental toughness and positive mental health, and longitudinal intervention research could also offer more definitive conclusions.

Despite some limited positive contributions, there is other research and anecdotal reports suggesting that mental toughness might be in conflict with physical health and well-being. Gucciardi et al. (2017) reported that athletes typically underutilize mental health services because of the perceived stigma that might emanate from others. Thus, it is plausible that being known as a mentally tough player would likely just exacerbate the feeling that they would be perceived as mentally weak (especially by teammates and coaches) if they sought out psychological help. It is clear that this is one area in need of empirical research, and further understanding the reasons athletes often underutilize mental health services and whether mental toughness plays a mediating role is a starting point.

In a related line of physical health and well-being research, questions continue to be raised on whether mentally tough athletes are more likely to play through injury and pain because this is one important behavior that signals that an athlete is mentally tough. Indeed, Coulter, Mallett, and Singer (2016) explored mental toughness in the Australian Football League and found that players who played through injury, pain, and fatigue were seen as mentally tough and were held in high esteem compared to those players who did not conform to these standards. However, empirical research is limited in this area and it is also possible that other personality and/or external factors influence whether an athlete tries to participate while injured. Along these lines, it is also important to consider the culture surrounding specific sports. Specifically, in relation to Australian football, Gucciardi and colleagues (2017) noted the extent to which subcultural beliefs, norms, and values of being mentally tough foster an idealized form of hypermasculinity and make it less likely that athletes will seek out professional psychological help. It is possible that this sort of competitive culture will likely provide norms to which athletes of different ages and gender adhere, as well as athletes playing sports varying in physical contact (e.g., football vs. tennis). Collectively, from reviewing the literature available, there is clearly a need for further empirical research to be conducted on mental toughness, sport culture, and athletes performing while feeling mentally well. Overall, research findings do emphasize that mental toughness (e.g., self-belief, focus, handling pressure, competitiveness) is an important psychological characteristic for athletes to develop, and this is supported across the wide range of literature focused on developing talented athletes. Future research should consider exploring optimal environments specific to sports and how these environments can appropriately engender mental toughness attributes at various athlete career stages.

5. Methodological Question: How to Identify Mental Toughness?

The final issue in mental toughness research where questions remain relates to measuring mental toughness and identifying who is mentally tough. While qualitative research has typically focused on determining what constitutes mental toughness and generating applied and often sport-specific frameworks, it is on the quantitative measurement (questionnaires) and, more specifically, the psychometric rigor of these measures that questions continue to be raised.

One generic measure that has been used more than others but is also one that is often criticized is the Mental Toughness Questionnaire-48 (MTQ-48; Clough et al., 2002). The MTQ-48 was developed in conjunction with the 4Cs framework (as discussed earlier in this chapter) and as such was generated from the construct of hardiness in health psychology, with the addition of confidence. One of the main concerns raised regarding the 4Cs framework was its suitability for use in the sport setting and thus the validity of the MTQ-48 was questioned. Nonetheless, the MTQ-48 has been used in research within academic (e.g., Stock et al., 2018) and sport settings (e.g., Slack et al., 2015). However, while the MTQ-48 shows promise as a measure of mental toughness, future research utilizing appropriate larger samples and confirmatory factor analysis processes is advised. With equivocal findings surrounding the MTQ-48, alternative measures could be considered for future research. Two such measures offering potential include the Mental Toughness Inventory (MTI) (cf. Middleton et al., 2011) and the Sport Mental

Toughness Questionnaire (SMTQ; Sheard et al., 2009). The SMTQ was designed and tested with a range of athletes and could well be suited for research with athletes of varying abilities (i.e., development, collegiate), while the MTI, following preliminary construct validation results, seems most suitable for research with elite athletes. The MTI is certainly considered a more robust measure than the early Psychological Performance Inventory (PPI; Loehr, 1986), which was also designed with elite athletes in mind, but research examining the PPI psychometric properties has not yet supported its factorial validity (e.g., Golby et al., 2007).

As an alternative to generic measures discussed previously, some researchers have developed sport-specific measures. As discussed earlier in this chapter, one question remains as to whether some of the mental toughness attributes are sport specific and therefore require a sport-specific quantitative measure. With this in mind, Gucciardi and colleagues have developed the Australian football Mental Toughness Inventory (AfMTI; Gucciardi et al., 2009b) as well as the Cricket Mental Toughness Inventory (CMTI; Gucciardi & Gordon, 2009). Both measures demonstrate the applied benefits of capturing sport-specific dimensions of mental toughness, and future research might consider developing more context-specific measures especially given the limitations of existing generic measures available. Nonetheless, the concern for these sport-specific measures is whether or not they are appropriate outside of that context. Thus, further development and testing are needed to perhaps identify whether sport-specific measures can be adapted to other similar sports (e.g., invasion games vs. aesthetic sports). It is also possible that a mixed approach can be taken to measuring mental toughness in the future so that a generic measure is not used on its own. As one example, mental toughness behaviors can be observed and measured in addition to using one of the multidimensional measures such as the MTQ-48 or the MTI. Bell, Hardy, and Beattie (2013) utilized this approach in their study with elite cricketers, which involved developing and measuring mental toughness behaviors. Originally a 15-item scale was developed and then statistically (factor analysis) it was reduced to an 8-item scale measuring specific behaviors (as opposed to psychological qualities). These behaviors related to maintaining a high level of performance when a match is particularly tight, when the conditions are difficult, when teammates are relying on one player to perform well, when a player is struggling with an injury, and when there are a large number of spectators present.

Conclusion

Although we have learned a lot about mental toughness from empirical data, there is still a great deal that needs to be done to better understand the different aspects of mental toughness. The purpose of this chapter was to highlight consistent areas of research regarding mental toughness as well as areas that need further research and clarification. Specific areas for future study were offered to help move the field forward in terms of both research and practice. Hopefully, this chapter will stimulate researchers to continue to study the many aspects of mental toughness that need further clarification so both researchers and practitioners can better understand the cognitions, affects, and behaviors that are associated with mental toughness.

References

Anthony, D., Gordon, S., Gucciardi, D., & Dawson, B. (2018). Adapting a behavioral coaching framework for mental toughness development. *Journal of Sport Psychology in Action, 9*, 1–32. doi:10.1080/21520704.2017.1323058

Arthur, A., Fitzwater, J., Hardy, L., Beattie, S., & Bell, J. (2015). Development and validation of a military training mental toughness inventory. *Military Psychology, 27*, 232–241.

Bauman, N. (2016). The stigma of mental health in athletes: Are mental toughness and mental health seen as contradictory in elite sport? *British Journal of Sports Medicine, 50*, 135–136.

Bell, J., Hardy, L., & Beattie, S. (2013). Enhancing mental toughness and performance under pressure in elite young cricketers: A 2-year longitudinal intervention. *Sport, Exercise & Performance Psychology, 2*, 281–297. doi:10.1037/a0033129

Bull, S., Shambrook, C., James, W., & Brooks, J. (2005). Towards an understanding of mental toughness in elite English cricketers. *Journal of Applied Sport Psychology, 17*, 209–227.

Clough, P., Earle, K., & Sewell, D. (2002). Mental toughness: The concept and its measurement. In I. Cockerill (Ed.), *Solutions in sport psychology* (pp. 32–45). Thomson.

Connaughton, D., Hanton, S., Jones, G., & Wadey, R. (2008). The development and maintenance of mental toughness: Perceptions of elite performers. *Journal of Sport Sciences, 28*, 699–716.

Coulter, T., Mallett, C., & Singer, J. (2016). A subculture of mental toughness in an Australian football league. *Psychology of Sport and Exercise, 22*, 98–113.

Crust, L., & Clough, P. (2005). Relationship between mental toughness and physical endurance. *Perceptual and Motor Skills, 100*, 192–194.

Dienstbier, R. (1991). Behavioral correlates of sympathoadrenal reactivity: The toughness model. *Medicine and Science in Sports and Exercise, 23*, 846–852.

Golby, J., Sheard, M., & Van Wersch, A. (2007). Evaluating the factor structure of the psychological performance inventory. *Perceptual and Motor Skills, 105,* 309–325.

Gucciardi, D. (2017). Mental toughness: Progress and prospects. *Current Opinion in Psychology, 16,* 17–23.

Gucciardi, D., & Gordon, S. (2009). Development and preliminary validation of the cricket mental toughness inventory. *Journal of Sport Sciences, 27,* 1293–1310.

Gucciardi, D., Gordon, S., & Dimmock, J. (2008). Towards an understanding of mental toughness in Australian football. *Journal of Applied Sport Psychology, 20,* 261–281.

Gucciardi, D., Gordon, S., & Dimmock, J. (2009a). Advancing mental toughness research using personal construct psychology. *International Review of Sport and Exercise Psychology, 2,* 54–72.

Gucciardi, D., Gordon, S., & Dimmock, J. (2009b). Development and preliminary validation of a mental toughness inventory for Australian football. *Psychology of Sport and Exercise, 10,* 201–209.

Gucciardi, D., Hanton, S., & Fleming, S. (2017). Are mental toughness and mental health contradictory concepts in elite sport? A narrative review of theory and evidence. *Journal of Science and Medicine in Sport, 20,* 307–311.

Gucciardi, D., & Jones, M. (2012). Beyond optimal performance: Mental toughness profiles and development success in adolescent cricketers. *Journal of Sport and Exercise Psychology, 34,* 16–36.

Hardy, L., Bell, J., & Beattie, S. (2014). Preliminary evidence for a neuropsychological model of mentally tough behavior. *Journal of Personality, 82,* 69–81.

Harmison, R. (2011). A social-cognitive framework for understanding and developing mental toughness in sport. In D. Gucciardi & S. Gordon (Eds.), *Mental toughness in sport: Developments in theory and research.* Routledge.

Horsburgh, V., Schermer, J., Veselka, L., & Verson, P. (2009). A behavioral genetic study of mental toughness and personality. *Personality and Individual Differences, 46,* 100–105.

Jones, G., Hanton, S., & Connaughton, D. (2002). What is this thing called mental toughness?: An examination of elite sport performers. *Sport Psychologist, 14,* 205–218.

Loehr, J. E. (1986). *Mental Toughness Training for Sports: Achieving Athletic Excellence.* Lexington, MA: Stephen Greene Press.

Middleton, S., Martin, A., & Marsh, H. (2011). Development and validation of the mental toughness inventory. In D. Gucciardi & S. Gordon (Eds.), *Mental toughness in sport: Developments in theory and research* (pp. 91–107). Routledge.

Sheard, M., Golby, J., & Van Wersch, A. (2009). Progress toward construct validation of the sport mental toughness questionnaire (SMTQ). *European Journal of Psychological Assessment, 25,* 186–193.

Slack, L. A., Butt, J., Maynard, I. W., & Olusoga, P. (2014). Understanding mental toughness in elite football officiating: Perceptions of English Premier League referees. *Sport and Exercise Psychology Review, 10,* 4–24.

Slack, L. A., Maynard, I. W., Butt, J., & Olusoga, P. (2015). An evaluation of a mental toughness education and training program for early-career English Premier League referees. *Sport Psychologist, 29,* 237–257.

Stock, R., Lynam, S., & Cachia, M. (2018). Academic success: The role of mental toughness in predicting and creating success. *Higher Education Pedagogies, 3,* 429–433.

Stoker, M., Maynard, I. W., Butt, J., Hays, K., & Hughes, P. (2019). The effect of manipulating individual consequences and training demands on experiences of pressure with elite disability shooters. *Sport Psychologist, 33,* 1–26.

Strycharczyk, D., & Clough, P. (2015). *Developing mental toughness: Coaching strategies to improve performance, resilience and wellbeing* (2nd ed.). Kogan Page Ltd.

Thelwell, R., Weston, N., & Greenlees, I. (2005). Defining and understanding mental toughness within soccer. *Journal of Applied Sport Psychology, 17*, 326–332.

Weinberg, R., Butt, J., & Culp, B. (2011). Coaches' view of mental toughness and how to build it. *International Journal of Sport and Exercise Psychology, 9*, 156–172.

Weinberg, R., Butt, J., Mellano, K., & Harmison, R. (2017). The stability of mental toughness across situations: Taking a social-cognitive approach. *International Journal of Sport Psychology, 48*, 1–23.

Weinberg, R., & Gould, D. (2019). *Foundations of sport and exercise psychology*. Human Kinetics.

7

Expert Performance

Joe Baker and Brad Young

Where does exceptionality begin? How do we define and measure it? What is the role of the environment in promoting or inhibiting the development of expertise? Despite being critical elements of philosophy for at least two millennia, empirical examinations of the origins and development of human exceptionality are relatively recent. It was not until Francis Galton's work in the mid-1800s that discussions of genius, talent, and, eventually, expertise evolved from hypothetical and theoretical arguments to well-defined hypotheses. The rise of empiricism, especially in areas of measurement, experimentation, and statistics, meant these hypotheses could now be tested. Sport eventually became a ripe domain for questions related to precursors, determinants, developmental conditions, and mechanisms attributed to talented performance.

State of the Art

As a field of study, expertise (i.e., the study of those who have attained the highest levels of attainment) has expanded nearly exponentially since it was founded (arguably, Chase & Simon, 1973, represents the first study in this field). It is not possible to adequately summarize the current developments in this field, so instead, we will direct the reader to key texts that summarize this research (e.g., Baker & Farrow, 2015; Ericsson et al., 2018). This field is incredibly active, ranging from evaluations of different applied perceptual-cognitive training interventions for fast-tracking skill acquisition in athletes (Schorer et al., 2015) to assessments of diverse forms of athletic engagement during extensive periods of talent development (Memmert et al., 2010).

Joe Baker and Brad Young, *Expert Performance* In: *Sport, Exercise and Performance Psychology.*
Edited by: Edson Filho and Itay Basevitch, Oxford University Press. © Oxford University Press 2021.
DOI: 10.1093/oso/9780197512494.003.0007

In the sections that follow, we explore notable and current questions from the field of expert performance in sport, ranging from (a) theoretical issues such as how best to conceptualize the influence of myriad nature-and-nurture variables on athlete development, to (b) measurement issues including how to best determine the value of specific forms of practice or replicate the unique constraints of the performance environment in laboratory settings, to (c) practical issues regarding how to best engage athlete development stakeholders to research the next series of "unknowns" in expert performance. Table 7.1 offers a list of key articles relating to these questions that provide further reading.

Table 7.1 Five Key Readings in the Science of Expert Performance

Authors	Methodological Design	Key Findings
Baker et al. (2020)	Conceptual review	There are limits to the deliberate practice framework (e.g., the need for clear operational definitions and more sophisticated conceptual models) that need to be acknowledged and overcome if it is going to be a comprehensive approach to expert performance.
Johnston et al. (2018)	Systematic review	Our understanding of talent is incomplete due to limited evidence regarding predictors of talent identification and the relevance of these factors in long-term talent development.
Macnamara, et al. (2016)	Meta-analysis	The value of deliberate practice and early specialization, as stated in the deliberate practice framework, has been overstated. Other factors need to be explored in models of expertise development.
McCardle, et al. (2019)	Systematic review	Self-regulated learning may play a key role in understanding how and why experts devote extensive time and energy to practice.
Pinder et al. (2011)	Conceptual review	Proposes and explains the notion of "representative learning design" (i.e., creating practice environments that closely reflect learning requirements of the competition setting) as a critical element in skill acquisition and expert performance.

Questions to Move the Field Forward

1. Theoretical Question: What Is Talent, and Is It Relevant for Understanding Expert Performance?

Although seemingly straightforward, this question belies real difficulties in how researchers, practitioners, and policymakers see the concept of talent (see Baker et al., 2019). Yet, operationally and empirically defining talent is central to understanding expert performance. In its simplest form, talent is seen as referring to "nature" in the nature-versus-nurture dichotomy and reflects biological predispositions to attain achievement (conversely, the nurture side reflects the determining role of the environment). From this perspective, talent is a highly stable variable whose influence does not change much over time. Early discussions of the development of perceptual-motor behavior and athletic performance focused on the role of latent "abilities" in determining success (Fleishman, 1958; McCloy, 1934), which were generally thought to represent talent-like capacities (i.e., fixed, stable predictors of performance). In the 1950s, the popular concept of a "general motor ability" similarly reflected the notion that individuals have different, innate capacities to perform motor activities like sports. This notion was akin to the concept of intelligence, which is widely described as reflecting an individual's general potential for cognitive activities.

Despite the appeal of the general motor ability concept and the notion that stable abilities might underpin an individual's capacity to develop sporting expertise, the evidence for these positions is not strong. In a classic study, Drowatzky and Zuccato (1967) examined performances within and between individuals on six different balance tasks. Correlations among the balance tests indicated little association even across tests derived from the same skill set (i.e., balancing), defying the notion of a singular ability. Fleishman and Rich (1963) were able to identify and group abilities that correlated with overall performance on various motor tasks (that involved manipulating types of apparatus), implying that particular individual differences in patterns of abilities should facilitate performance on some criterion tasks (sports) more than others. The ease of such an implication, however, was largely confounded by findings revealing that the pattern of abilities important to performance success changes over the course of practice, over time, and with increasing skill. This changing pattern is likely different for every type of criterion performance, and correlations of abilities with criterion performance are often quite low. They also noted that, over time, less variance in a criterion performance was attributed to fixed abilities, but instead to experience or practice at a criterion task. Further evidence against a strict interpretation of the abilities perspective comes from research on the specificity of perceptual-cognitive adaptations emphasizing that adaptations are highly specific to the type of training and experience undertaken by developing athletes (e.g., see Loffling et al., 2012).

Evidence for the nurture argument appears stronger. For instance, the deliberate practice framework (Ericsson, 2003; Ericsson et al., 1993) emphasizes the singular importance of high-quality training for explaining skill differences between individuals. The relationship between practice and skill is one of the strongest ever found in psychology, and the deliberate practice framework brings the importance of "nurture" back to the forefront of discussions of expertise. That said, it still positions practice and experience at one end of a dichotomy, with biological, ability, or nature-related factors at the other end. This dichotomy is almost certainly too simple to adequately explain the factors affecting the long-term skill acquisition that lead to expertise. More recent conceptions have focused on talent as emergent over time and highly influential to environmental influences. This would reconcile the disparate research areas that highlight the genetic influences on performance (e.g., Eynon et al., 2013) with the psychological research on the importance of practice (Ericsson et al., 1993). The notion of abilities has not disappeared—indeed, there is research that suggests abilities are fundamental to precocious performance and early interest in an achievement domain, and that individual differences in patterns of abilities may limit the ultimate performance that aspiring performers might reach (e.g., Ackerman, 2014). For example, following experimental laboratory work involving various memory tasks, Campitelli and Gobet (2011) suggested that patterns of abilities could predict performance above and beyond variance explained by deliberate practice, and that not all individuals benefit equally from deliberate practice. Although these notions insinuate a role for abilities, only prospective, longitudinal examinations of practice behaviors will ultimately inform our understanding of the interplay of practice and individual differences over time and at escalating levels of expertise.

2. Applied Question: Can We Identify Who Will Be Successful in the Future?

The evidence suggests that, up to now, we are poor evaluators of future success. From the perspective discussed previously, talent is highly unstable and emergent, which makes predicting it extremely difficult. This jibes with research evaluating the accuracy of talent predictions (Koz et al., 2012). The issue may be that traditional approaches focus on modeling variables as if they are stable and direct influences (e.g., Johnston et al., 2018), with few studies considering how these variables change over time and/or interact with other variables.

The solution may require a different approach to conceptualizing talent. Instead of focusing on single or limited lists of variables, approaches should consider collections of variables that could interact to result in an outcome. For instance, recent work on athlete development has focused on understanding the complexity of psychological factors underpinning long-term and/or optimal engagement in practice (Baker et al., 2017; Tedesqui & Young, 2018). If we can understand the range of variables that predict an individual's engagement in high-quality, intensive practice for extensive durations, we might be able to predict their likelihood of future success. One variable that is emerging is an individual's capability to self-regulate their own learning. Self-regulated learning (SRL) relates to the extent to which athletes actively control activities during their own practice, by enacting pertinent metacognitive and motivational processes to optimize skill acquisition. In two different studies (Jonker et al., 2010; Toering et al., 2009), SRL was found to differentiate between skilled and less skilled groups of athletes. More recent works by Bartulovic et al. (2017) and McCardle et al. (2017, 2018) show how SRL processes can distinguish skill groups, with particular emphasis on the role of specific self-processes (e.g., self-monitoring), and focus on understanding how they discriminate between groups on challenging tasks during practice.

Ultimately, focusing on variables that might predict one's engagement over time shifts the focus from looking at talent as a stable, fixed, and unidimensional factor to ones that evolve across development. This promotes a focus on constructing the optimal developmental environment that ensures athletes' needs are met and that appropriate challenge, support, and feedback are being integrated into training activities. Such integration likely involves self-appraisal and self-integration by athletes to complement the traditional notion that astute coaches heavily inform athletes' developmental process.

3. Theoretical and Methodological Question: Does Practice Need to Always Be Deliberate?

After the emergence of the deliberate practice framework, a body of sport literature attempted to understand how cumulative amounts of practice related to skill level status. Generally, research supported the notion that escalating skill groups (i.e., provincial versus national versus international level) could be significantly distinguished by amounts of training that approximated deliberate practice (for a review see Baker & Young, 2014). However, almost none of the studies portending to assess deliberate practice were quantifying deliberate practice per se. According to its definition, deliberate practice is a highly explicit form of practice that requires focused attention on the task, cognitive processes of error detection and correction, oftentimes with support/feedback from a coach. However, the proxy measure for deliberate practice used in most of those studies related to amounts of technical and/or tactical, sport-specific training. Other studies used indices that were operationalized in a hodgepodge of ways (e.g., see MacNamara et al., 2016, p. 336). The lack of a consistently operationalized definition of deliberate practice, and the failure to use a valid definition as the measurement in studies of amounts of practice, is a vulnerability in deliberate practice research. True understanding of the effects of amounts of deliberate practice depends on a more critical interrogation of its assessment in self-report (Tedesqui et al., 2018) and alternative methodologies (e.g., Coughlan et al., 2013), commensurate with a consensual definition.

There are many unanswered questions: How will this definition remain consistent so that it can be used across samples in different sports/achievement domains? At the same time, how will this definition remain sufficiently agile (i.e., temporally valid) so that it can be applied for measurement purposes over the course of a developmental trajectory? In other words, how can the characteristics of deliberate practice that are assessed remain operationally constant while the content (i.e., the constituent activities) comprising it changes across context or over time?

The dialogue around deliberate practice has begun to evolve, with increasing calls for determining *qualities* of practice and their effects on skill acquisition, rather than focusing on practice amounts. Moreover, in contrast to the definition of deliberate practice, literature on implicit learning suggests athletes can learn very effectively without attention directed to facets of a task, with little knowledge of rule structures governing mechanics of movements, and with only very broad scaffolding from a coach (Masters, 2000). Abernethy et al. (2003) noted that implicit learning may be the norm, and explicit learning like deliberate practice may actually be the exception for the acquisition of movement skills.

This leads to questions such as how much of expert skill acquisition can be attributed to implicit learning, and how does one design a research protocol to begin to disentangle explicit versus implicit learning to inform conditions of expert development? In essence, there remains the question of *how much practice needs to be deliberate?* Intertwined with this is the question of how does deliberate practice effectively translate to automatic processing in a competitive arena? If the ultimate competitive arena where a performer must apply their skills is pressured (by time/environmental factors), will deliberate practice have created a habitual form of explicit, cognitive processing of one's actions that could impede the free-flowing, automatic processing and execution required of expert competitors? If athletes are switched on to explicit processing during deliberate practice, how do they toggle to an "off" switch to automatically execute during competition? Thus, there remains the question of *when and how do expert transition from explicit to automatic processing* in service of learning and competitive application, respectively?

There is also the question of whether play can serve as a deliberate form of preparation that facilitates skill acquisition. Proponents of "deliberate play" have suggested it critically contributes to expertise development, directly at younger stages of athlete development, and latently, by setting the foundation for internalized perceptions of fun that direct athletes through more difficult training later in their trajectory (Hornig et al., 2016). Furthermore, in sporting roles that require motor creativity or tactical improvisation, deliberate play may be the very type of preparation needed to reach the highest performance levels (Memmert et al., 2010).

Finally, there is an important need to address whether incidental learning occurs from engaging in different sport activity contexts, and whether acquired mechanisms underpinning expertise in a target domain (e.g., soccer) can be refined by or transferred from sampling other sports (e.g., athletics, cycling, tennis). Research pertaining to team sport players in Australia showed that more sport sampling in the early years of development was associated with less requisite deliberate practice to achieve the most elite status (Baker et al., 2003). Côté and Fraser-Thomas's (2011) modeling of developmental trajectories in youth sport posited that the likelihood of acquiring elite performance was enhanced by involvement in several sports up to age 12, and delayed focus on one sport until age 15. Recent popular discourse in bestsellers like *Range* (Epstein, 2019) has favored notions of sport diversification, epitomized by Roger Federer, over early sport specialization (i.e., in one sport), epitomized by Tiger Woods. In light of this, and prevailing anti-early specialization sentiment encapsulated in many long-term athlete development guides, we need to better understand specialization versus diversification trends as they relate to eventual expert status. Such research would be timely considering contrarian works that suggest (a) early intensive investment in one sport may be beneficial for expertise as long as it does not preclude recreational involvement in other activities (Ford et al., 2009), and (b) links between specialized sport activity and burnout could be overstated, and that presence of an autonomy-supportive context may be more important (Larson et al., 2019).

If expertise research is to inform praxis related to coaching and programming of practice, the next frontier of research will need to interrogate the aforementioned questions related to explicit versus implicit learning, the role of play and competition, how different qualities and types of practice are effectively afforded to athletes, and the contribution of specialized and diversified activity.

4. Methodological Question: Can We Recreate the Expert Performance Environment in the Lab?

Much of the work discussed previously makes the assumption that we adequately capture the essential nuances of expert performance in empirical or experimental settings. However, the very act of attempting to divide an expert's performance into its component parts (e.g., by separating the act of anticipating an opponent's serve from the action required to intercept it) may compromise some elements of expertise. For example, the expert performance approach (Ericsson, 2003; Ericsson & Smith, 1991) guiding many lab-based efforts has adequate internal validity for the mechanistic examination of elite athletes' various modes of perceiving, deciding, and acting in notable (i.e., replicable) sport-specific scenarios. It does a satisfactory job of dictating procedures for how to discriminate elites from less skilled peers on indices of information processing and other cognitively informed aspects of performance. However, it is unclear whether such a mechanistic approach can account for expert performances in novel (i.e., not necessarily replicable) circumstances, for example, when a pre-eminent performer surprises, surpasses, recreates, or deceives in their manufacture of responses.

The relevant issue here is external validity (particularly, ecological validity—the extent to which a study's results apply in "real world" contexts) in the way representative tasks are set up in measurement settings. Discussions have focused on issues such as the need for "perception-action coupling" (i.e., the need to couple the specific perceptual-cognitive demands with motor execution elements of the task), which is essential in most sporting tasks. As pointed out by Mann et al. (2007, p. 180), "when perception and action are combined, the complexity of the interaction induces different effects to when cognition is detached from motor performance."

The rise of "ecological dynamics" centers on the notion that performers are inseparable from the environments in which they perform (Pinder et al., 2011). It posits that performers respond in unconscious ways to constraints and conditions in their surrounding environment, with little to no cognitive address of cues or schema/representations. In keeping with considerations of automaticity mentioned in the prior section, this begs the question: if expert performance is more than what is accessed in working memory, or more than what experts can be reliably prompted to think about, then why does the field of expert performance continue to rely extensively on cognition-based models for assessment? There is a need for more fulsome consideration of ecological approaches that contrast expert with less expert cohorts in settings that faithfully represents the constraints of actual execution.

Finally, much of the work on individual differences in practice amounts and/or personality variables has relied on self-report. Self-report data relating to a person's disclosure on a phenomenon/construct are then submitted to analyses for expert-novice discrimination. With the advent of new technologies and big data capture approaches, it remains to be seen how algorithms (formulae for understanding behavioral data and demographic profiling indices inherent in large datasets) will affect studies of expertise, particularly on efforts to identify key markers, conditions, and behaviors that forecast talent.

5. Applied Question: Are the Pursuit of Expertise and the Processes Driving Talent Identification Ethically Defendable?

One of the most significant changes over the past half century relates to how sport, and high-performance sport in particular, is viewed in most countries worldwide. The increased professionalization of sport from youth to elite levels reflects the increased cultural, political, and individual value it has compared to other vocations or leisure pursuits. Commensurately, the past decade has seen increased attention to issues of athlete maltreatment (Kerr & Stirling, 2017) and mental health (Poucher et al., 2019) among other concerns (International Olympic Committee, 2005). In light of these examples of prominent studies of negative developmental facets of elite participation, it may be important to scrutinize whether expertise and the processes driving elite sport systems (e.g., talent identification) are ethically justifiable.

It could be contended that expertise broadly holds less cache and/or is misunderstood in contemporary study. For example, expertise and excellencism are often unfairly misappropriated as perfectionism, and this conflation perpetuates among the general public and influences praxis (Gaudreau, 2019). This type of misunderstanding makes it easier for academics and stakeholders to shun expertise research. This is further compounded by the fact that the sport systems in most countries can reasonably be described as exclusionary, because they involve the deselection of the majority of youth from elite development programs so that a small minority can be retained. This landscape is the backdrop against which the value of sport expertise is judged. Indeed, when research on the precursors and developmental conditions of expertise is conveyed to policymakers and stakeholders, the end users may very well (and justifiably) ask whether application will compromise efforts at inclusion.

The realm of expertise is inherently exclusive—not everyone can reach a mantle among the very best. Expertise is the study of *inequalities*. That said, developmental conditions associated with expertise need not be *inequitable*, though in practice they are. Studies of talent development hold promise for underscoring pertinent and timely access to resources, infrastructure, coaching, and supports for expertise, and are critical for highlighting inequities associated with such supports. A way forward may be treating empirical perspectives on expertise to interrogate which groups are unfairly advantaged (and to socially critique privilege), and determining the interactions of inequities with practice effects. Two prospective goals are (a) to adequately account for inequitable opportunities to privilege in order to determine the extent to which individual strivings are uniquely responsible for high-level development in an achievement domain and (b) modeling the landscape of expert development (i.e., developmental trajectories, broadly with cohorts) should early inequities regarding access to resources/supports be resolved. Testing the first goal would empirically treat the objectivist tenant, to explain an individual's capacity in reaching their ultimate potential by pursuing self-rationalized and self-interested ends. Modeling the second goal would test the assumption of what would happen if everyone could have equal and free access to the expertise "marketplace."

What makes this a critical "next step question" is that there has been comparatively little discussion of the value of the pursuit of expertise. It is not possible to weigh the negatives without some comparison to the perceived positives of this pursuit. There are important social considerations associated with this issue, evidenced in parallel discussions for whether a focus on experts during the Olympics affects mass participation through "trickle down" effects (e.g., Potwarka & Leatherdale, 2016). Moreover, there are potentially positive social implications if the narrative on early talent identification switches from it being a conduit for directing young people to a focus on early specialization to a conduit for directing young people to avenues for which they will self-actualize and be highly competent, while swaying them from pursuits where they may be constrained.

More broadly, many questions about our species can only be answered by understanding the process of expertise development. For instance, what is the ultimate level of performance to which we can aspire? How does our environment affect the development of this performance? These questions and many others can only be explored using expert performance paradigms. In sum, it is important that discussions of athlete development are framed using knowledge of both positives and negatives. In our experience, such nuanced discussions are rare in the sport literature.

Conclusion

The past few decades have seen tremendous growth in our understanding of expert performance. However, key questions remain, from specific methodological challenges (e.g., how to replicate performance environments in controlled settings) to broader philosophical questions (e.g., whether the pursuit of expertise is ethically defensible). Most of the questions we have reviewed are not new, but recent advances in technology and theory suggest solutions or at least resolution may be close. This is an exciting time, as reflected in the growth of work in this area.

References

Abernethy, B., Farrow, D., & Berry, J. (2003). Constraints and issues in the development of a general theory of expert perceptual-motor performance: A critique of the deliberate practice framework. In J. L. Starkes & K. A. Ericsson (Eds.), *Expert performance in sports: Advances in research on sport expertise* (pp. 349–370). Human Kinetics.

Ackerman, P. L. (2014). Nonsense, common sense, and science of expert performance: Talent and individual differences. *Intelligence, 45*, 6–17.

Baker, J., Côté, J., & Abernethy, B. (2003). Sport specific training, deliberate practice and the development of expertise in team ball sports. *Journal of Applied Sport Psychology, 15*, 12–25.

Baker, J., & Farrow, D. (2015). *The Routledge handbook of sport expertise*. Routledge.

Baker, J., Wattie, J., & Schorer, J. (2019). A proposed conceptualization of talent in sport: The first step in a long and winding road. *Psychology of Sport & Exercise, 43*, 27–33.

Baker, J., & Young, B. W. (2014). 20 years later: Deliberate practice and the development of expertise in sport. *International Review of Sport & Exercise Psychology, 7*, 135–157.

Baker, J., Young, B. W., & Mann, D. (2017). Advances in athlete development: Understanding conditions of and constraints on optimal practice. *Current Opinion in Psychology, 16*(August), 24–27.

Baker, J., Young, B. W., Tedesqui, R. A. B., & McCardle, L. (2020). New perspectives on deliberate practice and the development of sport expertise. In R. Ecklund & G. Tenenbaum (Eds.), *Handbook of sport psychology* (4th ed., pp. 556–577). Wiley.

Bartulovic, D., Young, B. W., & Baker, J. (2017). Self-regulated learning predicts skill group differences in developing athletes. *Psychology of Sport & Exercise, 31*, 61–69.

Campitelli, G., & Gobet, F. (2011). Deliberate practice: Necessary but not sufficient. *Current Directions in Psychological Science, 20*, 280–285.

Chase, W. G., & Simon, H. A. (1973). Perception in chess. *Cognitive Psychology, 4*, 55–81.

Côté, J., & Fraser-Thomas, J. (2011). Youth involvement and positive youth development in sport. In P. Crocker (Ed.). *Sport psychology: A Canadian perspective*. Pearson.

Coughlan, E. K., Williams, A. M., McRobert, A. P., & Ford, P. R. (2013). How experts practice: A novel test of deliberate practice theory. *Journal of Experimental Psychology: Learning, Memory, & Cognition, 40*, 449–458.

Drowatzky, J. N., & Zuccato, F. C. (1967). Interrelationships between selected measures of static and dynamic balance. *Research Quarterly, 38*, 509–510.

Epstein, D. (2019). *Range: Why generalists triumph in a specialized world*. Riverhead Books.

Ericsson, K. A. (2003). Development of elite performance and deliberate practice: An update from the perspective of the Expert Performance Approach. In J. L. Starkes & K. A. Ericsson (Eds.), *Expert performance in sports: Advances in research on sport expertise* (pp. 49–83). Human Kinetics.

Ericsson, K. A., Hoffman, R. R., Kozbelt, A., & Williams, A. M. (2018). *The Cambridge handbook of expertise and expert performance* (2nd ed.). Cambridge University Press.

Ericsson, K. A., Krampe, R. T., & Tesch-Römer, C. (1993). The role of deliberate practice in the acquisition of expert performance. *Psychological Review, 100*, 363–406.

Ericsson, K. A., & Smith, J. (1991). Prospects and limits of the empirical study of expertise: An introduction. In K. A. Ericsson & J. Smith (Eds.), *Toward a general theory of expertise: Prospects and limits* (pp. 1–38). Cambridge University Press.

Eynon, N., Hanson, E. D., Lucia, A., Houweling, P. J., Garton, F., North, K. N., & Bishop, D. J. (2013). Genes for elite power and sprint performance: ACTN3 leads the way. *Sports Medicine, 43*, 803–817.

Fleishman, E. A. (1958). Dimensional analysis of movement reactions. *Journal of Experimental Psychology, 55*, 438–453.

Fleishman, E. A., & Rich, S. (1963). Role of kinesthetic and spatial-visual abilities in perceptual-motor learning. *Journal of Experimental Psychology, 66*, 6–11.

Ford, P. R., Ward, P., Hodges, N. J., & Williams, A. M. (2009). The role of deliberate practice and play in career progression in sport: The early engagement hypothesis. *High Ability Studies, 20*, 65–75.

Gaudreau, P. (2019). On the distinction between personal standards perfectionism and excellencism: A theory elaboration and a research agenda. *Perspectives on Psychological Science, 14*, 197–215.

Hornig, M., Aust, F., & Güllich, A. (2016). Practice and play in the development of German top-level professional football players. *European Journal of Sport Science, 16*, 96–105.

International Olympic Committee. (2005). *IOC consensus statement on training the elite child athlete*. Retrieved January 14, 2006, from multimedia.olympic.org/pdf/en_report_1016.pdf

Johnson, K., Wattie, N., Schorer, J., & Baker, J. (2018). Talent identification in sport: A systematic review. *Sports Medicine, 48*, 97–109.

Jonker, L., Elferink-Gemser, M. T., & Visscher, C. (2010). Differences in self-regulatory skills among talented athletes: The significance of competitive level and type of sport. *Journal of Sports Sciences, 28*, 901–908.

Kerr, G., & Stirling, A. (2017). Issues of maltreatment in high performance athlete development: Mental toughness as a threat to athlete welfare. In J. Baker, S. Cobley, J. Schorer, & N. Wattie (Eds.), *Routledge handbook of talent identification and development in sport* (pp. 409–420). Routledge.

Koz, D., Fraser-Thomas, J., & Baker, J. (2012). Accuracy of professional sports drafts in predicting career potential. *Scandinavian Journal of Medicine & Science in Sports, 22*, e64–e69.

Larson, H. K., Young, B. W., McHugh, T. L. F., & Rodgers, W. M. (2019). Markers of early specialization and their relationships with burnout and dropout in swimming. *Journal of Sport & Exercise Psychology, 41*, 46–54.

Loffing, F., Schorer, J., Hagemann, N., Lotz, S., & Baker, J. (2012). On the advantage of being left-handed in volleyball: Further evidence of the specificity of skilled visual perception. *Attention, Perception & Psychophysics, 74*, 446–453.

Macnamara, B. N., Moreau, D., & Hambrick, D. Z. (2016). The relationship between deliberate practice and performance in sports: A meta-analysis. *Perspectives on Psychological Science, 11*, 333–350.

Mann, D. T., Williams, A. M., Ward, P., & Janelle, C. M. (2007). Perceptual-cognitive expertise in sport: A meta-analysis. *Journal of Sport & Exercise Psychology, 29*, 457–478.

Masters, R. S. W. (2000). Theoretical aspects of implicit learning in sport. *International Journal of Sport Psychology, 31*, 530–541.

McCardle, L., Young, B. W., & Baker, J. (2017). Self-regulated learning and expertise development in sport: Current status, challenges, and future opportunities. *International Review of Sport & Exercise Psychology, 12*, 112–138.

McCardle, L., Young, B. W., & Baker, J. (2018). Two-phase evaluation of the validity of a measure for self-regulated learning in sport practice. *Frontiers in Psychology: Movement Science & Sport Psychology, 9*, 2641.

McCloy, C. H. (1934). The measurement of general motor capacity and general motor ability. *Research Quarterly, 5*(Supp. 1), 46–61.

Memmert, D., Baker, J., & Bertsch, C. (2010). Play and practice in the development of sport-specific creativity in team ball sports. *High Ability Studies, 21*, 3–18.

Pinder, R. A., Davids, K., Renshaw, I., & Araújo, D. (2011). Representative learning design and functionality of research and practice in sport. *Journal of Sport & Exercise Psychology, 33*, 146–155.

Potwarka, L. R., & Leatherdale, S. T. (2016). The Vancouver 2010 Olympics and leisure-time physical activity rates among youth in Canada: Any evidence of a trickle-down effect? *Leisure Studies, 35*, 241–257.

Poucher, Z., Tamminen, K. A., Kerr, G., & Cairney, J. (2019). A commentary on mental health research in elite sport. *Journal of Applied Sport Psychology, 33*, 60–82.

Schorer, J., Loffing, F., Rienhoff, R., & Hagemann, N. (2015). Efficacy of training interventions for acquiring perceptual-cognitive skill. In J. Baker & D. Farrow (Eds.), *Routledge handbook of sport expertise* (pp. 456–464). Routledge.

Tedesqui, R. A. B., McCardle, L., Bartulovic, D., & Young, B. W. (2018). Toward a more critical dialogue for enhancing self-report surveys in sport expertise and deliberate practice research. *Movement & Sport Sciences—Science & Motricité, 102*, 5–18.

Tedesqui, R. A. B., & Young, B. W. (2018). Comparing the contribution of conscientiousness, self-control, and grit to key criteria of sport expertise development. *Psychology of Sport & Exercise, 34*, 110–118.

Toering, T. T., Elferink-Gemser, M. T., Jordet, G., & Visscher, C. (2009). Self-regulation and performance level of elite and non-elite youth soccer players. *Journal of Sports Sciences, 27*, 1509–1517.

8

Decision-Making

Itay Basevitch and Gershon Tenenbaum

State of the Art

Decision-making (DM) is the act of selecting an action from several action possibilities (Tenenbaum, 2003). DM plays a crucial role in achieving goals proficiently and is one of the main determinants of reaching expertise (Araújo et al.; Bar-Eli et al., 2011; Raab et al., 2019).

Several approaches in studying DM in sport were carried out contrasting deterministic versus probabilistic in nature (see Bar-Eli et al., 2011) and static versus dynamic in temporal character (Araújo et al., 2011). However, research in DM in sport must consider a more dynamic perspective accounting for both cognition and action (Bar-Eli & Raab, 2009), particularly when the DM process is complex and dynamic in nature (Araújo et al., 2006). Thus, one of the critical challenges in the study of DM in sport is to capture the task constraints and conditions that validly represent the essential characteristics of various skill performances within specific sport contexts (Ericsson, 2020), and the functional patterns of behavior that emerge during performance (Davids & Araújo, 2010). Moreover, the reliability, validity, and representativeness of capturing DM have been of great concern in recent years (Ericsson, 2020).

Though DM refers to the action choice and its execution in the form of motor action, most of the DM researchers referred to the perceptual, cognitive, and constraint characteristics that precede DM and its manifestation in a motor action. In this vein, Tenenbaum (2003) introduced a conceptual model whereby DM refers to several perceptual-cognitive components such as *visual attention* (i.e., attention allocation), *selective attention* (i.e., which environmental cues to pay attention and which to ignore), *anticipation* (i.e., what events are expected to follow given the current constrains; what the associated probabilities are for such events), *information processing* (i.e., which units of information to forward for elaboration and response retrieval),

Itay Basevitch and Gershon Tenenbaum, *Decision-Making* In: *Sport, Exercise and Performance Psychology.*
Edited by: Edson Filho and Itay Basevitch, Oxford University Press. © Oxford University Press 2021.
DOI: 10.1093/oso/9780197512494.003.0008

long-term working memory (*LTWM*; how much information can be delivered, stored, and retrieved via working memory), *response selection* (i.e., DM), *temporal and special considerations* (i.e., where to place the body and the timing of DM execution), and *decision alteration* (the capability to make changes under extremely demanding temporal conditions when the preferred DM option has been made). Most of these components were considered as facets of DM and were extensively researched separately as eliciting the novice-expert perceptual-cognitive differences and as determinants and prerequisites of skill-level performance (Mann et al., 2007).

An additional aspect of DM in sport that was not given enough attention was the linkage between the DM process and emotions, which evidently affects DM quality. DM was studied in isolation from the stressful and emotion-evoking context in which it had been taking place. To close this gap, Tenenbaum et al. (2009) introduced a unified conceptual framework, which integrates the structural components of human performance, such as affective processes (i.e., feelings, mood), cognition (e.g., knowledge architecture, long-term working memory), motor processes (e.g., coordination), and the neurophysiologic foundation of these structural components (i.e., activation of cortical areas). The unified conceptual framework refers to a complex integration among the systems that operate harmonically and automatically under given circumstances by high-skill-level performers who in some cases "choke" under constraints, which interferes with the system's adaptation to the environmental conditions.

Tenenbaum et al. (2009) compiled concepts and research findings from various fields, such as intelligence, problem solving, emotions and emotion regulation, action and the motor system, and expertise, and made comprehensive claims regarding the underlying mechanisms of human performance. Specifically, Tenenbaum et al. (2009) claimed that once these mechanisms are uncovered, applied guidelines can be advanced to enhance performance. The authors maintained that response selection depends on the capacity to solve problems and consequently adapt to the environment. Cognitive processes and mental operations are used for this purpose. The effectiveness of these processes consists of the richness and variety of perceptions processed at a given time, that is, the system's capacity to *encode* (i.e., *store* and *represent*) and *access* (i.e., *retrieve*) information relevant to the task being performed (Tenenbaum, 2003). The perceptual-cognitive process develops via the accumulation of task-specific knowledge. The knowledge is stored in the long-term memory in the form of four levels: mental representation, mental control, sensorimotor representations, and sensori-motor control. Each of these levels maintains a specific function in producing motor actions (Schack, 2004). Mental control is induced intentionally, while sensorimotor control is induced perceptually. Thus, perception-action cou-pling runs automatically and is self-organized, but mental control relies on mental representations governing the perceptual-cognitive sequence that precedes DM and the decision execution.

According to Tenenbaum et al. (2009), emotions are a form of mental state whereby they can motivate, organize, and guide perception and thought pro-cesses, and mobilize action toward a behavioral purpose. Positive or pleasant emotions expand the behavioral and thought repertoire to face a given sit-uation (Fredrickson, 1998), which enhances the perceptual-cognitive pro-cess along with expanding the action possibilities and intellectual and social resources preceding DM. In contrast, negative emotions such as anxiety can result in both positive and negative outcomes (Carver & Scheier, 1988). Anxiety can alert the system but can negatively affect the perceptual and cog-nitive systems (e.g., attention narrowing and thought interference) and in-terfere with the operational function. The linkage between specific emotions and DM is not yet clear enough and must be comprehensively studied. Moreover, the effect of DM *self-efficacy* is related to the emotional state of the performer and has a substantial effect on the DM and execution phases of the motor action (for a review see Tenenbaum, 2003). In fact, DM self-efficacy is the confidence one maintains in scanning the environment, selecting the relevant cues, processing the information, retrieving the right response, and executing it. Thus, self-efficacy must be studied as a mediator between perceptual-cognitive skills and the motor system actions.

The perceptual-cognitive processes of the performer are reflected by the cerebral cortical activity during skilled visuo-motor performance. The more skillful the performer is, the more relaxed are the nonessential areas of the brain and the less is the communication between the thinking and the motor regions of the brain (Hatfield, 2018). Similarly, Haufler et al. (2000) observed less activation in the frontal, central, temporal, parietal, and occipital regions in expert shooters relative to novices. The skill difference was of greatest mag-nitude in the left temporal region and revealed a temporal asymmetry in the experts. The relationship between skill level, cortical activation, and order formation in long-term memory is of outmost importance. To learn more about these interactions and networks, one must combine the neurophysi-ological methods, like electroencephalography (EEG)-coherence measures

(Deeny et al., 2003), and methods for measuring the structure of mental representation (Schack, 2004), and integrate them into a meaningful operational system. Systematic study of cortical activation in perception of object and motor action must shed more light on the perception-action linkage. The growing research on the linkage among the emotional-perceptual-cognitive-motor systems will shed more light on the underlying mechanisms that account for the expert performance, which is so much dependent on the DM process and outcome. A review of current and important literature in the domain for further reading is presented in Table 8.1.

Table 8.1 Five Key Readings in Decision-Making

Authors	Methodological Design	Key Findings
Basevitch et al. (2020)	Expert-novice paradigm, between (i.e., skill level) and within (i.e., temporal occlusion and cued/noncued conditions) group analyses	The authors examined skill-level differences of anticipation and situational assessment skills using the temporal occlusion paradigm in soccer. Higher level players anticipated the action more accurately and generated less irrelevant options compared to lower level players. Furthermore, anticipation and situational assessment skills were positively and moderately correlated.
Hadlow et al. (2018)	Narrative review of the literature	A review of paradigms and technology used to train perceptual-cognitive skills is presented, emphasizing their strengths and limitations. Based on the review, a modified perceptual training framework is presented with the purpose of identifying the most efficient training methods based on three continuums: (a) the perceptual-cognitive skill (i.e., lower order to higher order), (b) stimuli presentation (i.e., general-domain specific), and (c) response format (i.e., general-domain specific).
Raab et al. (2019)	Review and future directions	A historical overview of judgment and decision-making research in the past 50 years in the sport domain is presented. Specifically, four theoretical perspectives (i.e., cognitive, ecological dynamics, economical, and social-cognitive) that have shaped and guided research in the domain are explored and future challenges are identified.

Continued

Table 8.1 *Continued*

Authors	Methodological Design	Key Findings
Tenenbaum et al. (2009)	Theoretical framework	A multilevel and integrated conceptual framework (i.e., the emotion-cognition-linkage model) is developed and presented consisting of emotional, cognitive, motor, and neural processes. Furthermore, the relationships among the various levels of processes are examined to provide a holistic and unified perspective on human performance emphasizing the regulation and representation of these processes.
Wimshurst et al. (2016)	Expert-novice paradigm, between (i.e., skill level) and within (i.e., occlusion time and sport type) group analyses	The authors examined behavioral (i.e., response) and brain activity (i.e., fMRI) differences using the occlusion paradigm of hockey and nonhockey players on a video-based occlusion paradigm anticipation task that included hockey (i.e., domain-specific) and badminton (i.e., domain-general) scenes. Findings indicated that hockey players anticipated better than nonhockey players only on the domain-specific (i.e., hockey) task. The fMRI data revealed main effects for expertise across tasks. Specifically, hockey players recruited more brain areas, and more activity was identified in a few regions such as the rostral inferior parietal lobule and left posterior cingulate.

fMRI, functional magnetic resonance imaging.

Questions to Move the Field Forward

1. Theoretical Question: What Can We Learn From the Neurophysiological Level of Analysis About the Decision-Making Process in Sports?

What. Most of the researchers examining DM in sports considered a cognitive and/or behavioral perspective (Araújo et al., 2006). Some of the leading theories and models in the area adopted either an information processing, ecological dynamic, or economic approach (Raab et al., 2019). These theories vary on a continuum that consists of high- (e.g., perceptual-cognitive processes) to low-level (e.g., self-organization and perception-action coupling) brain processes. However, research measuring the neural and bi-ological components of the brain (i.e., the neurophysiological level) during the DM process in sports and performance domains is relatively scarce (Hatfield, 2018).

Why. It is important to examine the various levels of analysis of the DM process to better capture the underlying mechanisms leading to expert DM (Raab et al., 2019). Findings from previous research in the area indicated that some of the main underlying mechanisms leading to expert DM include (a) a large and efficiently organized knowledge base, (b) the ability to attend to crucial cues in the environment, (c) advanced anticipation skills character-ized by early and accurate predictive abilities, and (d) generation of fewer irrelevant options, thus reducing "brain busyness" (i.e., quiescence state) and leading to quicker and better DM (Basevitch et al., 2020; Hatfield, 2018; Mann et al., 2007). Some of the brain activities related to these processes have been studied in various performance domains, such as identifying the areas of the brain that are active when a pattern has been recognized in chess (Bilalić et al., 2010), the speed at which the stimuli presented elicits a brain response in fencers (e.g., event-related potential [ERP]; Taddei et al., 2012), and the changes in the neurophysiological patterns of DM with experience and as players develop in field hockey (Wimshurst et al., 2016).

How. With the advancement of technology in neurophysiology, the ability to measure brain waves and activity in specific brain regions has developed and is more accessible and mobile. With the use of technology such as EEG and functional magnetic resonance imaging (fMRI), these variables can be measured, detected, and interpreted with relatively minor noise and more automated systems. Thus, with EEG technology, the speed of identifying a fa-miliar situation (e.g., patterns of players in soccer) and the ERP can be meas-ured and contrasted among players of different levels. Furthermore, with the development of mobile dry EEGs, brain waves can be measured during the DM process in real-world situations, such as during a golf swing or during a penalty situation (Stone et al., 2019). Another area to examine is the brain ac-tivity that takes place in various brain regions when making quick decisions under time pressure, compared to analytical decisions when more time is available (Basevitch et al., 2020). With the use of fMRI and consideration of the expert-novice paradigm, brain activity (i.e., spatial and temporal activa-tion of brain areas) can be examined and linked to various DM-related pro-cesses, such as anticipation and detection of deceptive actions (Bishop et al., 2013). However, fMRI measures are less ecologically valid than typical EEG measures, and researchers using fMRI will be required to use video-based paradigms (or similar lab-based methods).

2. Theoretical Question: What Processes Are Involved in Team Decision-Making and How Are They Developed?

What. Most of the athletes compete in team sports, where the market size and viewership is the largest (https://www.grandviewresearch.com). However, research in the sport science domain (e.g., athlete development) centered merely on individual athletes (Ward et al., 2008). Interestingly, the study of the developmental processes in teams, specifically related to DM, remains limited (Basevitch et al., 2020).

Why. Most of the DM research was devoted to individual sports (e.g., tennis) or individual events within team sports (e.g., penalty in hockey or soccer; Ward et al., 2008). Thus, the generalization of these findings to the team unit of analysis is limited. Team processes that are essential for the team's function must be further studied (e.g., communication and coordination among teammates). For example, findings from individual settings indicate that sometimes, under time pressure situations, decisions are made intuitively (Raab & Johnson, 2007). Does this finding transfer to team sports, where a decision of a player (e.g., such as a pass in soccer) is part of a larger team process? Thus, examining how teams make decisions in sync is essential for capturing the team DM process and its implementation.

How. Methods that have been used to examine DM in individual settings can be adapted to team settings. For example, a process tracing method that has been examined extensively in individual settings, such as penalty kicking in soccer, is gaze behavior (Kredel et al., 2017). Findings indicate that expert and successful goal keepers gaze at different body parts (and at different temporal points) of the player kicking the penalty than lower level and less successful goal keepers (Kredel et al., 2017). Adapting this research method to the team setting, it would be imperative to study gaze behavior of two or more teammates (as well as the opponent) from both attacking and defensive perspectives. Similarly, spatial and temporal occlusion paradigms (Ward et al., 2009) can be used in team settings by asking several players to simultaneously anticipate upcoming events (i.e., an anticipation measure) either from the perspective of the player who makes the decision or from the perspective of the teammate's playing position (e.g., the player receiving the pass). In addition to adapting individual research methods to the team setting, including team process measures such as agreement level among teammates and team mental models (e.g., shared and distributed knowledge; Filho et al., 2014) can provide a more comprehensive understanding of team DM. Additional variables of interest are team demographic factors such as time playing together, position of players throughout their career, and cultural (e.g., variability of nationalities) and age (e.g., young team) characteristics.

3. Applied Question: What Are the Most Effective Methods to Train and Develop Decision-Making Skills?

What. Most of the research pertaining to the DM domain centered on *measuring* various DM skills (e.g., anticipation and situational assessment; Mann et al., 2007). Research findings examining the *development* and *training* of DM skills indicated that experience and specifically practice (e.g., deliberate practice) are necessary for acquiring advanced DM skills (Ward et al., 2009). However, knowledge on how to accelerate the acquisition of DM skills and the type of practice that is the most beneficial in each domain remains scarce.

Why. One must examine and develop *measurement* and *assessment* tools prior to investigating *training* and *development* methods (Ward et al., 2009). To measure skills accurately, validly, and reliably requires capturing the developmental processes over time (e.g., compare baseline to posttraining measures; Ward et al., 2008). Although some studies focused on *training* DM skills, the majority focused on *measuring* these skills (Mann et al., 2007; Ward et al., 2009). There are various methods that capture anticipation, option generation, and DM skills reliably and validly such as the occlusion paradigm (Basevitch et al., 2020). Following this rationale, we must move the field forward and further examine the development and training of these skills.

How. Several limitations must be addressed to expand the research of training DM skills, including (a) increasing ecological validity, (b) improving training paradigms, (c) exploring expert training, and (d) bridging the gap between research and practice. Regarding ecological validity in DM research, to date, most of the measurement and training tools are video and/or lab based (Ward et al., 2009). The transfer of findings to the field and real-world environment has rarely been examined (for an exception see Williams et al., 2002). Furthermore, innovative methods deemed to measure and train DM skills on the field, in addition to more efficient use of advanced technology (e.g., virtual reality) where the presentation of and response to stimuli are more realistic must be implemented (Hadlow et al., 2018).

With respect to enhancing DM training methods, findings from the expert-novice paradigm have shaped the field. Specifically, the strategies used by experts (e.g., gaze behavior) were used to train novice and intermediate athletes (e.g., the expert performance approach; Ward et al., 2009). However, we cannot assume that designing expert-type training is efficient for training novice athletes. Thus, other paradigms must be examined for training DM skills. For example, studying the strategies of expert athletes retrospectively at different stages of their development and using those strategies for training novice athletes should be investigated.

Furthermore, exploring expert training is vital given that most of the training literature in DM focuses on the development of novice and intermediate athletes' skills and ignores training skills once athletes reach the level of expertise. In addition, the expert-novice paradigm assumes that the expert skills are the most refined. This might be true in most cases, but more research must examine methods aimed to improve and stretch the limits of expert skills like the innovative Fosbury jump technique, which expanded the limits of the high jump)Bar-Eli et al., 2008). Finally, there is a large body of literature on theoretical, measurement, and applied aspects of DM skills. However, there are very few coaches, clubs, and organizations that implement the knowledge in the area in their practices, training, and analytics in a systematic and effective manner. More applied research (e.g., Shipherd et al., 2018) must be devoted to move the DM field forward.

4. Methodological Question: How Can We Effectively Measure Creativity and Improvisation in the Sport Domain?

What. Creativity is the ability to perform a task in a unique and effective manner (Memmert, 2011). Improvisation is considered a creativity dimension and consists of motor tasks that are performed spontaneously (Coste et al., 2019). Creativity was studied extensively in various domains such as science, music, and business (Csikszentmihalyi, 2015; Memmert, 2011), while improvisation has been studied mostly in the performing arts (e.g., jazz; Coste et al., 2019). Both creativity and improvisation were given less attention in the sport domain (Coste et al., 2019).

Why. Advanced DM skills provide a major advantage in performing motor tasks (Tenenbaum, 2003). Although decisions of experts are efficient and lead to successful actions, a creative decision is a specific type of DM skill that only few players possess and by definition is rare and unique (Memmert, 2011). An interaction between the player and the environment is required for a creative decision to be made (Vaughan et al., 2019), and thus constraining and limiting the environment (as opposed to providing freedom) can help develop creativity and improvisation skills (Torrents et al., 2021). However, more research must be conducted to capture the essence of creativity in players such as Messi in soccer and Rondo in basketball.

How. A widely used method in many domains (e.g., education) to measure creativity skill is the divergent thinking task (Fürst, 2020). Tasks incorporating video clips, similar to the occlusion paradigm, were used to measure divergent thinking. Accordingly, a developing play is stopped at a certain point in the sequence and players must generate possible action options (Memmert, 2011). Fluency (i.e., number of options), flexibility (i.e., variability of options), and originality (i.e., uniqueness of the options) are assessed by experts in the area and a creativity score is generated. One of the criticisms of this method relates to the lack of distinction between creative cognitive (e.g., a through pass that crosses several defenders) and motor (e.g., a heel touch) decisions (Coste et al., 2019). Furthermore, a measure of how much the situation (as opposed to the player) lends itself to creative decisions is also important to obtain (Vaughan et al., 2019). Thus, studies in the sport domain must adjust the divergent thinking task by including both cognitive and motor creative measures and assessing the situation (i.e., the environment), while considering the interaction between the player and the situation.

5. Theoretical and Methodological Question: How Do Coaches Make Effective Decisions and How Can We Assess Their Decisions?

What. Most of the research on DM skills centered on athletes (Vergeer & Lyle, 2009). Only recently has research been extended to other sports personnel such as officials (Samuel et al., 2019). A missing area of research on DM are coaches (Vergeer & Lyle, 2009). Specifically, more research must be devoted to capture how coaches make effective decisions during the game (or a break in the game), such as changing tactics and knowing what to say to the players (and when and how to provide feedback in an effective manner; Ford et al., 2009).

Why. Coaches play an important role in individual and team performances during a game/match (Cloes et al., 2001). The limited research on coaches' DM skills varies from examining decisions related to injured players (Vergeer & Lyle, 2009) to exploring DM styles during practices (Kaya, 2014). Furthermore, coaches prepare the players and the team for games by setting a strategy, making substitutions and tactical changes during the game, and analyzing the game while providing feedback to the players (Cloes et al., 2001). However, only few researchers have examined the DM of coaches in general and specifically, during a game.

How. Theoretical frameworks have been proposed for coaching effectiveness and proficient DM (Cloes et al., 2001; Côté & Gilbert, 2009; Ford et al., 2009). One of the proposed frameworks follows the expert performance approach, which was initially developed to examine players' expertise and DM skills. Specifically, according to this approach, one must identify and measure DM skills that are representative of coaches' real-world tasks (e.g., what decisions coaches make during the game and when). Next, the underlying mechanisms leading to successful DM and expertise must be identified and explored (e.g., knowledge of the game, tactical creativity). Finally, how DM skills develop and how best to train them are processes that must be studied (e.g., looking at practice histories; Côté & Gilbert, 2009). Furthermore, studies that use the occlusion paradigm must be conducted to explore coaches' DM by asking coaches what instructions or feedback (e.g., tactical) they would provide at a certain moment and comparing their instructions to what actually happened in addition to examining expert-novice differences of instructions (Basevitch et al., 2018).

Conclusion

DM has been examined for more than half a century in the sport domain (Raab et al., 2019), mainly in individual settings. Future research in the domain must be directed to avenues that will move the field forward and extend the boundaries of current experts. Specifically, research must be directed to the applied area and evidence-based training paradigms developed that can and will likely be used by coaches. Furthermore, theoretical research examining the mechanisms and processes related to team performance and to the neurophysiology level of analysis is needed to expand our understanding of the complexity of team dynamics and brain processes during the DM process. Research on creativity and improvisation in natural settings can identify the underlying mechanisms leading to such rare and unique DM skills and, importantly, provide knowledge on how best to implement training methods required for developing these skills. Finally, a shift in research is also needed in the scope of personnel, specifically, focusing on coaches who play a major role in determining players' and teams' DM and performance.

References

Araújo, R., Afonso, J., & Mesquita, I. (2011). Procedural knowledge, decision-making and game performance analysis in Female Volleyball's attack according to the player's experience and competitive success. *International Journal of Performance Analysis in Sport*, *11*(1), 1–13.

Araújo, D., Davids, K., & Hristovski, R. (2006). The ecological dynamics of decision making in sport. *Psychology of Sport and Exercise*, *7*, 653–676.

Bar-Eli, M., Lowengart, O., Tsukahara, M., & Fosbury, R. D. (2008). Tsukahara's vault and Fosbury's flop: A comparative analysis of two great inventions. *International Journal of Innovation Management*, *12*, 21–39.

Bar-Eli, M., Plessner, H., & Raab, M. (2011). *Judgment, decision-making and success in sport*. John Wiley & Sons.

Bar-Eli, M., & Raab, M. (2009). Judgment and decision making in sport and exercise: A concise history and present and future perspectives. In D. Araujo, H. Ripoll & M. Raab (Eds.), *Perspectives on Cognition and Action in Sport:* Nova Science Publishers, Inc.

Basevitch, I., Prosoli, R., Budnik-Przybylska, D., & Rossato, C. (2018). Anticipation and imagery skill level differences of judo coaches. In *Movement: Journal of Physical Education and Sports Sciences: The 5th International Congress of Exercise and Sport Sciences: Book of Abstracts* (pp. 228–229). Academic College at Wingate.

Basevitch, I., Tenenbaum, G., Filho, E., Razon, S., Boiangin, N., & Ward, P. (2020). Anticipation and situation assessment skills in soccer under varying degrees of informational constraint. *Journal of Sport and Exercise Psychology*, *42*, 59–69.

Bilalić, M., Langner, R., Erb, M., & Grodd, W. (2010). Mechanisms and neural basis of object and pattern recognition: A study with chess experts. *Journal of Experimental Psychology: General*, *139*, 728–742.

Bishop, D. T., Wright, M. J., Jackson, R. C., & Abernethy, B. (2013). Neural bases for anticipation skill in soccer: An fMRI study. *Journal of Sport and Exercise Psychology*, *35*, 98–109.

Carver, C. S., & Scheier, M. F. (1988). A control-process perspective on anxiety. *Anxiety Research*, *1*, 17–22.

Cloes, M., Bavier, K., & Piéron, M. (2001). Coaches' thinking process: Analysis of decisions related to tactics during sports games. In M. Chin, L. Hensley, & Y. Liu (Eds.), *Innovation and application of physical education and sports science in the new millennium - An Asia-Pacific perspective* (pp. 329–341). Hong Kong Institute of Education Publisher.

Coste, A., Bardy, B. G., & Marin, L. (2019). Towards an embodied signature of improvisation skills. *Frontiers in Psychology, 10*, 2441.

Côté, J., & Gilbert, W. (2009). An integrative definition of coaching effectiveness and expertise. *International Journal of Sports Science and Coaching, 4*, 307–323.

Csikszentmihalyi, M. (2015). *The systems model of creativity. The collected works of Mihaly Csikszentmihalyi.* Springer.

Davids, K., & Araújo, D. (2010). The concept of "organismic asymmetry" in sport science. *Journal of Science and Medicine in Sport, 13*, 633–640.

Deeny, S. P., Hillman, C. H., Janelle, C. M., & Hatfield, B. D. (2003). Cortico-cortical communication and superior performance in skilled marksmen: An EEG coherence analysis. *Journal of Sport and Exercise Psychology, 25*, 188–204.

Ericsson, K. A. (2020). Towards a science of the acquisition of expert performance in sports: Clarifying the differences between deliberate practice and other types of practice. *Journal of Sports Sciences, 38*, 159–176.

Filho, E., Gershgoren, L., Basevitch, I., & Tenenbaum, G. (2014). Profile of high-performing college soccer teams: An exploratory multi-level analysis. *Psychology of Sport and Exercise, 15*, 559–568.

Ford, P., Coughlan, E., & Williams, M. (2009). The expert-performance approach as a framework for understanding and enhancing coaching performance, expertise and learning. *International Journal of Sports Science and Coaching, 4*, 451–463.

Fredrickson, B. (1998). What good are positive emotions? *Review of General Psychology, 3*, 300–319.

Fürst, G. (2020). Measuring creativity with planned missing data. *Journal of Creative Behavior, 54*(1), 150–164.

Hadlow, S. M., Panchuk, D., Mann, D. L., Portus, M. R., & Abernethy, B. (2018). Modified perceptual training in sport: A new classification framework. *Journal of Science and Medicine in Sport, 21*, 950–958.

Hatfield, B. D. (2018). Brain dynamics and motor behavior: A case for efficiency and refinement for superior performance. *Kinesiology Review, 7*, 42–50.

Haufler, A. J., Spalding, T. W., Santa Maria, D. L., & Hatfield, B. D. (2000). Neuro-cognitive activity during self-paced visuospatial task: Comparative EEG profiles in marksmen and novice shooters. *Biological Psychology, 53*, 131–160.

Kaya, A. (2014). Decision making by coaches and athletes in sport. *Procedia-Social and Behavioral Sciences, 152*, 333–338.

Kredel, R., Vater, C., Klostermann, A., & Hossner, E. J. (2017). Eye-tracking technology and the dynamics of natural gaze behavior in sports: A systematic review of 40 years of research. *Frontiers in Psychology, 8*, 1845.

Mann, D. T., Williams, A. M., Ward, P., & Janelle, C. M. (2007). Perceptual-cognitive expertise in sport: A meta-analysis. *Journal of Sport and Exercise Psychology, 29*, 457–478.

Memmert, D. (2011). Sports and creativity. In M. Runco & S. Pritzker (Eds.), *Encyclopedia of creativity* (2nd ed.). Elsevier Academic Press.

Raab, M., Bar-Eli, M., Plessner, H., & Araújo, D. (2019). The past, present and future of research on judgment and decision making in sport. *Psychology of Sport and Exercise, 42*, 25–32.

Raab, M., & Johnson, J. G. (2007). Expertise-based differences in search and option-generation strategies. *Journal of Experimental Psychology: Applied, 13*, 158–170.

Samuel, R. D., Galily, Y., Guy, O., Sharoni, E., & Tenenbaum, G. (2019). A decision-making simulator for soccer referees. *International Journal of Sports Science and Coaching*, *14*, 480–489.

Schack, T. (2004). The cognitive architecture of complex movement. *International Journal of Sport and Exercise Psychology*, *2*, 403–438.

Shipherd, A. M., Basevitch, I., Filho, E., & Gershgoren, L. (2018). A scientist–practitioner approach to an on-field assessment of mental skills in collegiate soccer student-athletes. *Journal of Sport Psychology in Action*, *9*, 1–10.

Stone, D. B., Tamburro, G., Filho, E., Robazza, C., Bertollo, M., & Comani, S. (2019). Hyperscanning of interactive juggling: Expertise influence on source level functional connectivity. *Frontiers in Human Neuroscience*, *13*, 321.

Taddei, F., Bultrini, A., Spinelli, D., & Di Russo, F. (2012). Neural correlates of attentional and executive processing in middle-age fencers. *Medicine and Science in Sports and Exercise*, *44*, 1057–1066.

Tenenbaum, G. (2003). An integrated approach to decision making. In J. L. Starkes & K. A. Ericsson (Eds.), *Expert performance in sport: Advances in research on sport expertise* (pp. 191–218). Human Kinetics.

Tenenbaum, G., Hatfield, B. D., Eklund, R. C., Land, W. M., Calmeiro, L., Razon, S., & Schack, T. (2009). A conceptual framework for studying emotions–cognitions–performance linkage under conditions that vary in perceived pressure. *Progress in Brain Research*, *174*, 159–178.

Torrents, C., Balagué, N., Ric, Á., & Hristovski, R. (2021). The motor creativity paradox: Constraining to release degrees of freedom. *Psychology of Aesthetics, Creativity, and the Arts*, *15*, 340–351

Vaughan, J., Mallett, C. J., Davids, K., Potrac, P., & López-Felip, M. A. (2019). Developing creativity to enhance human potential in sport: A wicked transdisciplinary challenge. *Frontiers in Psychology*, *10*, 2090.

Vergeer, I., & Lyle, J. (2009). Coaching experience: Examining its role in coaches' decision making. *International Journal of Sport and Exercise Psychology*, *7*, 431–449.

Ward, P., Farrow, D., Harris, K. R., Williams, A. M., Eccles, D. W., & Ericsson, K. A. (2008). Training perceptual-cognitive skills: Can sport psychology research inform military decision training? *Military Psychology*, *20*, S71–S102.

Ward, P., Suss, J., & Basevitch, I. (2009). Expertise and expert performance-based training (ExPerT) in complex domains. *Technology, Instruction, Cognition and Learning*, *7*, 121–145.

Williams, A. M., Ward, P., Knowles, J., & Smeeton, N. J. (2002). Anticipation skill in a real-world task: Measurement, training, and transfer in tennis. *Journal of Experimental Psychology: Applied*, *8*, 259–270.

Wimshurst, Z. L., Sowden, P. T., & Wright, M. (2016). Expert–novice differences in brain function of field hockey players. *Neuroscience*, *315*, 31–44.

9

Mind-Body Interaction
in Sport Psychophysiology

Maurizio Bertollo, Marika Berchicci, and Selenia di Fronso

State of the Art

"The elucidation of the relationships between psychological states, physiological responses, and human behaviour remains the discipline's core mission of psychophysiology" (Cooke & Ring, 2019, p 1). To understand the mind-body relationship, it is crucial to study brain-heart and brain-muscle interactions. These interactions can be assessed investigating functional connectivity between the brain activity (i.e., electroencephalography [EEG]) and peripheral electrophysiological activity (i.e., electrocardiography [ECG] and electromyography [EMG]) underlying a specific performance, especially in ecological settings (di Fronso et al., 2017; Teques et al., 2017).

Psychophysiological monitoring and intervention in sport has a long tradition in lab settings. However, recent investigations in the applied field of sport, exercise, and performance have improved our knowledge of the mind-body dynamics during actual performance. Moreover, the adoption of ecological tasks and the use of advanced brain-body technologies in practice have helped to elucidate the underlying cognitive and brain processes (e.g., attention, self-regulation, neural efficiency) involved in performance execution (Bertollo et al., 2020). Nowadays, when adopting a psychophysiological perspective, objective physiological measures (e.g., autonomic, cortical, somatic) can be recorded using dry electrodes and lightweight wireless amplifiers during sport performance (di Fronso et al., 2019). Consequently, modern psychophysiology has been used to conduct rigorous ecological research aimed at capturing the complex processes underpinning behavior in sport, exercise, and performance settings.

Maurizio Bertollo, Marika Berchicci, and Selenia di Fronso, *Mind-Body Interaction in Sport Psychophysiology* In: *Sport, Exercise and Performance Psychology*. Edited by: Edson Filho and Itay Basevitch, Oxford University Press. © Oxford University Press 2021. DOI: 10.1093/oso/9780197512494.003.0009

Historically, the first psychophysiological studies in sport were based on the framework of cardiovascular psychophysiology and investigated the cognitive processes (e.g., arousal and the cardiovascular activity modulated by attention) related to cardiac deceleration during performance (Lacey, 1969). To this purpose, Lacey and Lacey (1978) developed the *stimulus intake-rejection hypothesis*: predicting that stimulus intake (focused attention) is associated with cardiac deceleration (bradycardia), while stimulus rejection (cognitive function excluding distracting or aversive environmental stimuli) is accompanied by cardiac acceleration (tachycardia). Specifically, the first studies on this topic date back to the 1960s and 1970s with the foundation of the Society for Psychophysiological Research and the publication of its official journal: *Psychophysiology*. In the first issue of this journal, according to John Stern (1964, p. 90), psychophysiology was defined as the field "where behavioural variables are manipulated, and the effects of these independent variables are observed on physiological measures as dependent variables." Differently, previous articles in the last decades of the 19th and the first half of the 20th century distinguished the psychophysiological approach based on the topic of the studies, as follows: (a) electro-dermal responses and their sensitivity to psychological processes, (b) emotion and autonomic control, and (c) conditioning of autonomic and visceral responses (for a review see Cooke & Ring, 2019). During the last three decades of the 20th century, there has been a growing interest for the discipline of sport psychophysiology, especially because neuroscience became a useful approach to study the mind-body relationship. Nowadays, the main interest is represented by the investigation of higher level cognitive and psychological processes associated with peak (optimal) performance (Hatfield, 2018).

Peak (optimal) sport performance is the ultimate goal that athletes and applied sport psychologists strive to achieve and maintain. The main questions related to performance optimization (see Table 9.1), and addressed using the psychophysiological approach, concern (a) the neural efficiency and proficiency in experts, that is, reduced and specialized neural activity (Bertollo et al., 2016; Hatfield, 2018); (b) the neural markers of sport performance (Cheron et al., 2016); (c) both cortical and cardiac indices of preparation for action in sport (Cooke, 2013); and (d) the cortico-muscular and the cortico-cardiac coherence (Martínez-Aguilar & Gutiérrez, 2019). A closely related field pertains to bio- and neurofeedback interventions and the trans-electrical stimulation of brain regions. These intervention approaches have been developed to enhance performance, particularly through the increase of awareness and self-regulation in athletes (for a review see Bertollo et al., 2020).

One of the unexplored links in sport science and, more specifically, in sport psychology is the heart-brain interaction (for a general review see Thayer & Lane, 2009), despite the early work by Lacey and Lacey (1978) and the application of idiosyncratic approaches in elite athletes (Bertollo et al., 2012). Indeed, the bidirectional communication between the heart and the brain is of great importance and represents the prominent ground for many of the psychophysiological theories today. With the aim to better study optimal performance and its mechanisms, the following five major questions could move the field of heart-brain interaction/integration forward.

Table 9.1 Five Key Readings in Brain-Body Communication in Sport Settings

Authors	Methodological Design	Key Findings
Bertollo et al. (2016)	Within subjects	Proficiency is an active and qualitative process that involves the interaction between the efficiency of human processing and the efficacy of performance. Event-related synchronization brain activity is mainly associated with optimal-automatic performance in accordance with the neural efficiency hypothesis. Event-related desynchronization is more related to optimal-controlled performance in conditions reflecting neural adaptability and proficient use of cortical resources.
Cheron et al. (2016)	Review	Theta band (4–8 Hz) can serve as a biomarker of eye-head-body movement, navigation, episodic memory, sensorimotor integration, goal setting, network coordination, motor control, emotion, and dream recall. Alpha band (8–15 Hz) can serve as a biomarker of a global resting state, selective attention, cognitive performance, inhibition and gating, and consolidation of new motor sequences. Beta band (15–30 Hz) can serve as a biomarker of binding, sensorimotor association, sensory discrimination, fatigue, ANS regulation, and motor imagery.

Table 9.1 *Continued*

Authors	Methodological Design	Key Findings
Cooke (2013)	Review	Superior performance of experts in golf can be explained by experts engaging in greater external information processing than their less skilled counterparts, which is reflected by a greater heart rate deceleration and may also be associated with a greater negative amplitude of the readiness potential and reduced EEG alpha power during aiming.
		The increased accuracy of experts compared to novices in both shooting and golf may be further explained by a reduction in verbal-analytic information processing during preparation for action. This could be reflected by a progressive increase in EEG alpha power during preparation for the trigger pull in shooting and a reduction in EEG alpha power coherence between the left temporal and frontal midline regions of the brain during preparation for action in both shooting and golf.
Hatfield (2018)	Review	According to the psychomotor efficiency hypothesis, the association of areas of the cerebral cortex become progressively quiescent with practice and enhanced skill level.
		Expert brain processes reveal the recruitment of fewer resources compared to novices when they accomplish the same task.
		Cognitive load of the brain processes progressively diminishes with motor skill acquisition.
		Brain activation is cautiously recruited in the best performers even when the overall level of performance is rising.
		LORETA analyses confirmed noisy brain during performance under competitive stress and suggest elevated source activations and influential interactions between motor and nonmotor areas.
Martínez-Aguilar & Gutiérrez (2019)	Within subjects	Significant changes exist in the maximum cortico-muscular coherence in the beta brain rhythm as the exercise progresses and fatigue develops.
		Significant changes exist in the maximum cortico-cardiac coherence in the beta band, from the beginning to the end of an exercise protocol in cycling.

ANS, autonomic nervous system; EEG, electroencephalography; LORETA, low resolution electromagnetic tomography.

Questions to Move the Field Forward

1. Methodological Question: How Can We Collect Reliable Psychophysiological Measures on the Heart-Brain Relationship, Especially in Ecologically Valid Environments?

In ecologic and dynamic settings, one of the most used techniques to quantify brain activities is the EEG. Scientists mainly investigated brain rhythms (i.e., delta, theta, alpha, beta, gamma) when the onset of the movement was difficult to define and detect, like during cyclic and continuous movements (e.g., cycling, running, walking); when brain activities can be triggered to a specific event, like during discrete movements (e.g., shooting and throwing), event-related potential (ERP) and event-related desynchronization analyses are performed. A class of ERPs linking brain and heart is called heartbeat-evoked potentials (HEPs), because this biosignal is measured by time-locking the ERP to the R-wave spikes of the ECG waveform. Thus, to calculate the HEP, a simultaneous recording of both EEG and ECG is needed. Most of the paradigms used to investigate HEP have implicated heart-related attention (e.g., counting, tapping, and synchronizing attention to heartbeats), as this potential represents the cortical processing of the heartbeats and a neural correlate of interoception (Petzschner et al., 2019). Another measure taken from the ECG and related to the heart-brain relation is the heart rate variability (HRV), which is the sequence of time intervals between heartbeats. HRV was also proposed as a measure of the organic capacity to functionally and flexibly adapt to the environment (see Thayer & Lane, 2009).

The employment of heart-brain measures is needed to determine the cortical and subcortical regions implicated in skilled motor performance during differ+ent cardiovascular loads and its contribution during the recovery period to develop idiosyncratic behavioral and integrated mind-body interventions. Indeed, experimental and clinical studies have illustrated a complex network, known as the central autonomic network (Benarroch, 1997), characterized by several highly interconnected cortices, subcortical forebrain structures, and brain stem areas (Tahsili-Fahadan & Geocadin, 2017), which together process and control cardiovascular function. Key regions are the insula, the amygdala, and the prefrontal cortex (PFC): the insula is implicated in physiological regulation during exercise and the cognitive representation of perceptions (i.e., visual, auditory, bodily); the amygdala seems to modulate the effects of emotional stimuli on the heart; the

PFC regulates the vagally mediated cardiac functions (HRV) and, at the same time, the executive function and the affective processing (Thayer & Lane, 2009).

Physiological measures able to quantify the degree to which central and autonomous systems are orchestrated and modulated by specific sport training are warranted. Nowadays, by means of new mobile devices and dry electrodes, it is feasible to integrate heart-brain data in the same amplifier during dynamic tasks in the real-world environment. Collecting data in the field setting would allow monitoring the contribution provided by both systems to sport performance. Following this approach, objective psychophysiological measures will be developed to improve and inform motor skills training. For example, if the motor performance is affected by enhanced activity of the PFC and high HRV, then training these physiological processes underpinning executive functions would benefit the athlete. Again, if the insula is implicated during recovery, then the modulation of this activity together with heartbeats by means of mind-body interventions would decrease the time to recovery. Further mind-body interventions based on psychophysiological recordings are needed to improve the provision of tailored skill-training programs for athletes.

2. Theoretical Question: How Can Heart-Brain Interactions Explain Both Self-Regulation Processes in Athletes and the Arousal-Emotion-Attention-Performance Linkage?

Understanding the arousal-emotion-attention-performance linkage and self-regulation processes related to performance optimization have been some of the main challenges in sport psychology. Self-regulation involves a complex mix of behavioral, emotional, and cognitive processes, which in turn influence the physiological processes underpinning optimal performance states. Moreover, arousal is the physiological and psychological state of activation, involving both the central and the autonomous nervous systems; it is a condition of sensory alertness, mobility, and readiness to respond (e.g., Weinberg, 2019, p. 16). For this reason, arousal is important in regulating attention, alertness, and information processing during performance in sport settings. Moreover, according to the attentional control theory, arousal is modulated by the attentional control in the context of anxiety and cognitive performance (Eysenck et al., 2007). Therefore, it is important for athletes to find their individual zones of optimal functioning so that they can learn to self-regulate (by using biofeedback methods) their psychophysiological states, including heart-brain interactions. Furthermore, self-regulation is related to HRV, and arousal induction can affect the cortical processing of heartbeats (Luft & Bhattacharya, 2015). Therefore, investigating the interaction between the brain and heart is essential to advance research on performance optimization and self-regulation processes in sports.

Different models proposed that self-regulation processes—involving cognition, emotion, and arousal—influence performance. For instance, the neurovisceral integration model (Thayer & Lane, 2009) proposes that cognitive, affective, and physiological regulation processes may be related to each other in the service of goal-directed behavior. Another model, the predictive coding (Seth et al., 2012), suggests that the perception of the body and the world—interoception and exteroception—involves intertwined processes of inference, learning, and prediction. The intertwined nature of exteroceptive and interoceptive processes is based on the assumption that the brain actively constructs a generative model of its sensory inputs (from its external environment or from its own body), inverts this model to determine the causes of its sensations (inference), continuously updates the model (learning) based on new sensory information, and forecasts future inputs (prediction). In this framework, Petzschner et al. (2019) showed that the focus of attention can modulate HEP, as attention gates the influence of sensory information on perception. These authors observed that the HEP is significantly higher during interoceptive compared to exteroceptive attention, suggesting that it is modulated by pure attention. In future studies, especially in precision sport contexts, HEP should be adopted as a neural correlate of interoceptive predictive errors, and its amplitude modulation should be employed to understand when attention is directed toward or away from the heart (Petzschner et al., 2019).

Furthermore, Ribeiro and Castelo-Branco (2019) identified an association between neural modulation of the heart and other cognitive processes, such as perceptual decision-making. Drawing on this association, future studies should envisage protocols enhancing the complexity of sport performance tasks by increasing the number of possible responses. This procedure would also increase the amplitude of the preparatory cardiac deceleration. Such studies would allow verifying, in the sport context, whether the modulation of preparatory cardiac deceleration by the manipulation of task demands can predict the ability to maintain responses and facilitate decision-making as well as attentional control.

3. Theoretical Question: How Can the Heart-Brain Connection Explain Interoception and Neuromuscular Fatigue?

Interoception provides the representation of the physiological condition coming from the body and combining the crosstalk between the central and autonomous nervous systems (Tahsili-Fahadan & Geocadin, 2017). Thus, interoceptive signals play a crucial role in homeostatic regulation during sport performance, enabling peak performance in different kinds of disciplines. Interoceptive abilities (e.g., accuracy, sensitivity, and awareness) benefit from sport and, at the same time, facilitate the regulation of emotion and behavior during sport performance (Georgiou et al., 2015). As mentioned earlier, a reliable measure of interoceptive sensitivity is the HEP. Interoception is then related to homeostatic regulation and decision-making, which is a cognitive processing under the PFC control and highly implicated in motor performance (Craig, 2002). In high-stress situations, for example, when neuromuscular fatigue occurs, both interoception and decision-making are affected. Indeed, neuromuscular fatigue is a multidimensional concept combining psychophysiological and psychological aspects; it is an individual's experience that includes altered sensations about tasks being more difficult or taking more effort than expected (Søgaard et al., 2006).

Moreover, individuals' perception of effort is thought to be modulated by the potential motivation, which is the maximum amount of effort that a person is willing to exert to succeed in the task (de Morree et al., 20125). Motivation drive states are generated by a core set of neural structures, particularly within the medial PFC (Thayer & Lane, 2009). They allow for a successful adaptation to the changing environment and to psychophysiological demands (integration between the internal homeostasis and signals from the environment). Indeed, it was proposed that during prolonged physical exercise, the neuromuscular integrity is managed by brain mechanisms using the symptoms of fatigue as key regulators to ensure that the exercise is completed without threatening the homeostatic stability (Noakes, 2012). Available neuroimaging data (Hilty et al., 2011) showed an increased thalamo-insular activation during fatiguing tasks, which was interpreted as a central mechanism mediating the termination of the task to protect the integrity of the organism. Indeed, the thalamus, the anterior cingulate cortex, the insular cortex, and the medial PFC are involved in sensations of discomfort; these brain areas alert the organism to urgent homeostatic imbalance, thus playing a key role in the regulation of autonomic states and in the regulation of efforts during prolonged physical exercise (Noakes, 2012). These brain regions are the link between psychological stress (mind) and health-related physiology (body) (see Gianaros & Wager, 2015).

Future studies should investigate the dynamic interaction between the heart and brain during different stress-induced cardiovascular situations, like prolonged physical exercise, marathon, altitude, underwater, and heat. Indeed, in these conditions the heart-brain interaction needs to be highly flexible to adapt to the demands of the environment and could be an important reference for improving sport training. For example, how is the PFC activity modulated by increasing efforts and cardiovascular loads? Do the central and autonomic systems recover at the same time? Is there a relationship between HEP and insula activity? The response to these and other related questions would advance current knowledge on the psychophysiological processes underpinning recovery after exhaustion. Thus, the capacity to manage interoception and neuromuscular fatigue and to provide mind-body interventions is essential to reach and sustain peak performance.

4. Applied Question: Which Applied Interventions Integrating the Heart and Brain Are Useful to Improve and/or Optimize Performance?

The development of useful interventions for modulating HEP is at the core of an applied point of view for sport psychology/psychophysiology experts. For example, attention to interoceptive stimuli (i.e., attention directed toward the heart) could play a prominent role in the precision of interosensory information, thereby increasing the likelihood of error detection and prediction, in comparison to an attentional focus on exteroceptive stimuli (Auksztulewicz & Friston, 2015; Petzschner et al., 2019). Accordingly, attention training and HEP recordings could turn into useful tools to better study anxiety and performance-related anxiety. Indeed, some forms of anxiety (e.g., generalized anxiety disorder) are related to overly salient sensory signals from the body. HEP is also sensitive to arousal. Specifically, situations or conditions with higher intrinsic levels of arousal, both cognitive and physiological, are associated with a larger HEP (Petzschner et al., 2019). This effect is especially evident over the right temporoparietal regions, which play a key role in modulating autonomic and behavioral aspects of emotion-related arousal. Consequently, future studies and interventions should use arousal induction methods to promote emotion regulation, which is one of the most important factors for successful performance in sport (e.g., di Fronso et al., 2020).

Furthermore, when using emotion induction processes in association with HRV biofeedback, HEPs can be used to identify the specific mechanism of afferent input from the heart to the brain. These afferent inputs could have an impact on the activity of higher brain centers involved in perceptual, cognitive, and emotional processing, thereby affecting several aspects of motor performance experiences (McCraty et al., 2009). Moreover, the same inputs may affect the homeostatic regulatory centers in the brain, such as the central autonomic network, which is connected to other brain networks devoted to the modulation of executive functions, affective responses, and attentional-oriented behavior. A common reciprocal inhibitory cortico-subcortical neural circuit contributes to regulate not only autonomic but also emotional and cognitive functions. Despite being more invasive, the use of vagal nerve stimulation (VNS) in association with HRV biofeedback and HEP can be considered as a further potential intervention to target the function of the afferent pathways of the autonomic nervous system. Specifically, VNS may serve as a useful tool to better study the neuromodulation of cognitive processes (e.g., emotional memory) that can be crucial to explain how individuals reach and sustain optimal performance. VNS (or neurofeedback) can also be used to stimulate brain areas related to cardiac deceleration (e.g., frontal areas) and serve as a technique to improve, for example, aiming or simple balance performance. Also, the integrated use of EEG/ECG would allow to better investigate sympathetic/parasympathetic balance, which is important for both sport and health reasons. To this purpose, scholars could use EEG electrodes positioned in and around the ear, while heartbeat artifacts generally present in EEG recordings (e.g., R waves of the QRS complex) could be used to simultaneously record ECG data and to analyze HRV. This methodological approach provides accurate measures also during movements (as opposed to static data collection), and it is characterized by a portable technology that is comfortable to participants performing daily activities and, most importantly, allows for fast and integrated biofeedback interventions (Bleichner & Debener, 2017).

5. Applied Question: How Can Neuro-Visceral-Cognitive Interventions Enhance Performance?

The best neuro-visceral-cognitive interventions that can improve performance are represented by bio- and neurofeedback training. Specific protocols (e.g., cardiac modulation, EEG cortical asymmetries) can help individuals to self-regulate, thereby creating physiological coherence, a scientifically measurable state characterized by increased order and harmony in our mind, emotions, and body (McCraty et al., 2009). Moreover, virtual reality can enrich the perception of the actual environment, as individuals can be immersed in different scenarios and be involved in the three types of illusions of virtual reality: place illusion, plausibility illusion, and embodiment (Colombetti & Thompson, 2008). More precisely, place illusion is the sensation of being in a real place, plausibility illusion is the illusion that the scenario depicted is actually occurring, and embodiment refers to the sense of concrete representation of the scenario (e.g., di Fronso et al., 2020). In the context of virtual reality, it is possible to include also psychophysiological indices derived from EEG (e.g., alpha peak frequency) and ECG (e.g., HRV indices); thus, individuals can interact with ecological scenarios, learning how to modulate heart-brain interactions during induced cognitive and emotional states, with the aim of improving performance. From an applied point of view, for example, the use of specific smart glasses can simultaneously display real-time performance data (e.g., speed and pacing), ocular metrics (e.g., fixation, saccades, and gaze), brain rhythms (e.g., alpha and theta waves), and cardiovascular responses (e.g., HRV). In other words, smart glasses can lead to an augmented reality, while enhancing the measurement and trainability of neurocognitive components, emotional responses, and individual performance metrics. Also, specific helmets or visors (e.g., Oculus rift) that provide 3D feedback modulated by brain and heart activities could be useful in increasing heart-brain interaction/integration.

The main challenge for the future is to implement heart-brain coherence protocols that can be integrated within brain-computer interface (BCI) systems. In turn, BCI systems can be integrated into new software like neuromore (https://www.neuromore.com), which is a platform enabling anyone to create connected and emotionally intelligent applications. The use of other neurocognitive tools, such as NeuroTracker (https://neurotracker.net/), can be used to further enhance cognitive processes related to attention and performance, thereby also influencing heart-brain interaction. Furthermore, it has been demonstrated that heart-brain interactions and executive functions can be modulated by cardiovascular load (Crowe et al., 2020). This could be essential to the development of novel performance optimization training protocols, especially in sports like biathlon or modern pentathlon, which combine high precision in shooting and endurance during skiing (biathlon) or running (pentathlon).

Regarding endurance sports, it has been suggested that brain endurance training could be considered as a further neurocognitive visceral intervention for performance optimization (Marcora et al., 2015). According to this kind of training, developed within the psychobiological model of fatigue framework (see de Morree & Marcora, 2015), practitioners could use acute mental fatigue as a stimulus to induce chronic reduction in fatigue during physical tasks. For instance, cognitive tasks, such as the Flanker or Stroop test, could be administered during cycling practice. In this way, sport professionals could cautiously increase training load in endurance athletes without compromising their musculoskeletal system.

All the technologies and interventions mentioned need to be integrated into a holistic perspective including different methodologies, such as mindfulness, yoga, or other behavioral techniques aimed at developing and/or enhancing adaptable self-regulation strategies and heart-brain interaction/integration.

Conclusion

The investigation of mind-body interaction/integration can benefit from recent psychophysiology and neuroscience developments. From a methodological point of view, the miniaturization of devices and the development of new algorithms for studying neurovisceral functional connectivity can contribute to the creation of new ecological paradigms in which scholars can study the psychophysiological features underpinning athletes' expert behavior by using a holistic approach. From a theoretical point of view, it is important to understand not only the role played by heart-brain communication in self-regulation and attentional control but also the role of interoception in optimal performance experiences. From an applied point of view, integrated interventions targeting heart-brain interactions can help athletes learning how to up/down-regulate peripheral (e.g., HRV) and central (brain rhythms) physiological responses linked to optimal performance in sports.

In conclusion, a better understanding of the mind-body-behavior communication can advance interventions for performance optimization in the field of sport psychology. Specifically, going back to the future, heart-brain integration in sport performance should be investigated.

References

Auksztulewicz, R., & Friston, K. (2015). Attentional enhancement of auditory mismatch responses: A DCM/MEG study. *Cerebral Cortex, 25*(11), 4273–4283. http://doi.org/10.1093/cercor/bhu323

Benarroch, E. E. (1997). *Central autonomic network: Functional organization and clinical correlations.* Futura Publishing Company.

Bertollo, M., Di Fronso, S., Filho, E., Conforto, S., Schmid, M., Bortoli, L., & Robazza, C. (2016). Proficient brain for optimal performance: The MAP model perspective. *PeerJ, 4,* e2082. https://doi.org/10.7717/peerj.2082

Bertollo, M., Doppelmayr M., & Robazza C. (2020). Using brain technology in practice. In G. Tenembaum & R. Eklund (Eds.), *Handbook of sport psychology* (pp 666–693), 4th edition. Hoboken, NJ: Wiley & Blackwell.

Bertollo, M., Robazza, C., Falasca, W. N., Stocchi, M., Babiloni, C., Del Percio, C., Marzano, N., Iacoboni, M., Infarinato, F., Vecchio, F., Limatola, C., & Comani, S. (2012). Temporal pattern of pre-shooting psycho-physiological states in elite athletes: A probabilistic approach. *Psychology of Sport and Exercise, 13*(2), 91–98. https://doi.org/10.1016/j.psychsport.2011.09.005

Bleichner, M. G., & Debener, S. (2017). Concealed, unobtrusive ear-centered EEG acquisition: CEEGrids for transparent EEG. *Frontiers in Human Neuroscience, 11,* 163. https://doi:10.3389/fnhum.2017.00163

Cheron, G., Petit, G., Cheron, J., Leroy, A., Cebolla, A., Cevallos, C., Petieau, M., Hoellinger, T., Zarka, D., Clarinval, A.-M., & Dan, B. (2016). Brain oscillations in sport: Toward EEG biomarkers of performance. *Frontiers in Psychology, 7,* 246. https://doi.org/10.3389/fpsyg.2016.00246

Colombetti, G., & Thompson, E. (2008) The feeling body: Towards an enactive approach to emotion. In W. F. Overton, U. Müller, & J. Newman (Eds.), *Developmental perspectives on embodiment and consciousness* (p. 4568). Lawrence Erlbaum.

Cooke, A. (2013). Readying the head and steadying the heart: A review of cortical and cardiac studies of preparation for action in sport. *International Review of Sport and Exercise Psychology, 6*(1), 122–138. https://doi.org/10.1080/1750984X.2012.724438

Cooke, A., & Ring, C. (2019). Psychophysiology of sport, exercise, and performance: Past, present, and future. *Sport, Exercise, and Performance Psychology, 8*(1), 1–6. https://doi.org/10.1037/spy0000156

Craig, A. D. (2002). How do you feel? Interoception: The sense of the physiological condition of the body. *Nature Reviews: Neuroscience, 3*(8), 655–666. https://doi.org/10.1038/nrn894

Crowe, E. M., Wilson, M. R., Harris, D. J., & Vine, S. J. (2020). Eye tracking and cardiovascular measurement to assess and improve sporting performance. In M. Bertollo, P. Terry, & E. Filho (Eds.), *Advancements in mental skill training* (pp. 135–148). Routledge.

de Morree, H. M., Klein, C., & Marcora, S. M. (2012). Perception of effort reflects central motor command during movement execution. *Psychophysiology, 49*, 1242–1253. https://doi.org/10.1111/j.1469-8986.2012.01399.x

de Morree, H. M., & Marcora, S. M. (2015). Psychobiology of perceived effort during physical tasks. In G. Gendolla, M. Tops, & K. Sander (Eds.), *Handbook of biobehavioral approaches to self-regulation* (pp. 255–270). Springer doi:10.1007/978-1-4939-1236-0_17

di Fronso, S., Fiedler, P., Tamburro, G., Haueisen, J., Bertollo, M., & Comani, S. (2019). Dry EEG in sports sciences: A fast and reliable tool to assess individual alpha peak frequency changes induced by physical effort. *Frontiers in Neuroscience, 13*, 982. https://doi.org/10.3389/fnins.2019.00982

di Fronso, S., Robazza, C., Bortoli, L., & Bertollo, M. (2017). Performance optimization in sport: A psychophysiological approach. *Motriz: Revista de Educação Física, 23*(4), e1017138. https://doi.org/10.1590/s1980-6574201700040001

di Fronso, S., Werthner, P., Christie, S., & Bertollo, M. (2020). Using technology for self-regulation in sport. In M. C. Ruiz & C. Robazza (Eds.), *Feelings in sport theory, research, and practical implications for performance and well-being.* Taylor & Francis.

Eysenck, M. W., Derakshan, N., Santos, R., & Calvo, M. G. (2007). Anxiety and cognitive performance: Attentional control theory. *Emotion, 7*, 336–353. https://doi.org/10.1037/1528-3542.7.2.336

Georgiou, E., Matthias, E., Kobel, S., Kettner, S., Dreyhaupt, J., Steinacker, J. M., & Pollatos, O. (2015). Interaction of physical activity and interoception in children. *Frontiers in Psychology, 6*, 502. https://doi.org/10.3389/fpsyg.2015.00502

Gianaros, P. J., & Wager, T. D. (2015). Brain-body pathways linking psychological stress and physical health. *Current Directions in Psychological Science, 24*(4), 313–321. https://doi.org/10.1177/0963721415581476

Hatfield, B. D. (2018). Brain dynamics and motor behavior: A case for efficiency and refinement for superior performance. *Kinesiology Review, 7*(1), 42–50. https://doi.org/10.1123/kr.2017-0056

Hilty, L., Jäncke, L., Luechinger, R., Boutellier, U., & Lutz, K. (2011). Limitation of physical performance in a muscle fatiguing handgrip exercise is mediated by thalamo-insular activity. *Human Brain Mapping, 32*, 2151–2160.

Lacey, B. C., & Lacey, J. I. (1978). Two-way communication between the heart and the brain: Significance of time within the cardiac cycle. *American Psychologist, 33*, 99–113. https://doi.org/10.1037/0003-066X.33.2.99

Lacey, J. I. (1969). Autonomic indices of attention, readiness, and rejection of the external environment. In D.P. Kimble (Ed.), *Readiness to remember* (pp. 511–610). Gordon & Breach.

Luft, C. D. B., & Bhattacharya, J. (2015). Aroused with heart: Modulation of heartbeat evoked potential by arousal induction and its oscillatory correlates. *Scientific Reports, 5*, 15717. https://doi.org/10.1038/srep15717

Marcora, S. M., Staiano, W., & Merlini, M. (2015). A randomised controlled trial of Brain Endurance Training (BET) to reduce fatigue during endurance exercise. *Medicine & Science in Sports & Exercise, 47*(5S), 198. doi:10.1249/01.mss.0000476967.03579.44.

Martínez-Aguilar, G. M., & Gutiérrez, D. (2019). Using cortico-muscular and cortico-cardiac coherence to study the role of the brain in the development of muscular fatigue. *Biomedical Signal Processing and Control, 48*, 153–160. https://doi.org/10.1016/j.bspc.2018.10.011

McCraty, R., Atkinson, M., Tomasino, D., & Bradley, R. T. (2009). The coherent heart: Heart-brain interactions, psychophysiological coherence, and the emergence of system-wide order. *Integral Review: A Transdisciplinary & Transcultural Journal for New Thought, Research, & Praxis, 5*(2), 11–115.

Noakes, T. D. (2012). Fatigue is a brain-derived emotion that regulates the exercise behavior to ensure the protection of whole body homeostasis. *Frontiers in Physiology, 3*, 82. https://doi.org/10.3389/fphys.2012.00082

Petzschner, F. H., Weber, L. A., Wellstein, K. V., Paolini, G., Do, C. T., & Stephan, K. E. (2019). Focus of attention modulates the heartbeat evoked potential. *Neuroimage, 186*, 595–606. https://doi.org/10.1016/j.neuroimage.2018.11.037

Ribeiro, M. J., & Castelo-Branco, M. (2019). Neural correlates of anticipatory cardiac deceleration and its association with the speed of perceptual decision-making, in young and older adults. *Neuroimage, 199*, 521–533. https://doi.org/10.1016/j.neuroimage.2019.06.004

Seth, A. K., Suzuki, K., & Critchley, H. D. (2012). An interoceptive predictive coding model of conscious presence. *Frontiers in Psychology, 2*, 395. https://doi.org/10.3389/fpsyg.2011.00395

Søgaard, K., Gandevia, S. C., Todd, G., Petersen, N. T., & Taylor, J. L. (2006). The effect of sustained low-intensity contractions on supraspinal fatigue in human elbow flexor muscle. *Journal of Physiology, 573*, 511–523. https://doi.org/10.1113/jphysiol.2005.103598

Stern, J. A. (1964). Toward a definition of psychophysiology. *Psychophysiology, 1*(1), 90–91. https://doi.org/10.1111/j.1469-8986.1964.tb02626.x

Tahsili-Fahadan, P., & Geocadin, R. G. (2017). Heart-brain axis. Effects of neurologic injury on cardiovascular function. *Circulation Research, 120*, 559–572. https://doi.org/10.1161/CIRCRESAHA.116.308446

Teques, P., Araújo, D., Seifert, L., del Campo, V. L., & Davids, K. (2017). The resonant system: Linking brain–body–environment in sport performance. In M. R. Wilson, V. Walsh, & B. Parkin (Eds.), *Progress in brain research* (pp. 33–52). Elsevier. https://doi.org/10.1016/bs.pbr.2017.06.001

Thayer, J. F., & Lane, R. D. (2009). Claude Bernard and the heart-brain connection: Further elaboration of a model of neurovisceral integration. *Neuroscience and Biobehavioral Reviews, 33*(2), 81–88. https://doi.org/10.1016/j.neubiorev.2008.08.004

Weinberg, R. (2019). Arousal. In D. Hackfort, R. J. Schinke, & B. Strauss (Eds.), *Dictionary of sport psychology: Sport, exercise, and performing arts* (p. 337). Academic Press.

10

Genetics

Sigal Ben Zaken

In the year 1896, Gregor Mandel, the founding father of genetics, was deceased and terms such as *gene*, *DNA*, and *chromosomes* were nonexistent. Yet, at the 1896 Olympic Games, humanity admired sport performance at its finest. Today, more than 120 years later, genetic knowledge has been vastly developed, the human genome is decoded, and advanced applications in genetic engineering have been developed. Yet, many questions regarding the genetic basis of sport, exercise, and performance remain unanswered.

Genetics is the study of genes, genetic variation, and heredity in living organisms. Most human traits, including psychological and behavioral traits, are heritable and are based on biological mechanisms. The heritability of traits such as mental toughness, motivation, and self-regulation, which are important concepts in sport psychology, is approximately 50% to 60% (Li et al., 2019; Lin et al., 2017; Willems et al., 2019), meaning that 50% to 60% of the variability seen in these traits may be attributed to genetic variability. Yet, these heritability estimations are based on research conducted on the general population and have not necessarily been applied to sport, exercise, and physical activity. Research on the heritability of mental toughness, motivation, and self-regulation in relation to sport and exercise are rare. Heritability studies are common in the field of *behavioral genetics*. Behavioral genetics investigate the nature and origins of individual differences in behavior mainly by using twin and family research paradigms.

While heritability estimates the proportion of variability attributed to genetics, *molecular genetics* is the field that explores the sources of genetic variability by studying the structure and function of genes at a molecular level. The study of molecular genetics in the physiological domain of sport, exercise, and performance has made large progress during the last decades along with the general progress in molecular genetic methods. However, parallel progress in the psychological domain of sport and exercise has not been made. Thus, it is only natural to assume that behavioral genetics and

Sigal Ben Zaken, *Genetics* In: *Sport, Exercise and Performance Psychology.* Edited by: Edson Filho and Itay Basevitch,
Oxford University Press. © Oxford University Press 2021. DOI: 10.1093/oso/9780197512494.003.0010

molecular genetics will meet at the sport, exercise, and performance domain, which combines both psychological and physiological traits. However, this integration has not happened yet, leaving many research questions open. The present chapter will review some of these questions and possible future directions.

State of the Art

The whole is greater than the sum of its parts.

—Aristotle

Sport Performance: More Than the Sum of Traits

Every time we witness an athlete score a goal, win a trophy, or perform an extraordinary drill of physical prowess, we find ourselves asking the question: how? What makes this individual great? Is this achievable by ordinary individuals or is it a God-given gift? Questions such as these encompass the ancient argument of nature versus nurture as it pertains to competitive sports and athletic performance (Davids & Baker, 2007; Johnson & Tenenbaum, 2006; Tucker & Collins, 2012).

The "nurture" side of the debate claims that performance is inseparable from training, repetition, and perseverance as described in the *deliberate practice theory* (Ericsson, 2007). The direct derivative from this theory is that, fundamentally, any individual (given enough time) who is willing to "put in the time" can achieve greatness should they pursue a correct training regime. However, the "nature" point of view advocates that this is not a realistic possibility, as people are fundamentally different from one another in many traits (e.g., height, flexibility, mental toughness, training responsiveness) that show distribution across the population regardless of their individual efforts. This defining variability of the human race stems, at least partially, from interpersonal genetic variability.

In this sense, one must point out that athletic performance is not an attribute, a quality, or a trait. Performance, such as winning a competition, scoring a goal, and so forth, is more of an "occurrence." For an athlete to achieve this occurrence, several conditions must be met, and the athlete needs a specific combination of skills, attributes, and traits. Yet, sport performance is too dynamic, multidimensional, and complex (Tenenbaum et al., 2009) and cannot be simplified as the sum of traits.

The sport performance model that we have previously suggested (Ben-Zaken et al., 2019) is composed of four layers: (a) the genotype layer represents the *genetic predisposition* determined at fertilization and is unchanged during life; (b) the trait layer represents the level of a *specific trait* (out of many) related to performance, with the level of the trait representing a gene-environment interaction that might vary in time; (c) the *environment* layer can range from supportive to nonsupportive; and (d) the *performance layer* is the outcome of all other layers. All the layers interact in a dynamic way, enabling various pathways that can lead to high performance.

Basic Terms: Learn the Biological Language

You can never understand one language until you understand at least two.

—Geoffrey Willans

As in every scientific field, genetics has its own language. In this sense it is important to emphasize the difference between several interrelated terms such as *trait, inheritance, genetic, DNA,* and *chromosomes*. A trait is a distinct characteristic variant of an organism; it may be internal or external, physiological or psychological (Violle et al., 2007). Traits can be categorized in many ways, for example, "body related" versus "mind related," or "inherited" versus "acquired." Two main constructs compose the field of genetics: (a) heredity/inheritance, the study of passing traits from parents to offspring, and (b) molecular genetics, which centers on the genes' structure and function and on the way genes and genetic variants result in traits and trait variability.

Other important terms are *gene expression* and *epigenetics*. Gene expression is the process by which information from a gene is used in the synthesis of a functional gene product, mainly protein. Epigenetics is the study of heritable changes in gene expression (active versus inactive genes) that do not involve changes to the underlying DNA, which in turn affect how cells read the genes. When it comes to the discussion about the role of genetics in sport performance, one must keep in mind the following:

1. Most human traits, including psychological and behavioral traits, are multifactorial traits and result from the complex combination of genetic factors, environmental factors, and the interaction between them (Rice & Reich, 1985).
2. Almost every trait, including psychological traits, relies on biological mechanisms (Kosslyn et al., 2002) and is facilitated by proteins (such as transporters, neurotransmitters, and receptors). Therefore, genes play a pivotal role in determining the trait, and genetic variability may result in trait variability, and hence performance variability.
3. Athletic performance–related traits are sport dependent. Agility, for instance, may be critical in a certain field and irrelevant in another. While the anatomical/biomechanical/motoric demands vary from one sport to another, mental requirements such as motivation, grit, and determination pertain to most if not all sports.
4. Adaption to training is characterized by changes at the cellular and molecular levels, and therefore by changes in protein synthesis. However, adaption to training is characterized not only by physiological changes but also by the subjective-affective experience of training and the psychosocially conditioned training motivation (Bryan et al., 2011). Therefore, changes in gene expression might be expected also in psychological mechanisms related to initiation, acceptance, and maintenance of training.

Why Are Genetics and Sport Psychology Mutually Estranged?

Gregor Mendel (1822–1884) and Sir Francis Galton (1822–1911) were born in the same year but never met and were not aware of the works of each other. In our day, with the perspective views of their tremendous work, it is clear that the integration of their domains is necessary to forward research in the psychology of sport performance to the next level.

Gregor Mendel followed the inheritance of seven traits in pea plants for 8 years before he described his conclusions in a two-part paper, "Experiments on Plant Hybridization" (Mendel, 1865). Mendel's conclusions were largely ignored until they were rediscovered decades after his death and he was crowned as the founding father of modern genetics (Henig, 2000). Detailed descriptions of his experiments can be found in every genetic textbook, and his three foundational principles of inheritance—the law of segregation, law of independent assortment, and law of dominance—laid the foundation to what later became known as modern genetics.

Galton, the founding father of eugenics and behavioral genetics (Gillham, 2001), coined the famous phrase "nature vs. nurture" (Gillham, 2001) and was influenced by the book *On the Origin of Species* written by his half-cousin, Charles Darwin (Fancher, 2009). The book, dealing with the diversity and evolution of life on Earth, led Galton to be interested in the factors that determine what he called human "talent and character" and its hereditary basis. He constructed his own theory of inheritance in which nature and not nurture plays the leading role. Ironically, Galton and Darwin were not aware that their contemporary, Gregor Mendel, had already solved the problem that puzzled Darwin the most—the lack of an explanation for heredity.

From that point on, these two domains evolved almost separately, with only few intersection points. While molecular genetics employs methods of molecular biology and provides insight into genetic variation, behavioral genetics uses family and twin models to investigate the nature and origins of individual differences in behavior. While the name "behavioral genetics" connotes a focus on genetic influences, the field broadly investigates genetic and environmental influences.

It is only natural to assume that behavioral genetics and molecular genetics will meet at the athletic performance domain. Athletic/sport performance is a field coalescing both psychological and physiological traits influenced by the interrelated relations and interactions of genetic and environmental factors. However, integration of behavioral genetics and molecular genetics in the study of sport performance is scarce.

The research on the genetic basis of human athletic performance has increased dramatically since the early 1990s, as can be seen in the yearly human gene map for performance and health-related fitness phenotypes, which was first published in 2001(Rankinen et al., 2001) and has been published almost yearly since then (Sarzynski et al., 2016). Parallel to the extensive research conducted to identify specific genes and genetic variants related to *physiological traits* of sport performance, the research aimed at identifying the genetic basis of *psychological traits* of sport performance is substantially meager. The lack of genetic research in the psychological-behavioral domain of sport and exercise is surprising considering the extensive research in general (Munafò et al., 2003) and in clinical psychology (Noble, 2000). Variables/traits such as motivation, emotion regulation, information processing, decision-making, and other psychological traits are crucial for athletic performance and yet not sufficiently studied.

Suggested Reading

To fully capture the complexity and multidimensional character of questions regarding the genetics and psychology of motor performance, I suggest the readings listed in Table 10.1, although many others might be enlightening as well.

Table 10.1 Five Key Readings in Genetics in the Sport, Exercise, and Performance Psychology Domain

Authors	Methodological Design	Key Findings
Wang et al. (2016)	Review; summarizes current and future directions in exercise genetics and genomics	Hypothesis-free genome-wide approaches will provide comprehensive coverage and in-depth understanding of the biology underlying sports-related traits and related genetic mechanisms. Large, collaborative projects with sound experimental designs (e.g., clearly defined phenotypes, considerations and controls for sources of variability, and necessary replications) are required to produce meaningful results.
Valeeva & Rees (2019)	Book chapter; prospective view of the up-to-date genetic polymorphisms related to psychological traits among athletes	To date, 16 psychogenetics-specific genetic markers have been reported to be associated with predisposition to specific sports (via case-control designs), and 12 markers have been linked with personality traits (via genotype-phenotype designs) in athletes. Future genetic research with large cohorts of athletes, with further validation and replication, will substantially contribute to the discovery of causal genetic variants, which may partly explain the heritability of athlete status and related psychological phenotypes.
Johnson et al. (2016)	Original research, association study; explores relations between genetic polymorphisms and behavioral inhibition system/behavioral activation system (BIS/BAS)	Though this research is not sport oriented, it provides one of the first polygenic examinations of behavioral traits. Its main finding is that *BDNF* is related to threat sensitivity, and *OPRM1* is related to reward sensitivity. The findings support the merit of a combined psychological and genetic approach.

Table 10.1 *Continued*

Authors	Methodological Design	Key Findings
Gottschling et al. (2016)	Original research, twin study; comparison between monozygotic and dizygotic twins	Though this research is not sport oriented, it emphasizes that genetic mediation analyses can contribute to our understanding of phenotypic mediation in personal and self-regulation, and the relationship between neuroticism and stress resistance
Ben-Zaken et al. (2019)	Book chapter; narrative view on the gene-environment paradigm	The chapter contributes to the ongoing nature-nurture debate by emphasizing the role of genetics in expertise development and suggests a dynamic model for the gene-environment paradigm in sport expertise.

Questions to Move the Field Forward

1. Theoretical and Applied Question: How Can We Optimize Personalized Training With the Help of Genetic Knowledge?

The 21st century has been characterized by a constant push toward genetic knowledge–based personalization in medicine (Hamburg & Collins, 2010) and nutrition (Drabsch & Holzapfel, 2019). It is just natural to assume that sport and exercise training will also be part of this paradigm. Evidence has emerged that large interindividual variation exists regarding the magnitude and direction of adaption following exercise (Bamman et al., 2007; Hubal et al., 2005). Yet, only a small number of studies have been conducted to identify biological/genetic factors responsible for interpersonal variability in training responses.

The goal of most training programs is to maximize the dose/response specific to the long-term objective(s). A number of studies have revealed important aspects of how cells respond to exercise (Neufer et al., 2015), but very little is known as to how these molecular responses ultimately translate to the individual's physiological, metabolic, and behavioral response. This in turn limits the ability to prescribe the desired dose required for optimal long-term outcomes. Nevertheless, the variation in psychological aspects related to training responsiveness is usually ignored, though it is well established that both cognition and mental factors contribute to performance.

Recently, several research findings indicated that individual trainability can change during the life course due to external factors such as nutrition or stress (Mann, Lamberts, & Lambert, 2014). This is where epigenetics comes into play. Again, epigenetics deals with processes that alter gene expression patterns without affecting the DNA sequence. Though individualization is a well-established key principle in periodization of sports training, to date, this kind of individualization does not incorporate genetic variables into the individualization procedure. Therefore, future interdisciplinary work in the field of individualized training will have to integrate epigenetics, sociology, and psychology into reasonable research programs.

Therefore, future research in the field of genetically based individualized training needs to take into account two main aspects: intraindividual repetition of measurements including the systematic combination of group-based and individual information and the joint consideration of multiple explanatory variables including psychological, genetic, and epigenetic variables. While these two fundamental considerations are based on statistical principles, their full implementation is beset with many practical difficulties. Therefore, from an applied perspective, the ways of implementing personalized training will differ considerably depending on the specific task and the framework conditions (Hecksteden & Meyer, 2018).

2. Applied and Methodological Question: How Can We Bridge the Gap Between Biology and Psychology Scaling?

One of the reasons that genetics and psychology evolved as separated domains is the scale differences. While genetic researchers focus on genes, which are fractures of cells, psychology researchers focus primarily on human behavior. It seems that biology and psychology stand at opposite ends of a continuum scale ranging from molecular to behavioral. This continuum can be seen from two perspectives: as a transformational system and as a reactive system. According to the transformational system approach, the genomic DNA information is translated into a diversity of expressed proteins (the proteome). The proteome then fashions the traits that define the functioning organism. The genome, from such a viewpoint, appears as the master plan that encodes the organism (Mayr, 1961). The explanation of the living system, from this viewpoint, is obtained by reducing its complexity to an orderly, sequential transformation of information from genes to traits (Cohen & Harel, 2007). According to the reactive system approach (Harel, 2004), the system does not behave according to a preprogrammed chain of linked instructions. Rather, such a system reacts in parallel to many concurrent inputs. A reactive system expresses a dynamic narrative in which the DNA code is one of the many formative inputs and the environment of the living system is a critical source of information (Cohen & Harel, 2007). To promote our understanding of behavior in general, and sport psychology in particular, we must shift from a transformational approach, in which biology and psychology represent two different scales, to a reactive approach, in which biology and psychology are parts of a holistic system.

An emergent property of a system is its behavior, taken as a whole, that is not expressed by any one of the lower scale components that compose it. Life, for example, is an emergent property; none of the molecule components of a cell are alive—only a whole cell is alive. Sport performance is also an emergent property, in which none of its components (e.g., motivation, muscle structure) is the sport performance per se. Therefore, sport performance emerges only when you step back—"zoom out"—and look at the performer at an appropriate scale (Cohen, 2000). Future research should take into consideration broad continuous scale measures including genomic, proteomic, and behavioral variables. This requires deep understanding of the biological mechanism underlying sport behavior as well as a multidisciplinary approach incorporating genetics, neuroscience, and behavior.

3. Applied and Methodological Question: How to Best Incorporate Genetics Into a Multidisciplinary Approach in the Study of Sport Performance?

Sport disciplines, such as biomechanics, performance analysis, physiology, psychology, and sociology, are interdisciplinary perspectives that provide a broad and in-depth view of the variables leading to successful performances. The European College of Sport Science (ECSS), which was founded in 1995, regards sport science as the integrator of knowledge of human movement acquired in all these disciplines and subdisciplines (Balagué et al., 2017). The search for minimum principles that explain the maximum number of phenomena is an implicit goal of all sciences, but tremendous growth in sport science has mostly produced further specialization and fragmentation

(Hristovski, 2013). This is because each discipline focuses on different levels of organization of matter. An interdisciplinary approach is defined as more than one area of sport and exercise science working together in an integrated and coordinated manner to solve a problem (MacLeod, 2018).

It is undeniable that a multidisciplinary approach to sport psychology is essential to move the field forward. When it comes to very different disciplines such as genetics and psychology, there is a need for multidisciplinary scientists from both disciplines not only to become familiar with the language of the other discipline but also to shift their point of view to a more holistic perspective (Carr, Loucks, & Blöschl, 2018). Moreover, interdisciplinary research does not occur automatically by bringing together several disciplines in a research project. Extra effort is needed to promote the formation of a cohesive research team involving researchers from different disciplines, to combine expertise from several knowledge domains, and to overcome communication problems among researchers from different disciplines (Tobi & Kampen, 2018). Future research designs should integrate insights from psychology, neuroscience, and genetic domains into increasingly complex and dynamic explanatory mechanisms gathered around a well-defined problem.

4. Theoretical and Methodological Question: How to Address the Complicated Interactions and Relations Between Genes and Environment?

All sport performance–related traits are multifactorial traits that result from a complex interplay between genetic and environmental factors. Specific genetic make-up does not necessarily ensure elite athletic performance, which results from the gene-environment interactions. The term *gene-environment interaction* refers to situations in which the effect of genes depends on the environment, and/or the effect of the environment depends on genotype (Halldorsdottir & Binder, 2017). Gene-environment interactions account for the reason people respond differently to environmental factors. In motor proficiency, gene-environment interactions account for people's variation in responding to exercise (Bouchard & Rankinen, 2001). Though this phenomenon is quite known in sport, it usually is attributed to physiological genetic predisposition.

Gene-environment interaction has two main meanings: *substantial meaning* and *statistical meaning*. The substantial meaning implies that when it comes to psychological, physiological, and other traits, both genes and the environment are important. In statistical terms, it means that there are main effects of the environment and main effects of genes, but the effect of one variable cannot be understood without taking into account the other variable, since their effects are not independent. Genes and the environment are interrelated entities. Although some environmental influences may be largely random, such as experiencing a natural disaster, many environmental influences are not entirely random (Kendler et al., 1993). For example, individuals are genetically predisposed toward sensation seeking, and this makes them more likely to be attracted to extreme sports such as skiing (a gene-environment interaction), which increases their chance to become an elite skier. Are the predisposing sensation-seeking genes or the environment the causal agent? In actuality, the question is debatable—they both play a role; it is much more informative to try to understand and model these interactive pathways than to ask whether the genes or the environment was the critical factor in the outcomes and behaviors. Therefore, future research should take into consideration the complex interactions between genes and the environment, and hence adopt the view that they are not separate entities. Accordingly, researchers and practitioners should move from traditional paradigms seeking the causes and the influence of genetic or environmental factors to new paradigms seeking the best pathways to improve and develop an interactive approach. Future research designs should take into consideration that every human being is a unique combination of genes and the environment that cannot be treated as separate factors.

5. Methodological Question: How to Design Research in the Relatively New and Upcoming Field of Sport Psychogenetics?

Behavioral genetics was based almost entirely on twin and family studies. Those studies made a strong case for the importance of genes in behavior, but the connection always remained loose and statistical. Moreover, those studies were conducted in the general population; therefore, their conclusions do not necessarily apply to the sport domain.

Only in rare cases could a direct connection between a particular gene or set of genes and a particular behavior be made. New research disciplines in the field of genetics such as bioinformatics and genetic engineering allow researchers to measure, analyze, and manipulate genetic material rapidly and easily. These techniques have changed the composition of the field of behavioral genetics, engaging the interest of new groups of researchers beyond psychology, such as molecular biologists, who had previously seen behavior as too slippery for biological research.

Today, it is clear that a single gene for a complex phenomenon such as sport performance is unlikely to exist, let alone be found, even with the most sophisticated methods. Complex behavioral traits, which are fundamental in the field of sport psychology, are influenced by tens if not hundreds of genes, each interacting with the environment and each other in unpredictable ways. Nonetheless, behavioral genetics continues to hold promise for a better understanding of the biological basis of behavior.

This flood of data accompanying the Human Genome Project means that the ability to gather, organize, and analyze biological information is increasingly critical. Therefore, incorporating bioinformatics in research design and results analysis is necessary. Moreover, case-control association study, which is the basic research design in the study of genetics and sport, is limited. However, it is important to keep in mind that even with the most advanced research techniques and designs, there is no simple answer to a complex question. The deeper scientists delve into the genetics of complex behaviors, the more they find that such behaviors are influenced by tens or hundreds of interacting genes, each accounting for only a small portion of the overall variance. Moreover, it is not genes alone, but rather genes in interaction with the environment that produce complex behaviors.

New techniques may help researchers overcome at least some of those challenges. One particularly promising area is the combination of behavioral genetics with visualization tools in biology. In living animals, including humans, functional magnetic resonance imaging and other brain imaging techniques are providing increasingly high-resolution maps of large-scale neural activity. Meanwhile, in cells, molecular techniques such as tagging enzymes with green fluorescent protein are allowing researchers to watch changes in gene expression as they occur. These techniques may bring behavioral geneticists one step closer to the very important goal: discovering how neurons, shaped by interactions between genes and the environment, give rise to behavior.

Conclusion

It seems that it is almost impossible to capture the complexity and multi-dimensionality of sport performance in a simplified way. Any study on the genetic basis of motor performance must incorporate the psychological domain and the complicated interaction between psychological and physiological traits as well as the continuous interaction with the environment.

References

Balagué, N., Torrents, C., Hristovski, R., & Kelso, J. A. S. (2017). Sport science integration: An evolutionary synthesis. *European Journal of Sport Science, 17*(1), 51–62. https://doi.org/10.1080/17461391.2016.1198422

Bamman, M. M., Petrella, J. K., Kim, J., Mayhew, D. L., & Cross, J. M. (2007). Cluster analysis tests the importance of myogenic gene expression during myofiber hypertrophy in humans. *Journal of Applied Physiology, 102*(6), 2232–2239. https://doi.org/10.1152/japplphysiol.00024.2007

Ben-Zaken, S., Richard, V., & Tenenbaum, G. (2019). *Genetics and the psychology of motor performance.* Routledge.

Bouchard, C., & Rankinen, T. (2001). Individual differences in response to regular physical activity. *Medicine and Science in Sports and Exercise, 33*(6 Suppl), S446–S451; discussion S452–S453. http://www.ncbi.nlm.nih.gov/pubmed/11427769

Bryan, A. D., Magnan, R. E., Nilsson, R., Marcus, B. H., Tompkins, S. A., & Hutchison, K. E. (2011). The big picture of individual differences in physical activity behavior change: A transdisciplinary approach. *Psychology of Sport and Exercise, 12*(1), 20–26. https://doi.org/10.1016/J.PSYCHSPORT.2010.05.002

Carr, G., Loucks, D. P., & Blöschl, G. (2018). Gaining insight into interdisciplinary research and education programmes: A framework for evaluation. *Research Policy, 47*(1), 35–48. https://doi.org/10.1016/j.respol.2017.09.010

Cohen, I. R. (2000). *Tending Adam's garden: Evolving the cognitive immune self.* Academic Press.

Cohen, I. R., & Harel, D. (2007). Explaining a complex living system: Dynamics, multi-scaling and emergence. *Journal of the Royal Society Interface, 4*(13), 175–182. https://doi.org/10.1098/rsif.2006.0173

Davids, K., & Baker, J. (2007). Genes, environment and sport performance: Why the nature-nurture dualism is no longer relevant. *Sports Medicine, 37*(11), 961–980. http://www.ncbi.nlm.nih.gov/pubmed/17953467

Drabsch, T., & Holzapfel, C. (2019). A scientific perspective of personalised gene-based dietary recommendations for weight management. *Nutrients, 11*(3), 617. https://doi.org/10.3390/nu11030617

Ericsson, K. A. (2007). Deliberate practice and the modifiability of body and mind: Toward a science of the structure and acquisition of expert and elite performance. *International Journal of Sport Psychology, 38.* https://pdfs.semanticscholar.org/3b1e/28f4b2b22f801e8bf2f4451a2f434bf3571e.pdf

Fancher, R. E. (2009). Scientific cousins: The relationship between Charles Darwin and Francis Galton. *American Psychologist, 64*(2), 84–92. https://doi.org/10.1037/a0013339

Gillham, N. W. (2001). Sir Francis Galton and the birth of eugenics. *Annual Review of Genetics*, 35(1), 83–101. https://doi.org/10.1146/annurev.genet.35.102401.090055

Gottschling, J., Hahn, E., Maas, H., & Spinath, F. M. (2016). Explaining the relationship between personality and coping with professional demands: Where and why do optimism, self-regulation, and self-efficacy matter? *Personality and Individual Differences*, 100, 49–55. https://doi.org/10.1016/J.PAID.2016.03.085

Halldorsdottir, T., & Binder, E. B. (2017). Gene × environment interactions: From molecular mechanisms to behavior. *Annual Review of Psychology*, 68(1), 215–241. https://doi.org/10.1146/annurev-psych-010416-044053

Hamburg, M. A., & Collins, F. S. (2010). The path to personalized medicine. *New England Journal of Medicine*, 363(4), 301–304. https://doi.org/10.1056/NEJMp1006304

Hecksteden, A., & Meyer, T. (2018). Personalized sports medicine – Principles and tailored implementations in preventive and competitive sports. *Deutsche Zeitschrift Für Sportmedizin*, 2018(3), 73–80. https://doi.org/10.5960/dzsm.2018.323

Henig, R. M. (2000). *The monk in the garden: The lost and found genius of Gregor Mendel, the father of genetics*. Houghton Mifflin.

Hristovski, R. (2013). Synthetic thinking in (sports) science: The self-organization of the scientific language. *Research in Physical Education Sport and Health*, 2(1), 27–34.

Hubal, M. J., Gordish-Dressman, H., Thompson, P. D., Price, T. B., Hoffman, E. P., Angelopoulos, T. J., Gordon, P. M., Moyna, N. M., Pescatello, L. S., Visich, P. S., Zoeller, R. F., Seip, R. L., & Clarkson, P. M. (2005). Variability in muscle size and strength gain after unilateral resistance training. *Medicine and Science in Sports and Exercise*, 37(6), 964–972. http://www.ncbi.nlm.nih.gov/pubmed/15947721

Johnson, M., & Tenenbaum, G. (2006). The roles of nature and nurture in expertise in sport. In D. Hackfort & G. Tenenbaum (Eds.), *Essential processes for attaining peak performance* (pp. 26–52). Meyer & Meyer Sport.

Johnson, S. L., Carver, C. S., Joormann, J., & Cuccaro, M. L. (2016). Genetic polymorphisms related to behavioral approach and behavioral inhibition scales. *Personality and Individual Differences*, 88, 251–255. https://doi.org/10.1016/J.PAID.2015.09.024

Kendler K.S., Neale M., Kessler R., Heath A., & Eaves L. (1993) A twin study of recent life events and difficulties. *Arch Gen Psychiatry*, 50(10), 789–796. doi:10.1001/archpsyc.1993.01820220041005. PMID: 8215803.

Kosslyn, S. M., Cacioppo, J. T., Davidson, R. J., Hugdahl, K., Lovallo, W. R., Spiegel, D., & Rose, R. (2002). Bridging psychology and biology: The analysis of individuals in groups. *American Psychologist*, 57(5), 341–351. https://doi.org/10.1037/0003-066X.57.5.341

Li, Z., Wang, Y., Yan, C., Cheung, E. F. C., Docherty, A. R., Sham, P. C., Gur, R. E., Gur, R. C., & Chan, R. C. K. (2019). Inheritance of neural substrates for motivation and pleasure. *Psychological Science*, 30(8), 1205–1217. https://doi.org/10.1177/0956797619859340

Lin, Y., Mutz, J., Clough, P. J., & Papageorgiou, K. A. (2017). Mental toughness and individual differences in learning, educational and work performance, psychological well-being, and personality: A systematic review. *Frontiers in Psychology*, 8, 1345. https://doi.org/10.3389/fpsyg.2017.01345

MacLeod, M. (2018). What makes interdisciplinarity difficult? Some consequences of domain specificity in interdisciplinary practice. *Synthese*, 195(2), 697–720. https://doi.org/10.1007/s11229-016-1236-4

Mann, T. N., Lamberts, R. P., & Lambert, M. I. (2014). High responders and low responders: Factors associated with individual variation in response to standardized training. *Sports Medicine*, 44(8), 1113–1124. https://doi.org/10.1007/s40279-014-0197-3

Mayr, E. (1961). Cause and effect in biology. *Science*, 134(3489), 1501–1506. https://doi.org/10.1126/science.134.3489.1501

Mendel, G. (1865). Experiments in plant hybridization P (1865). *Meetings of the Brünn Natural History Society*. http://www.netspace.org./MendelWeb/

Munafò, M. R., Clark, T. G., Moore, L. R., Payne, E., Walton, R., & Flint, J. (2003). Genetic polymorphisms and personality in healthy adults: A systematic review and meta-analysis. *Molecular Psychiatry, 8*(5), 471–484. https://doi.org/10.1038/sj.mp.4001326

Neufer, P. D., Bamman, M. M., Muoio, D. M., Bouchard, C., Cooper, D. M., Goodpaster, B. H., Booth, F. W., Kohrt, W. M., Gerszten, R. E., Mattson, M. P., Hepple, R. T., Kraus, W. E., Reid, M. B., Bodine, S. C., Jakicic, J. M., Fleg, J. L., Williams, J. P., Joseph, L., Evans, M., . . . Laughlin, M. R. (2015). Understanding the cellular and molecular mechanisms of physical activity-induced health benefits. *Cell Metabolism, 22*(1), 4–11. https://doi.org/10.1016/j.cmet.2015.05.011

Noble, E. P. (2000). Addiction and its reward process through polymorphisms of the D2 dopamine receptor gene: A review. *European Psychiatry, 15*(2), 79–89. https://doi.org/10.1016/S0924-9338(00)00208-X

Harel, D. (2004). A grand challenge for computing: Towards full reactive modeling of a multi-cellular animal. *Current Trends in Theoretical Computer Science*, 559–568.. https://doi.org/10.1142/9789812562494_0031

Rankinen T, Pérusse L, Rauramaa R, Rivera MA, Wolfarth B, Bouchard C. (2001). The human gene map for performance and health-related fitness phenotypes. *Medicine & Science in Sports & Exercise, 33*(6), 855–867. doi:10.1097/00005768-200106000-00001.

Rice, J., & Reich, T. (1985). Familial analysis of qualitative traits under multifactorial inheritance. *Genetic Epidemiology, 2*(3), 301–315. https://doi.org/10.1002/gepi.1370020307

Sarzynski, M. A., Loos, R. J. F., Lucia, A., Pérusse, L., Roth, S. M., Wolfarth, B., Rankinen, T., & Bouchard, C. (2016). Advances in exercise, fitness, and performance genomics in 2015. *Medicine and Science in Sports and Exercise, 48*(10), 1906–1916. https://doi.org/10.1249/MSS.0000000000000982

Tenenbaum, G., Hatfield, B., Eklund, R. C., Land, W., Camielo, L., Razon, S., & Schack, K. A. (2009). Conceptual framework for studying emotions-cognitions-performance linkage under conditions which vary in perceived pressure. In M. Raab, J. G. Johnson, & H. Heekeren (Eds.), *Progress in brain research: Mind and motion-The bidirectional link between thought and action* (pp. 159–178). Elsevier.

Tobi, H., & Kampen, J. K. (2018). Research design: The methodology for interdisciplinary research framework. *Quality and Quantity, 52*(3), 1209–1225. https://doi.org/10.1007/s11135-017-0513-8

Tucker, R., & Collins, M. (2012). What makes champions? A review of the relative contribution of genes and training to sporting success. *British Journal of Sports Medicine, 46*(8), 555–561. https://doi.org/10.1136/bjsports-2011-090548

Valeeva, E. V., & Rees, T. (2019). Psychogenetics and sport. In D. Barh & I. Ahmetov (Eds.), *Sports, exercise, and nutritional genomics* (pp. 147–165). Academic Press. https://doi.org/10.1016/B978-0-12-816193-7.00007-5

Violle, C., Navas, M. L., Vile, D., Kazakou, E., Fortunel, C., Hummel, I., & Garnier, E. (2007). Let the concept of trait be functional! *Oikos, 116*(5), 882–892. https://doi.org/10.1111/j.0030-1299.2007.15559.x

Wang, G., Tanaka, M., Eynon, N., North, K. N., Williams, A. G., Collins, M., Moran, C. N., Britton, S. L., Fuku, N., Ashley, E. A., Klissouras, V., Lucia, A., Ahmetov, I. I., de Geus, E., Alsayrafi, M., & Pitsiladis, Y. P. (2016). The future of genomic research in athletic performance and adaptation to training. *Medicine and Sport Science, 61*, 55–67. https://doi.org/10.1159/000445241

Willems, Y. E., Boesen, N., Li, J., Finkenauer, C., & Bartels, M. (2019). The heritability of self-control: A meta-analysis. *Neuroscience and Biobehavioral Reviews, 100*, 324–334. https://doi.org/10.1016/J.NEUBIOREV.2019.02.012

11

Group Dynamics

Edson Filho and Francisco Miguel Leo

State of the Art

Research on team dynamics in sport, exercise, and performance psychology is vast. Overall, scholars concur that team dynamics is a complex and multilayered process, as individual, team, and contextual factors interact and together influence the development of high-performing and resilient teams (Carron & Eys, 2012; Filho, 2019). Notably, previous research on team dynamics has revolved around theoretical inquiry and instrument development aimed at discriminating key team processes or attributes, including cohesion, collective efficacy, and team cognition variables. To this extent, the Group Environment Questionnaire (see Carron & Eys, 2012), which measures social and task cohesion at the individual and team level of analyses, and the Collective Efficacy Questionnaire for Sports (see Short et al., 2005), which measures efficacy beliefs at the team level, are among the most used instruments in the field. Regarding team cognition variables, a scale to measure transactive memory systems in sports (Leo et al., 2018), and conceptual frameworks on team coordination (Eccles, 2010) and team mental models (Filho & Tenenbaum, 2020) have been outlined in attempts to describe and explain how teammates "think as a team" and learn to be coordinated in space and time.

Recently, research on team dynamics has focused on meta-theoretical work. Specifically, scholars have tried to understand how (a) successful teamwork evolves and takes place in the natural world and (b) key team processes are intertwined in a systematic fashion. Regarding the former, McEwan and Beauchamp (2014) proposed the meta-theoretical idea of teamwork in sports, which develops over time (i.e., episodic cycles) and influences and is influenced by myriad individual, team, and contextual factors. Regarding the latter, Filho and colleagues (Filho, 2019; Filho et al., 2015; Leo et al., 2019) have been trying to evolve a parsimonious (best-fit) input-throughput-output

Edson Filho and Francisco Miguel Leo, *Group Dynamics* In: *Sport, Exercise and Performance Psychology.*
Edited by: Edson Filho and Itay Basevitch, Oxford University Press. © Oxford University Press 2021.
DOI: 10.1093/oso/9780197512494.003.0011

systemic theory of team dynamics by linking cohesion, collective efficacy, team mental models, coordination, and performance.

Contemporary research on team dynamics has also been focused on the notion of "team resilience," which pertains to the "dynamic, psychosocial process which protects a group of individuals from the potential negative effect of stressors they collectively encounter" (Morgan et al., 2013, p. 552). In other words, team resilience is a meta-theoretical ("umbrella") construct that encompasses several team attributes as well as individual team members' qualities. Accordingly, scholars have tried to understand the team-level and individual-level qualities that make a team resilient (Fletcher & Sarkar, 2016) and explore the factors that differentiate resilient (i.e., those capable of overcoming adversities) from vulnerable teams (Bowers et al., 2017; Sarkar & Fletcher, 2014).

Furthermore, research interest on big data analytics and the psychophysiological markers of team processes has grown substantially over the past decade. Specifically, scholars have been trying to analyze large data sets on different variables (e.g., historical, physiological, scouting, tracking) in order to study team dynamics and performance in sport and exercise settings (see Rein & Memmert, 2016). Scholars have also been trying to capture peripheral physiological (e.g., galvanic skin response, heart rate, heart rate variability) and central neural markers (e.g., alpha, beta, delta, and theta brain waves) of team processes (Hoyle et al., 2020; Thorson et al., 2018). In other words, it is important to understand latent variables, such as cohesion, team mental models, and other team processes (e.g., leadership), and whether they have physiological and measurable (manifest variables) neural correlates (e.g., Hoyle et al., 2020). Notably, this line of research has been operationalized through the study of dyadic teams, with previous research suggesting that changes in interbrain synchronization across different frequency bands is linked to leadership dynamics (leader-follower dichotomy) in duet guitar playing (e.g., Sänger et al., 2013) and the emergence of team mental models (activation of shared and complementary mental networks) in dyadic cooperative juggling (see Filho & Tenenbaum, 2020).

Overall, current research on team dynamics has been geared toward advancing (a) integrated (meta-theoretical) frameworks linking different levels of analyses and team processes, (b) our understanding of team resilience, and (c) big data analytics and the search for physiological and neural markers of team processes. We believe more research on these fronts is needed. Accordingly, we recommend a number of papers as a starting point to the interested reader (see Table 11.1) and propose five open questions on team dynamics in sport, exercise, and performance psychology.

Table 11.1 Five Key Readings in Team Dynamics

Authors	Methodological Design	Key Findings
Filho (2019)	Narrative review	This article outlines a generative class of models ("a model of models") linking cohesion, team mental models, coordination, collective efficacy, and team outcomes. Congruent with Popper's falsifiability principle, the author argues that scholars should test and try to falsify several alterative models linking the aforementioned team processes to evolve a parsimonious and integrated theory of team dynamics.
Leo et al. (2020)	Correlational-longitudinal study	The authors study how socialization tactics influence team structure variables and cohesion in sport teams. Using structural equation modeling, they showed that socialization tactics influence task cohesion, role clarity, and intentions to return to team. These findings revealed that socialization tactics relate to a range of key individual-level and team-level factors and highlight the importance of additional studies on the relations targeting team structure variables.
McEwan & Beauchamp (2014)	Narrative review	The authors reviewed 29 models of teamwork and proposed an integrated framework to inform research on teamwork and team effectiveness in sports. The proposed input-mediator-output model considers the role of different team processes, levels of analysis, and episodic cycles on teamwork and team effectiveness.
Morgan et al. (2019)	Qualitative (ethnography) study	The authors explored the psychosocial enablers and strategies associated with the development of team resilience within a high-level sports team. A season-long ethnography analysis revealed five categories for team resilience development, thus providing practitioners with a platform for designing team resilience interventions in sport settings.
Sänger et al. (2013)	Experimental (hyperbrain) study	This is a seminal study, wherein electroencephalography data from pairs of guitarists playing a duet music piece were simultaneously recorded. Data analysis of the between-brain couplings revealed that the guitarists' interbrain networks were amplified during coordination periods, and that the directionality of these interbrain networks predicted leader-follower dynamics (i.e., who leads and who follows) in guitar duets. These findings showed that hyperbrain methods of analyses can be used to capture the neural markers of team processes, such as team coordination and peer leadership.

Questions to Move the Field Forward

1. Theoretical Question: What Are the Antecedents of Cohesion and Other Team Processes?

Addressing this question will help advance our understanding of the mechanisms anteceding the development of key team attributes. Indeed, extant previous research has attested to the importance of cohesion and other team attributes to successful performance (Benson et al., 2016; Eys et al., 2019). In theory, a team showing high levels of cohesion, team mental models, coordination, and collective efficacy is more likely to be successful than a team lower on these team attributes (Filho, 2019). Hence, *if* we are able to understand and optimize the mechanisms that make it possible for a team to become cohesive, confident, and coordinated, *then* we can set the conditions for the development of high-performing teams (Leo et al., 2019). In this regard, Carron and Eys (2012) have outlined a series of background factors that precede cohesion, namely (a) *individual characteristics of the players*, (b) *group environment*, and (c) *team structure*.

Individual characteristics refer to the group composition (e.g., motor abilities, social status) or the quantity, variability, and compatibility of group resources (i.e., complementarity of skills between players). To this extent, there is a need to advance research on team diversity. Recent studies revealed that diversity in teams (e.g., number of players from different nationalities) is positively associated with task cohesion (Godfrey et al., 2020). Teammates with different backgrounds bring unique insights to the execution and problem-solving of team tasks (Filho & Rettig, 2018). Hence, further research is needed to understand the role of diversity in the development of team processes and outputs, especially because we are living in an increasingly globalized world wherein multicultural teams are becoming more and more prevalent in sports and other domains (Godfrey et al., 2020).

Group environment pertains to the contextual and group-level variables that might impact the emergence and development of cohesion and other team processes. To date, group size and competition level have been the most studied group environment factors (Carron & Eys, 2012). There is consensus that, as group size and competitive level increases, cohesion levels tend to decrease (see Carron & Eys, 2012). Therefore, future research should focus on other elements of group environment, including environmental pressure in matches (i.e., created by opponents, fans, or social media) and team and club structure (i.e., players' tenure/time in the team, role of managers or presidents, coach turnover), which have been found to influence performance in sports (Juravich et al., 2017).

Team structure has been operationalized through the assessment of coaches' behaviors and athletes' behaviors and roles (Eys et al., 2019). Noteworthy, different theoretical approaches have been used to examine the relationship between coach behaviors and team processes (Bosselut et al., 2018; Leo et al., 2021). Regardless of the theoretical background used to study team structure, scholars observed that cohesion levels depend, in part, on coaches' behaviors. Coaches who exhibit high task and social support (Leo et al., 2021) and transformational leadership styles are more likely to develop highly cohesive teams (Bosselut et al., 2018). Coaches who foster task-oriented motivational climates (García-Calvo et al., 2014) and who are perceived as competent and fair by their players are also successful in developing highly cohesive teams (García-Calvo et al., 2019). Considering this literature, we believe future research on this topic should focus on how different behavioral leadership styles influence other team processes (e.g., team mental models, team coordination) through intervention programs based on robust experimental studies.

Athlete leadership is also an important part of team structure (for a review see Cotterill & Fransen, 2016). Specifically, the quantity and quality of peer leaders within a team influence cohesion because peer leaders help to integrate newcomers (Leo et al., 2020) and to develop a task-oriented motivational climate (García-Calvo et al., 2014). Given that peer leaders foster the development of high-performing teams, future research on peer leadership should aim to develop intervention programs to capacity peer leaders (e.g., Mertens et al., 2020). Research on the relationship between peer leaders and team coaches might also yield new insights into the nature of high-performing teams.

Noteworthy, players' roles within the team have also been studied under the "team structure umbrella." Individuals with clear roles and who commit to their roles help to improve team dynamics (Bosselut et al., 2012; Coleman et al., 2020; Eys et al., 2020). To advance knowledge on this area, scholars should investigate how (a) the integration of new players occurs (e.g., how veteran players feel about the signings of new players) and (b) competition between players with the same role impacts team dynamics (see Leo et al., 2020). Noteworthy, research on these fronts should target the beginning of the season, as this phase is a crucial period during which team roles are established (Leo et al., 2020).

In summary, variables related to the individuals, the environment, and the structure of teams influence overall team functioning, performance, and satisfaction (Carron and Eys, 2012). Hence, it is important that scholars keep on asking questions about group structure to develop high-functioning teams, wherein myriad team processes (e.g., cohesion, collective efficacy, coordination, transactive memory systems, and team mental models) positively influence one another (Filho, 2019; Leo et al., 2019).

2. Theoretical Question: What Is the "Best Fit" Input-Throughput-Output Model Linking Team Processes and Outcomes?

Across domains, scholars work toward theoretical integration by combining models and testing for alternative solutions. Accordingly, to advance theory and practice in the field, we need to evolve an integrated model of team dynamics. Foremost, advancing an integrated theory of team dynamics would help to evolve best-practice guidelines for team building. Specifically, practitioners would be clear on the unique properties (i.e., discriminant validity) of cohesion, team mental models, and collective efficacy and understand the reciprocal linkages among these team processes. As such, Filho (2019) has urged scholars to test a series of models linking key team processes, namely cohesion, team mental models, coordination, collective efficacy, and team outcomes (e.g., performance and satisfaction).

Filho (2019) posits that scholars should test for alternative solutions until a best-fit and parsimonious model is reached. For instance, pursuing this research line would allow to clarify whether team cognition variables (e.g., team mental models and transactive memory systems) lead to the development of collective efficacy, or if team cognition and collective efficacy develop simultaneously (see Filho et al., 2015; Leo et al., 2019). Future research should also consider the role of moderating variables, representing different levels of analyses (e.g., age, gender, leadership behaviors), on the linkage among the aforementioned team processes and outcomes.

Multiwave data collection studies are also needed to advance our understanding of time effects on specific team processes (e.g., cohesion, collective efficacy) and team dynamics at large. Specifically, cross-lagged and longitudinal growth and modeling should be used to examine how the linkage among team processes and outcomes varies over time. Multicase studies comparing changes in the aforementioned team processes and across teams of different levels are also worth pursuing. Multicase studies can help to clarify (a) the role of contextual factors (e.g., club structure) in the development of high-performing teams and (b) how fluctuations in a given team process (e.g., cohesion) can yield different outcomes in different teams. Finally, experimental and quasi-experimental studies manipulating different team processes (e.g., team mental models, collective efficacy) are needed to clarify input-output relations among different team processes. Overall, working toward an integrated model of team dynamics will allow practitioners to develop high-performing and resilient teams.

3. Applied Question: What Are the Individual and Team-Level Mechanisms Associated With the Development of Resilient Teams?

Competitive sport teams must overcome numerous performance challenges, which inevitably influence team dynamics. Put plainly, for a team to be successful, it must be able to maintain a positive and self-reinforcing linkage among team processes (e.g., cohesion, team mental models, collective efficacy) during times of difficulty (Filho, 2019). That is, the ability to remain resilient in the face of difficulties is a characteristic of high-performing teams (López-Gajardo et al., 2020).

It follows that longitudinal studies targeting different sports and performance contexts are needed to clarify whether team processes are reflective indicators of team resilience (Bowers et al., 2017; Filho, 2019). In this regard, Bowers et al. (2017) proposed a theoretical model conceptualizing team resilience as a second-order emergent state. Specifically, Bowers et al. (2017) posited that team resilience is the combined result of several team-level emergent states, such as group cohesion, collective efficacy, and shared mental models. Filho (2019) has also suggested that team resilience is a meta-theoretical concept, encompassing a team's levels of cohesion, team mental models, collective efficacy, and team coordination. As such, multiwave studies are needed to clarify whether team resilience is indeed reflected by teammates' perceived levels of different team processes over the course of a season. Alternatively, and perhaps counterintuitively, high levels of some team processes (e.g., high social cohesion) might hinder rather than facilitate team resilience (i.e., "too much of a good thing effect"), as is the case with groupthink, for instance.

The synthesis of different theoretical models is another ripe area for future research on team resilience, especially given that several models of team resilience have been proposed recently. For instance, Gucciardi et al. (2018) identified nine key areas for development of team resilience, including individual, group, and contextual areas. Morgan et al. (2013) suggested that team resilience is composed of four subfactors (i.e., group structure, team learning, social capital, and collective efficacy) and related to transformational leadership, shared leadership, team learning, group social identity, and positive emotions. Morgan, Fletcher, and Sarkar (2019) have also suggested that team resilience is related to a series of "contextual enablers," including the development of a system of responsibility among the team members and a strong team identity. While we understand that team resilience is a multilevel and multidimensional construct (López-Gajardo et al., 2020), we echo the notion that scholars should work to falsify their models until an integrated and parsimonious model can be achieved.

We thus call scholars to juxtapose these several models of team resilience to evolve a parsimonious and integrated model of team resilience. This can be done through the use of structural equation modeling aimed at (a) capturing the reflective and formative indicators of team resilience and (b) contrasting alternative models of team resilience until a "best-fit model" is achieved. Advancing an integrated and parsimonious model of team resilience will allow for the development of evidence-based team building at large and team resilience in particular. Theoretical clarity on team resilience will also facilitate meta-analytical work on the relationship between team resilience and other team processes and outcomes.

4. Methodological Question: How Can We Use Big Data Analyses and Psychophysiological Monitoring to Study Team Processes and Outcomes?

To date, the bulk of research on team dynamics in sport, exercise, and performance psychology is based on cross-sectional and survey data and qualitative inquiries. A promising area of future research pertains to the use of big data methodologies and intrateam psychophysiological monitoring to study team processes and outcomes. Specifically, the use of tracking (e.g., GPS, online video analysis), physiological (e.g., heart rate and heart rate variability), and scouting data (e.g., percentage of successful passes, number of fouls) can help to explain team coordination and performance (see Rein & Memmert, 2016). For instance, Müller and Lindenberger (2011) have shown that the cardiovascular responses of choir members involved in cooperative singing tend to be synchronized, which in turn suggests that team coordination hinges on physiological synchronization. Previous research has also shown that big data analysis of historical events can be used to predict team performance in professional sports (e.g., Filho & Rettig, 2018).

Notably, scholars interested in using big data and psychophysiological monitoring methods to study team processes and outcomes must consider whether their data was collected *before*, *during*, or *after* team practice and performance (Thorson et al., 2018). Importantly, data collected during actual practice and performance must be "locked in time"; that is, the data from all participants must be collected simultaneously (for a review see Thorson et al., 2018). Regardless of the time window of interest, we encourage scholars to propose and test ways to use big data analytics and psychophysiological monitoring to understand emergent team processes and team dynamics. For instance, researchers can use GPS data to examine whether more cohesive and coordinated teams run more or better (i.e., distributed effort) than less cohesive teams. Similarly, more confident teams might show similar levels of heart rate variability before a "big match," in comparison to teams with lower levels of collective efficacy.

Overall, team processes are emergent states; that is, they emerge from "the team as a whole" rather than from individual team members (Filho & Tenenbaum, 2020; Thorson et al., 2018). As such, big data analytics and team-level psychophysiological monitoring can help to further understand well-studied team processes in sports (e.g., cohesion, collective efficacy), as well as other group-level constructs such as compliance, networking, and team fatigue and burnout, to name but a few. Intrateam psychophysiological monitoring can also shed light on the neural markers of team processes, as elaborated upon next.

5. Methodological Question: How Can We Use Hyperbrain Methods to Study Team Dynamics?

Research on hyperbrains (when two or more brains are measured simultaneously) is needed to move the field forward. In this regard, recent advancements in electroencephalography (EEG) methods, including the development of portable systems, have allowed for the simultaneous mon-itoring of two or more brains engaged in joint motor action. Previous re-search in this area has focused on hand-to-hand mimics, dyadic juggling, dyadic guitar playing, cooperative video-game playing, and simulated flights involving pilot and copilot interactions (for a review see Filho & Tenenbaum, 2020). We invite scholars to continue studying these joint motor tasks and to advance other experimental designs to advance know-ledge of interbrain interactions.

Advancing hyperbrain methodologies is essential to further our under-standing of the neural correlates of team processes and team learning. As aforementioned, previous research on interbrain interactions has been used to study coordination, team mental models, and leadership in dyadic teams (Filho & Tenenbaum, 2020; Hoyle et al., 2020). Hyperbrain research with dyadic teams is a good starting point because a dyad is the smallest team possible, and because every larger team can be broken down into subteams of two individuals (Filho, in press). Studying triads and quartets teams and subteams (e.g., spine players, including the goalkeeper, defender, center midfield, and offensive player in soccer; the center, quarterback, and wide receiver in American football) is a natural next step for research on this front.

Noteworthy, hyperbrain research with dyads and triads can also be used to study the recently proposed notion of the shared zones of optimal func-tioning (SZOF) framework (see Filho, in press). In a nutshell, the SZOF framework purports that dyadic teams or subteams share a psychophysio-logical state linked to optimal and suboptimal performance experiences. The synchronous monitoring of two or more brains engaged in joint motor action can put to test this theorizing and help develop shared bio- and neurofeedback interventions aimed at bringing teammates to a shared psy-chophysiological state linked to optimal performance.

Overall, by engaging in the simultaneous monitoring of multiple brains while manipulating individual (e.g., skill-level), team (e.g., historicity—time practicing together), task (e.g., complexity level), and context (e.g., high and low environmental pressure) variables, scholars can examine how within-brain and between-brain rhythms influence team dynamics and perfor-mance. Such research will most certainly move our field forward and lead to the development of bio- and neurofeedback interventions targeting the team level of analyses.

Conclusion

In summary, we believe that future research should explore the antecedents of key team processes and seek to evolve an integrated and parsimonious theory of team dynamics and team resilience. Furthermore, we suggest that novel research using big analytic and psychophysiological monitoring methods is needed to advance our understanding of physiological and neural markers of team processes and outcomes. Finally, we propose that advancing research on multibrain monitoring will allow for the development of shared (multiperson) bio- and neurofeedback interventions.

References

Benson, A. J., Šiška, P., Eys, M., Priklerová, S., & Slepička, P. (2016). A prospective multilevel examination of the relationship between cohesion and team performance in elite youth sport. *Psychology of Sport and Exercise, 27,* 39–46. doi:10.1016/j.psychsport.2016.07.009

Bosselut, G., Boiché, J., Salamé, B., Fouquereau, E., Guilbert, L., & Serrano, O. C. (2018). Transformational leadership and group cohesion in sport: Examining the mediating role of interactional justice using a within-and between-team approach. *International Journal of Sports Science and Coaching, 13,* 912–928. doi:10.1177/1747954118801156

Bosselut, G., McLaren, C. D., Eys, M. A., & Heuzé, J. P. (2012). Reciprocity of the relationship between role ambiguity and group cohesion in youth interdependent sport. *Psychology of Sport and Exercise, 13,* 341–348. doi:10.1016/j.psychsport.2011.09.002

Bowers, C., Kreutzer, C., Cannon-Bowers, J., & Lamb, J. (2017). Team resilience as a second-order emergent state: A theoretical model and research directions. *Frontiers in Psychology, 8,* 1360. doi:10.3389/fpsyg.2017.01360

Carron, A. V., & Eys, M. A. (2012). *Group dynamics in sport* (4th ed.). Morgantown, WV: Fitness Information Technology.

Coleman, T., Godfrey, M., López-Gajardo, M. A., Leo, F. M., & Eys, M. A. (2020). Do it for the team: Youth perceptions of team cohesion and role commitment in interdependent sport. *Sport, Exercise, and Performance Psychology.* Manuscript submitted for publication.

Cotterill, S. T., & Fransen, K. (2016). Athlete leadership in sport teams: Current understanding and future directions. *International Review of Sport and Exercise Psychology, 9,* 116–133. doi:10.1080/1750984X.2015.1124443

Eccles, D. (2010). The coordination of labour in sports teams. *International Review of Sport and Exercise Psychology, 3,* 154–170. doi:10.1080/1750984X.2010.519400

Eys, M. A., Beauchamp, M., Godfrey, M., Dawson, K., Loughead, T., & Schinke, R. (2020). Role commitment and acceptance in a sport context. *Journal of Sport and Exercise Psychology, 42,* 89–101. doi:10.1123/jsep.2019-0057

Eys, M. A., Bruner, M. W., & Martin, L. J. (2019). The dynamic group environment in sport and exercise. *Psychology of Sport and Exercise, 42,* 40–47. doi:10.1016/j.psychsport.2018.11.001

Filho, E. (2019). Team dynamics theory: Nomological network among cohesion, team mental models, coordination, and collective efficacy. *Sport Sciences for Health, 15*, 1–20. doi:10.1007/s11332-018-0519-1

Filho, E. (in press). Shared zones of optimal functioning (SZOF): A framework to capture peak performance, momentum, psycho-bio-social synchrony and leader-follower dynamics in teams. *Journal of Clinical Sport Psychology.*

Filho, E., & Rettig, J. (2018). The road to victory in the UEFA women's Champions League: A multi-level analysis of successful coaches, teams, and countries. *Psychology of Sport and Exercise, 39*, 132–146. oi:10.1016/j.psychsport.2018.07.012

Filho, E., & Tenenbaum, G. (2020). Team mental models: Theory, empirical evidence, and applied implications. In G. Tenenbaum, R. C. Eklund, & B. Nataniel (Eds.), *Handbook of sport psychology* (4th ed., pp. 611–631). John Wiley & Sons.

Filho, E., Tenenbaum, G., & Yang, Y. (2015). Cohesion, team mental models, and collective efficacy: Towards an integrated framework of team dynamics in sport. *Journal of Sports Sciences, 33*, 641–653. doi:10.1080/02640414.2014.957714

Fletcher, D., & Sarkar, M. (2016). Mental fortitude training: An evidence-based approach to developing psychological resilience for sustained success. *Journal of Sport Psychology in Action, 7*, 135–157. doi:10.1080/21520704.2016.1255496

García-Calvo, T., Leo, F. M., & González Ponce, I. (2019). Coach justice and competence in football. In E. Konter, J. Beckmann, & T. M. Loughead (Eds.), *Football psychology: From theory to practice* (pp. 138–149). Routledge.

García-Calvo, T., Leo, F. M., Gonzalez-Ponce, I., Sánchez-Miguel, P. A., Mouratidis, A., & Ntoumanis, N. (2014). Perceived coach-created and peer-created motivational climates and their associations with team cohesion and athlete satisfaction: Evidence from a longitudinal study. *Journal of Sports Sciences, 32*, 1738–1750. doi:10.1080/02640414.2014.918641

Godfrey, M., Kim, J., Eluère, M., & Eys, M. A. (2020). Diversity in cultural diversity research: A scoping review. *International Review of Sport and Exercise Psychology, 13*, 128–146. doi:10.1080–1750984x.2019.1616316

Gucciardi, D. F., Crane, M., Ntoumanis, N., Parker, S. K., Thøgersen-Ntoumani, C., Ducker, K. J., Peeling, P., Chapman, M. T., Quested, E., & Temby, P. (2018). The emergence of team resilience: A multilevel conceptual model of facilitating factors. *Journal of Occupational and Organizational Psychology, 91*, 729–768. doi:10.1111/joop.12237

Hoyle, B., Taylor, J., Zugic, L., & Filho, E. (2020). Coordination cost and super-efficiency in teamwork: The role of communication, psychological states, cardiovascular responses, and rhythms. *Applied Psychophysiology and Biofeedback, 45*, 323–341. doi:10.1007/s10484-020-09479-8

Juravich, M., Salaga, S., & Babiak, K. (2017). Upper echelons in professional sport: The impact of NBA general managers on team performance. *Journal of Sport Management, 31*, 466–479. doi:10.1123/jsm.2017-0044

Leo, F. M., González-Ponce, I., García-Calvo, T., Sánchez-Oliva, D., & Filho, E. (2019). The relationship among cohesion, transactive memory systems, and collective efficacy in professional soccer teams: A multilevel structural equation analysis. *Group Dynamics: Theory, Research, and Practice, 23*, 44–56. doi:10.1037/gdn0000097

Leo, F. M., González-Ponce, I., Pulido, J. J., López-Gajardo, M. A., & García-Calvo, T. (2021). Multilevel analysis of coach leadership, group cohesion and collective efficacy in semiprofessional football teams. *International Journal of Sport Psychology.*

Leo, F. M., González-Ponce, I., Sánchez-Oliva, D., Pulido, J. J., & García-Calvo, T. (2018). Adaptation and validation of the Transactive Memory System Scale in Sport (TMSS-S). *International Journal of Sports Science & Coaching, 13*, 1015–1022.

Leo, F. M., López-Gajardo, M. A., González-Ponce, I., García-Calvo, T., Benson, A. J., & Eys, M. (2020). How socialization tactics relate to role clarity, cohesion, and intentions to return in soccer teams. *Psychology of Sport and Exercise, 50*, 101735. doi:10.1016/j.psychsport.2020.101735

Lopez-Gajardo, M. A., Pulido, J. J., Flores-Cidoncha, A., Tapia-Serrano, M. A. & Leo, F. M. (2021). Do teams with greater characteristics of team resilience perceive higher performance at the end of the season? A multi-level analysis in sport teams. *Manuscript in preparation.*

McEwan, D., & Beauchamp, M. R. (2014). Teamwork in sport: a theoretical and integrative review. *International Review of Sport and Exercise Psychology, 7*(1), 229–250.

Mertens, N., Boen, F., Steffens, N. K., Cotterill, S. T., Haslam, S. A., & Fransen, K. (2020). Leading together towards a stronger "us": An experimental test of the effectiveness of the 5R Shared Leadership Program in basketball teams. *Journal of Science and Medicine in Sport, 23*, 770–775. doi:10.1016/j.jsams.2020.01.010

Morgan, P. B. C., Fletcher, D., & Sarkar, M. (2013). Defining and characterizing team resilience in elite sport. *Psychology of Sport and Exercise, 14*, 549–559. doi:10.1016/J.PSYCHSPORT.2013.01.004

Morgan, P. B. C., Fletcher, D., & Sarkar, M. (2019). Developing team resilience: A season-long study of psychosocial enablers and strategies in a high-level sports team. *Psychology of Sport and Exercise, 45*, 101543. doi:10.1016/j.psychsport.2019.101543

Müller, V., & Lindenberger, U. (2011). Cardiac and respiratory patterns synchronize between persons during choir singing. *PloS One, 6*(9), e24893.

Rein, R., & Memmert, D. (2016). Big data and tactical analysis in elite soccer: Future challenges and opportunities for sports science. *Springer Plus, 5*, 1410. doi:10.1186/s40064-016-3108-2

Sänger, J., Müller, V., & Lindenberger, U. (2013). Directionality in hyperbrain networks discriminates between leaders and followers in guitar duets. *Frontiers in Human Neuroscience, 7*, 1–14. doi:10.3389/fnhum.2013.00234

Sarkar, M., & Fletcher, D. (2014). Psychological resilience in sport performers: A review of stressors and protective factors. *Journal of Sports Sciences, 32*, 1419–1434. doi:10.1080/02640414.2014.901551

Short, S. E., Sullivan, P., & Feltz, D. L. (2005). Development and preliminary validation of the collective efficacy questionnaire for sports. *Measurement in Physical Education and Exercise Science, 9*, 181–202. doi:10.1207/s15327841mpee0903_3

Thorson, K. R., West, T. V., & Mendes, W. B. (2018). Measuring physiological influence in dyads: A guide to designing, implementing, and analyzing dyadic physiological studies. *Psychological Methods, 23*, 595–616. doi:10.1037/met0000166

12

Athlete Leadership

Todd M. Loughead, Krista J. Munroe-Chandler,
Matthieu M. Boisvert, and Katherine E. Hirsch

State of the Art

To those involved in sport, leadership is viewed as a key element to achieving team success. Coaches are often seen as *the leader* of their respective teams. This is not surprising since an important role of coaches as leaders is to assist their athletes in improving performance levels. Coaches have a plethora of duties to perform and may not be able to attend to all of their players' needs. Consequently, athletes also seek leadership from their teammates to help ensure that their needs are being satisfied. This source of leadership has been termed *athlete leadership*. Consequently, athlete leadership is defined as an athlete who occupies a formal or informal leadership role within the team and influences team members to achieve a common goal (Loughead et al., 2006). To some extent, this definition challenged the traditional characterization of leadership as a unidirectional, hierarchical system and replaced it with a fluid, inclusive, and interactive form of leadership. As such, the definition implies that multiple athletes can perform leadership. This is evidenced by the fact that athletes can occupy formal leadership roles (i.e., designated to a leadership position within a team such as a team captain) or an informal leadership role that emerges based on athletes' interactions and communications with their teammates. Therefore, athlete leadership can be viewed as a form of shared or distributed leadership among teammates. The terms *shared* and *distributed leadership* have been used interchangeably and refer to leadership emanating from those holding formal leadership roles but also enacted by multiple individuals on the team. For instance, team members can deliver leadership when they feel it is appropriate and warranted and then step back in other moments to allow others to lead. In doing so, athlete leadership becomes a shared dynamic team process composed of mutual

Todd M. Loughead, Krista J. Munroe-Chandler, Matthieu M. Boisvert, and Katherine E. Hirsch, *Athlete Leadership*
In: *Sport, Exercise and Performance Psychology.* Edited by: Edson Filho and Itay Basevitch, Oxford University Press.
© Oxford University Press 2021. DOI: 10.1093/oso/9780197512494.003.0012

influence and shared responsibility among team members, who lead each other toward the achievement of team goals (Loughead et al., 2019).

In the last 15 years, there has been a steady increase of research in the area of athlete leadership utilizing both qualitative and quantitative research designs (see Table 12.1 for key readings in this field). From a qualitative research perspective, a central research theme has been the characteristics required for effective athlete leadership. For instance, through the use of semistructured interviews, Bucci et al. (2012) found coaches viewed effective athlete leaders as those players who possessed a strong work ethic, were a positive role model for their teammates, and were able to follow the coaching staff's instructions. Other characteristics of effective athlete leaders were being generous, being honest, and showing a concern for teammates' well-being. Similarly, Dupuis, Bloom, and Loughead (2006) conducted semistructured interviews with six former intercollegiate male hockey captains that were viewed by their coaches as being exceptional athlete leaders. They showed that effective leaders needed to have emotional control, be strong communicators, remain positive in front of teammates, and be respectful toward both teammates and the coaching staff. Additional characteristics of effective athlete leaders include being trustworthy, generous, selfless, and respectful, and having good interpersonal skills. In addition to these characteristics, Camiré (2016) interviewed a professional hockey captain who believed that being an effective leader required him to be open to learning, be a positive role model, lead by example, have a strong work ethic, and work collectively with the other team leaders. In their examination of shared mental models, Filho et al. (2014) used a case study approach to investigate a volleyball captain's perceived leadership role at the individual and team levels. The captain noted that at the individual level, communicating both on and off the court, being a motivator to her teammates, and coordinating defensive roles were critical responsibilities for her to fulfill. At the team level, the captain believed that having team routine behaviors (pregame, after each point) mentally helped them be prepared. Further, the captain also felt that the team shared a similar match philosophy toward volleyball that included being committed to the team's game plan, having common team goals, and supporting each other during the game. Taken together, these studies highlight the numerous characteristics that are required for effective leadership.

When applying a quantitative research perspective, researchers have utilized two general approaches. The first approach has been the use of traditional self-report questionnaires such as the Leadership Scale for Sports

(LSS; Chelladurai & Saleh, 1980) and the Differentiated Transformational Leadership Inventory (DTLI; Callow et al., 2009) to measure the frequency of athlete leadership behaviors. The LSS measures five leadership behaviors that include *training and instruction* (teaches the skills and tactics of the sport), *democratic behavior* (encourages participation in the decision-making process), *autocratic behavior* (stresses personal authority), *social support* (shows concern for the welfare of teammates), and *positive feedback* (recognizes and rewards good performance). The DTLI assesses seven dimensions that include six transformational and one transactional leadership behaviors. The six transformational leadership dimensions are *inspirational motivation* (provides meaning and challenge to teammates), *individual consideration* (demonstrates acceptance of teammate differences, needs, and goals), *intellectual stimulation* (finds new ways to old problems), *appropriate role modeling* (leads by example), *fostering acceptance of group goals and promoting teamwork* (encourages cooperation among teammates toward a common goal), and *high-performance expectations* (creates an atmosphere by encouraging high-performance standards). The lone transactional leadership behavior is *contingent reward* (rewards teammates for performing well).

To date, numerous outcomes, at both the individual and team levels, have been examined in relation to athlete leadership behaviors. At the individual level, athlete transformational leadership behavior was positively related to the outcomes of sport enjoyment and intrinsic motivation (Price & Weiss, 2013). That is, athlete leaders who frequently used the leadership behaviors of inspiration, motivation, enhanced creativity, and problem-solving had teammates that enjoyed their sporting experience and were motivated to pursue challenging tasks and learn skills. At the team level, cohesion (i.e., teams sticking together and remaining united) is arguably the most studied construct. In their examination of intercollegiate athletes, Vincer and Loughead (2010) found the athlete leadership behaviors of social support and positive feedback (measured via the LSS) were associated to both task and social cohesion, while democratic behavior was positively related to task cohesion and autocratic behavior was negatively related to both task and social cohesion. Similarly, Callow et al. (2009), using the DTLI to measure athlete leadership behaviors, found that fostering acceptance of group goals and promoting teamwork, individual consideration, and high-performance expectations were positively related to task cohesion, while fostering acceptance of group goals and promoting teamwork were associated with social cohesion.

The second quantitative approach has been the use of social network analysis (SNA). The advantage of SNA, compared to questionnaires such as the LSS and DTLI, is that it assesses athlete leadership between team members. That is, SNA is a research method that aims to examine the relationships that individuals and teams form with each other. While there is a small number of studies that have used this quantitative approach, it can be said that (a) over the course of a season there were increases in the overall amount of task and social leadership (Duguay et al., 2020), (b) the leadership responsibilities on a team are shared by numerous athletes (Fransen et al., 2015a), (c) teammates feel more socially connected to their team when high-quality leadership is available (Fransen et al., 2015b), and (d) and having high-quality athlete leadership was positively associated with stronger feelings of team cohesion (Loughead et al., 2016).

Table 12.1 Five Key Readings in the Field of Athlete Leadership

Authors	Methodological Design	Key Findings
Callow et al. (2009)	Cross-sectional	Use of a transformational leadership inventory to measure athlete leadership behaviors. Found a positive relationship with task and social cohesion.
Duguay et al. (2016)	Intervention	A theoretically grounded, season-long athlete leadership development program that enhanced leadership behaviors, athlete satisfaction, and peer-motivational climate from pre- to postintervention.
Fransen et al. (2015a)	Social network analysis	This study highlighted the presence of shared athlete leadership. The shared nature of athlete leadership was distributed among formal and informal leaders.
Loughead & Hardy (2005)	Cross-sectional	One of the first studies to show that coaches and athlete leaders display varying amounts of leadership behaviors. Specifically, coaches and athlete leaders used differing amounts of the five leadership behaviors assessed by the Leadership Scale for Sports.
Loughead et al. (2006)	Cross-sectional	This study advanced a definition of athlete leadership. It found that athlete leaders performed task, social, and external leadership functions.

Questions to Move the Field Forward

1. Theoretical Question: Is There a Need to Advance an Athlete Leadership Framework?

To help answer this question, it is important to examine the frameworks that have been previously used to study athlete leadership. The two primary models emanate from sport coaching and organizational psychology. Chelladurai's (2007) multidimensional model of leadership (MML), from sport coaching, is a linear model composed of antecedent variables that influence the throughput of leadership behaviors, which in turn influence the consequences. The antecedents are categorized into three factors that include situational characteristics, leader characteristics, and member characteristics. The situational characteristics refer to factors such as group goals, task type (e.g., individual versus team, closed versus open tasks), and the social context of the team. The leader characteristics include personal characteristics of the leader such as age, gender, or experience. Lastly, member characteristics include factors such as personality (e.g., need for achievement, need for affiliation, cognitive structure) and ability to perform the specific task. According to Chelladurai, the throughput refers to leadership behaviors and is viewed along three types: required (leadership behaviors needed to meet the situational demands), actual (leadership behaviors that are displayed), and preferred (leadership behaviors favored by team members). The final component in the model is the consequences. Originally, Chelladurai identified two outcomes: satisfaction and performance. However, Chelladurai noted that the consequences could encapsulate more than these two identified outcomes.

Avolio's (1999) full range leadership model (FRLM) is another framework that has been used to study athlete leadership. Similar to the MML, this model encapsulates a broad range of leadership behaviors that can be classified from least to most effective: laissez-faire, transactional, and transformational forms of leadership. Laissez-faire is a form of leadership that is described as nonleadership or an absence of leadership (Avolio, 1999). Transactional leadership is characterized by an exchange relationship between the leader (e.g., athlete leader) and follower (e.g., teammates) to meet their own self-interests through the use of reward and recognition. While transactional leadership is an effective form of leadership through the use of positive and corrective forms of feedback, to evaluate followers to achieve more, leaders need to supplement these transactional behaviors with transformational leadership behaviors. Transformational leadership is about inducing the follower past their own self-interests, making followers more aware of the importance and values of task outcomes, and engaging them in thinking about the higher order needs for the good of the team. Augmenting these two theoretical frameworks (MML and FRLM), another useful paradigm that has been alluded to in several athlete leadership studies and in the definition of athlete leadership is the notion of shared leadership. Zhu et al. (2018) noted three key characteristics of shared leadership: (a) lateral influence among peers (i.e., teammates), (b) emergent team phenomenon (leadership roles are distributed among teammates), and (c) leadership roles and influence are distributed among team members (i.e., teammates). Based on these three characteristics, the sport team is a natural context for shared leadership to occur. Consequently, there is no unified theoretical model that explains the emergence and consequences of shared athlete leadership.

To help guide researchers in the field of athlete leadership, we advance a working framework drawing from the extant literature (see Figure 12.1). At the heart of the model is *shared athlete leadership,* wherein numerous athletes exhibit leadership and do so using a wide variety of behaviors (Duguay et al., 2018). Similar to other sport leadership models (Beauchamp et al., 2019; Chelladurai, 2007; Horn, 2008; Smoll & Smith, 1989), athlete leadership is also shaped by antecedent factors that include *characteristics of athlete leaders, teammates, and/or coaches* (e.g., age, experience, personality) as well as *situational characteristics* (e.g., task type, level of competition, practice,

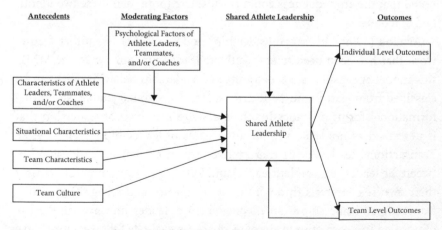

Figure 12.1. A working model for the study of athlete leadership.

competition), *team characteristics* (e.g., team size, ability, maturity, diversity), and *team culture* (e.g., values, beliefs). Further, the relationship between *characteristics of athlete leaders, teammates, and/or coaches* and *shared athlete leadership* will be moderated by the *psychological factors of athlete leaders, teammates, and/or coaches* (e.g., motivational orientation, efficacy beliefs, self-esteem, behavioral intentions). The *situational factors, team characteristics,* and *team culture* will directly impact shared athlete leadership. Shared athlete leadership will impact both individual (e.g., athlete satisfaction, motivational orientation, self-efficacy, individual performance) and team-level (e.g., cohesion, collective efficacy, intrateam communication, team performance) outcomes. There is a feedback loop from individual and team-level outcomes to shared athlete leadership. Athlete leaders are likely to alter their behaviors based on the relative achievement of the outcome variables.

2. Methodological Question: Is There a Need for an Athlete Leadership Behaviors–Specific Questionnaire?

As noted earlier, the LSS (Chelladurai & Saleh, 1980) and the DTLI (Callow et al., 2009) have been primarily used to measure athlete leadership behaviors. Both of these inventories were originally developed to assess sport coaching and military contexts, respectively. A comment that we have received from reviewers when publishing our research findings is whether these two inventories are appropriate when measuring athlete leadership behaviors. Confirmatory factor analysis of the LSS and DTLI have shown both inventories to be valid and reliable (see Callow et al., 2009; Vincer & Loughead, 2010). Further evidence supports the usefulness of measuring the athlete leadership behaviors contained in these two inventories. Specifically, Duguay et al. (2018) asked athletes to rate on a 5-point scale how important (higher scores reflect greater importance) it was for their athlete leaders to exhibit these leadership behaviors. For eight of the 11 leadership behaviors, scores were above 4, and the other three were above 3 on the 5-point scale. Taken together, the results showed that the leadership behaviors contained within the LSS and DTLI are important for athlete leaders to exhibit. However, two caveats should be noted. First, if the LSS and DTLI are retained as inventories, an analysis of the items should be conducted to determine whether they are appropriate for measuring athlete leadership. For instance, the LSS item "Encourages team members to make suggestions for ways of conducting practices" may be attributed more to coaches than athlete leaders since the latter may not have the ability or authority to dictate practices or training sessions. Second, Avolio (1999) noted that it is possible that other aspects of leadership have not yet been discovered. In fact, we have conducted in-depth interviews with athletes asking them about what behaviors would constitute effective athlete leadership. While these preliminary results have shown that the leadership behaviors from both the LSS and DTLI are present, we have found that other leadership behaviors unique to athlete leadership have emerged, such as fostering cohesion and team norms (Loughead & Munroe-Chandler, 2020). Thus, to capture the full extent of athlete leadership behaviors, a specific questionnaire should be developed by researchers.

3. Methodological Question: How Can the Field of Athlete Leadership Be Advanced in Terms of Research Methodology?

To answer this question, we must first look to the type of research published most often in the area. To say that most of the research has been cross-sectional in nature would be an understatement. A survey of the research conducted for this chapter showed that approximately 70% of the articles published in the area of athlete leadership have employed a cross-sectional design, thus allowing for adequate description and generalization. Through survey (e.g., Callow et al., 2009; Loughead & Hardy, 2005) and SNA methodologies (e.g., Fransen et al., 2015a; Loughead et al., 2016), various samples have been recruited with respect to sport, age, and gender (e.g., intercollegiate athletes, youth athletes, soccer players, frisbee players). However, these studies have provided a mere snapshot of athlete leadership at one moment in time. Granted, cross-sectional designs allow for many variables to be examined simultaneously (e.g., athlete leadership, cohesion, and athlete satisfaction) and are oftentimes more convenient to implement than longitudinal or experimental designs. Consequently, they fail to account for changes over time at the group and/or individual level, and it is difficult to determine causation.

Researchers (Duguay et al., 2020; Fransen et al., 2018) have used SNA to examine athlete leadership over time (longitudinal). Using this type of analysis, answers can be sought to such questions as (a) Does leadership change over the course of an athletic season? (b) What are the antecedents and consequences of these changes over time? (c) How do these changes over time impact team processes and outcomes such as cohesion and performance? Answers to these questions not only advance the literature on athlete leadership but also provide coaches and sport psychology practitioners with information leading to a better understanding of the leadership processes in teams.

To date (and to the authors' knowledge), there have been no studies in the area of athlete leadership that have used an experimental design. Several studies (e.g., Duguay et al., 2016; Voight, 2012) have delivered athlete leadership interventions with one team over the course of a season, but none have included a control group. Notwithstanding the time and the cost required to conduct experimental studies, it is often difficult to find coaches and athletes who are open to participating in a no-treatment control group. A researcher may consider using a matched experimental and control repeated-measures design wherein the control group will receive the intervention (e.g., leadership training) at the end of the study (waitlist control). Experimental studies are desperately needed to generate causal knowledge that will inform policy and applied practice.

4. Theoretical Question: What Can We Do to Disentangle the Use of "Leader" and "Leadership"?

As noted earlier, researchers have examined the characteristics of athlete leaders (e.g., ideal number of athlete leaders present on a team) and determinants of effective and ineffective leadership (e.g., being a positive role model). While the main responsibility of a leader is to provide effective leadership, a leader and leadership do not inherently produce the same behaviors and outcomes. Given the incongruence in behaviors and outcomes, researchers should be careful to use "leader" and "leadership" as distinct, noninterchangeable terms.

The distinction in verbiage may sound minor at first glance, but making the distinction between leader and leadership is necessary because a leader is a person, whereas leadership is a process. Leadership has been identified as a shared process among team members (Duguay et al., 2019) wherein it is exhibited by athletes who are informal or formal leaders. However, athlete leaders can behave in ways that are not characteristic of good leadership (e.g., being selfish), thereby demonstrating that mere presence of athlete leaders does not quantify the amount of effective leadership that is shown or present on a team. By disentangling "leader" and "leadership" terminology, we can better understand how leaders operate as individuals and how leadership functions as a process without confusing the person and the process.

As researchers and practitioners, we can take a number of steps to resolve this issue. First, be attentive of our own understanding and use of the terms *leader* and *leadership*. Second, be mindful of articles, studies, and questionnaires on leaders and leadership. It is important that the objective of the study (e.g., to analyze leadership) matches the survey tools to measure that objective (e.g., leadership behavior questionnaire) and that the language remains consistent throughout the manuscript such that *leader* language is used to describe a person exhibiting leadership or given the title as athlete leader. In contrast, *leadership* language should be used to describe the process of leaders' actions and thoughts as they affect the team. Third, improve the congruence between leaders and leadership on the team by developing leadership skills of all team members. When all team members possess effective leadership skills, the outcomes of having a high number of leaders who are doing leadership on a team will be similar.

5. Applied Question: What Must Be Addressed in the Field of Athlete Leadership Development?

Coaches and athletes alike have frequently identified a lack of leadership as a problem among athletes. For example, Voelker, Gould, and Crawford (2011) found that high school captains did not receive any type of leadership training, did not feel prepared to be a leader, and could not clearly articulate how they developed their leadership capabilities. This lack of focus on leadership can be attributed to the erroneous belief that sport participation automatically fosters leadership development (Extejt & Smith, 2009). While coaches recognize the importance of athlete leadership (Bucci et al., 2012), many coaches do not have the knowledge or the resources necessary to develop leadership in their athletes. In fact, Trottier and Robitaille (2014) interviewed 24 high school and community coaches and asked which life skills they felt comfortable teaching their athletes. Interestingly, only three coaches mentioned leadership. Given the importance attributed to leadership, there is a need to create additional learning opportunities that directly and explicitly target the development of leadership among athletes.

The research dedicated to the study of athlete leadership development is limited. To our knowledge, only eight published articles have reported on the development of athlete leadership behaviors. This lack of evaluation is surprising given the proliferation of empirical evidence (e.g., meta-analyses) on the effectiveness of leadership development in several general leadership studies (e.g., Avolio et al., 2009; Collins & Holton, 2004). Leadership interventions were found to have moderately positive effects regardless of organization type (i.e., profit, not for profit, military) and were beneficial regardless of the theories used in the leadership development intervention (i.e., operationalized as newer and traditional leadership theories). While the results from the general leadership literature are promising, research in sport should address the lack of knowledge and exposure to athlete leadership development.

Research examining leadership theories and models best suited for the study of athlete leadership development is currently lacking. Many of these articles simply stated that the program was grounded in leadership research without any insight or information into which theories were used to develop the leadership development program. The lack of studies on athlete leadership development is partly due to the fact that many of the athlete leadership development programs have been conducted face to face (i.e., researcher physically present). While this method of delivery has been effective (e.g., Cotterill, 2017; Gould & Voelker, 2010; Voight, 2012), it is limited in the number of athletes it can reach. When we have presented our research findings at conferences, the main recommendation from administrators, coaches, and athletes is to expand the access of leadership development programs to more athletes.

One way that we can expand accessibility is through the use of internet-based platforms. There are two types of communication for online learning, synchronous and asynchronous. Synchronous learning refers to real-time online communication that includes the use of technology (e.g., videoconferencing). Synchronous communication can enhance people's sense of social presence so that communication feels real, even though it is mediated by technology (McInnerney & Roberts, 2004). In contrast, asynchronous learning is commonly facilitated through media such as online learning modules when participants cannot be online at the same time. Asynchronous learning provides many benefits for learners (e.g., convenience and flexibility) but also has drawbacks (e.g., impersonal, lack of interaction with others such as the facilitator). Whether it is synchronous or asynchronous, these technologies offer significant advantages in terms of reach, convenience, cost savings, and eco-friendliness.

Conclusion

Although the field of athlete leadership is still in its infancy, researchers, over the last 15 years, have been steadily publishing research findings utilizing both qualitative and quantitative methodologies. The five questions forwarded in this chapter are important for advancing our knowledge in this field and are important for establishing athlete leadership as an emerging field of inquiry. The use of different methodologies has allowed for the examination of various research questions. We see this as a strength and encourage researchers to continue using a combination of methodologies in a quest to further understand the complexities of athlete leadership. To grow the field of athlete leadership, it will be important to use fundamentally sound theoretical frameworks. We have advanced a working framework to encourage researchers to examine the components of our model but more importantly stimulate thoughts and ideas on conceptualizing a framework that is unique to athlete leadership. To assist in the examination of the relationships contained within our working framework, the development of an athlete leadership–specific inventory is required. Further, we have distinguished between a leader and leadership, which can be used to assist researchers in clarifying the focus of their research questions. Is the focus of a particular study concerned with the leader or with elements of the leadership process? Finally, there are relatively few studies examining the development of athlete leadership. Typically, most interventions have used face-to-face methods of delivery, which can be limiting in terms of reach. To provide universal access, the use of online technologies should be examined to determine their effectiveness. By highlighting questions that require investigation, we hope this will encourage researchers to critically examine those questions with the goal of expanding knowledge and application.

References

Avolio, B. J. (1999). *Full leadership development: Building the vital forces in organizations.* Sage.

Avolio, B. J., Reichard, R. J., Hannah, S. T., Walumbwa, F. O., & Chan, A. (2009). A meta-analytic review of leadership impact research: Experimental and quasi-experimental studies. *The Leadership Quarterly, 20,* 764–784.

Beauchamp, M. R., Jackson, B., & Loughead, T. M. (2019). Leadership in physical activity contexts. In T. S. Horn & A. L. Smith (Eds.), *Advances in sport and exercise psychology* (4th ed., pp. 151–170). Human Kinetics.

Bucci, J., Bloom, G. A., Loughead, T. M., & Caron, J. (2012). Ice hockey perceptions of athlete leadership. *Journal of Applied Sport Psychology, 24*, 243–259.

Callow, N., Smith, M., Hardy, L., Arthur, C., & Hardy, J. (2009). Measurement of transformational leadership and its relationship with team cohesion and performance level. *Journal of Applied Sport Psychology, 21*, 395–412.

Camiré, M. (2016). Benefits, pressures, and challenges of leadership and captaincy in the National Hockey League. *Journal of Clinical Sport Psychology, 10*, 118–136.

Chelladurai, P. (2007). Leadership in sports. In G. Tenenbaum & R. C. Eklund (Eds.), *Handbook of sport psychology* (3rd ed., pp. 111–135). John Wiley and Sons.

Chelladurai, P., & Saleh, S. D. (1980). Dimensions of leader behavior in sports: Development of a leadership scale. *Journal of Sport Psychology, 2*, 34–45.

Collins, D. B., & Holton, E. F. (2004). The effectiveness of managerial leadership development programs: A meta-analysis of studies from 1982 to 2001. *Human Resource Development Quarterly, 15*, 217–248.

Cotterill, S. T. (2017). Developing leadership skills in sport: A case study of elite cricketers. *Case Studies in Sport and Exercise Psychology, 1*, 16–25.

Duguay, A. M., Hoffmann, M. D., Guerrero, M. D., & Loughead, T. M. (2020). An examination of the temporal nature of shared athlete leadership: A longitudinal case study of a competitive youth male ice hockey team. *International Journal of Sport and Exercise Psychology, 18*, 672–686.

Duguay, A. M., Loughead, T. M., & Cook, J. M. (2019). Athlete leadership as a shared process: Using a social network approach to examine athlete leadership in competitive female youth soccer teams. *The Sport Psychologist, 33*, 1–43.

Duguay, A. M., Loughead, T. M., & Munroe-Chandler, K. J. (2016). The development, implementation, and evaluation of an athlete leadership development program with female varsity athletes. *The Sport Psychologist, 30*, 154–166.

Duguay, A. M., Loughead, T. M., & Munroe-Chandler, K. J. (2018). Investigating the importance of athlete leadership behaviors and the impact of leader tenure. *Journal of Sport Behavior, 41*, 129–147.

Dupuis, M., Bloom, G. A., & Loughead, T. M. (2006). Team captains' perceptions of athlete leadership. *Journal of Sport Behavior, 29*, 60–78.

Extejt, M. M., & Smith, J. E. (2009). Leadership development through sports team participation. *Journal of Leadership Education, 8*, 224–237.

Filho, E., Gershgoren, L., Basevitch, I., Schinke, R., & Tenenbaum, G. (2014). Peer leadership and shared mental models in a college volleyball team: A season long case study. *Journal of Clinical Sport Psychology, 8*, 184–203.

Fransen, K., Delvaux, E., Mesquita, B., & Van Puyenbroeck, S. (2018). The emergence of shared leadership in newly formed teams with an initial structure of vertical leadership: A longitudinal analysis. *The Journal of Applied Behavioral Science, 54*, 140–170.

Fransen, K., Van Puyenbroeck, S., Loughead, T. M., Vanbeselaere, N., De Cuyper, B., Broek, G. V., & Boen, F. (2015a). Who takes the lead? Social network analysis as a pioneering tool to investigate shared leadership within sports teams. *Social Networks, 43*, 28–38.

Fransen, K., Van Puyenbroeck, S., Loughead, T. M., Vanbeselaere, N., De Cuyper, B., Broek, G. V., & Boen, F. (2015b). The art of athlete leadership: Identifying high-quality athlete leadership at the individual and team level through social network analysis. *Journal of Sport and Exercise Psychology, 37*, 274–290.

Gould, D., & Voelker, D. K. (2010). Youth sport leadership development: Leveraging the sports captaincy experience. *Journal of Sport Psychology in Action, 1*, 1–14.

Horn, T. S. (2008). Coaching effectiveness in the sport domain. In T. S. Horn (Ed.), *Advances in sport psychology* (3rd ed., pp. 239–267). Human Kinetics.

Loughead, T. M., Duguay, A. M., & Hoffmann, M. D. (2019). Athlete leadership in football. In E. Konter, J. Beckmann, & T. M. Loughead (Eds.), *Football psychology: From theory to practice* (pp. 91–100). Routledge.

Loughead, T. M., Fransen, K., Van Puyenbroeck, S., Hoffmann, M. D., De Cuyper, B., Vanbeselaere, N., & Boen, F. (2016). An examination of the relationship between athlete leadership and cohesion using social network analysis. *Journal of Sports Sciences, 34*, 2063–2073.

Loughead, T. M., & Hardy, J. (2005). An examination of coach and peer leader behaviors in sport. *Psychology of Sport and Exercise, 6*, 303–312.

Loughead, T. M., Hardy, J., & Eys, M. A. (2006). The nature of athlete leadership. *Journal of Sport Behavior, 29*, 142–159.

Loughead, T. M., & Munroe-Chandler, K. J. (2020). [Leadership behaviors used by athlete leaders]. Unpublished raw data.

McInnerney, J. M., & Roberts, T. S. (2004). Online learning: Social interaction and the creation of a sense of community. *Educational Technology and Society, 7*, 73–81.

Price, M. S., & Weiss, M. E. (2013). Relationships among coach leadership, peer leadership, and adolescent athletes' psychosocial and team outcomes: A test of transformational leadership theory. *Journal of Applied Sport Psychology, 25*, 265–279.

Smoll, F. L., & Smith, R. E. (1989). Leadership behaviors in sport: A theoretical model and research paradigm. *Journal of Applied Social Psychology, 19*, 1522–1551.

Trottier, C., & Robitaille, S. (2014). Fostering life skills development in high school and community sport: A comparative analysis of the coach's role. *The Sport Psychologist, 28*, 10–21.

Vincer, D. J. E., & Loughead, T. M. (2010). The relationship among athlete leadership behaviors and cohesion in team sports. *The Sport Psychologist, 24*, 448–467.

Voelker, D. K., Gould, D., & Crawford, M. J. (2011). Understanding the experience of high school sport captains. *The Sport Psychologist, 25*, 47–66.

Voight, M. (2012). A leadership development intervention program: A case study with two elite teams. *The Sport Psychologist, 26*, 604–623.

Zhu, J., Liao, Z., Yam, K. C., & Johnson, R. E. (2018). Shared leadership: A state-of-the-art review and future research agenda. *Journal of Organizational Behavior, 39*, 834–852.

SECTION 2
HEALTH AND WELL-BEING

13

Mental Health

Brad Donohue, Gavin Breslin, and Shane Murphy

The importance of systemically addressing athletes' mental health is increasingly being recognized around the globe. However, studies continue to show that athletes of all levels of competitiveness are rarely provided evidence-supported mental health programming, particularly programs that have been developed to fit sport culture (Breslin & Leavey, 2019). Poor adoption of mental health programming in sport appears to be influenced by a general lack of awareness of mental health issues, limitations in policy, availability of services, ethical guidelines, and legal requirements governing appropriate scope of practice in this area. This chapter underscores important scientific contributions to mental health in athletes, including answers to five critical questions that are specific to advancing mental health practice with athletes and highlighting exemplary studies that are likely to move the field forward (see Table 13.1).

Prevalence. The true prevalence of diagnosable psychiatric disorders in athletes is undetermined, particularly in youth athletes (Donohue, Gavrilova, & Strong, 2020). Adult athletes have usually been found to experience about the same severity of symptoms associated with depression, anxiety, and eating and substance use disorders relative to the general population (Rice et al., 2016). However, symptom severity rates vary greatly across studies due to differences in methodological rigor, population characteristics, study year, instrumentation, and so on. For instance, rates of symptoms associated with mood disorders have ranged from 4% (Schaal et al., 2011) to 68% (Hammond et al., 2013). Thus, well-designed studies specific to athletes' mental health disorder prevalence are warranted.

Mental health awareness programs. There is a need to enhance awareness of the continuum of mental health and its management in athletes, including psychological skills training aimed at reducing stigma and other barriers associated with the pursuit of mental health care and improving help-seeking behaviors. Implementation guidelines and evaluation of

Brad Donohue, Gavin Breslin, and Shane Murphy, *Mental Health* In: *Sport, Exercise and Performance Psychology*. Edited by: Edson Filho and Itay Basevitch, Oxford University Press. © Oxford University Press 2021.
DOI: 10.1093/oso/9780197512494.003.0013

mental health awareness programs in nonelite contexts are especially crucial because they are relevant to the vast majority of sport participants world-wide. Examples of these programs are summarized by Breslin and Leavey (2019), who highlighted considerable program heterogeneity in sports settings, athlete populations, mental health problems, and evaluations. As reported, awareness programs that are sensitive to sport culture are recommended. Notable awareness programs include *Ahead of the Game* (Liddle et al., 2019), *State of Mind Ireland* (Breslin et al., 2019), and online applications (Gulliver et al., 2012; for a systematic review see Breslin et al., 2017). These programs are innovative and often incorporate modern tech-nology. For instance, in one program video, case studies of former student-athletes struggling with mental illness are utilized to facilitate discussion of mental health (Kern et al., 2017). Van Raalte et al. (2015) developed an interactive multimedia website (http://www.supportforsport.org/) to assist athletes in making mental health referrals and improving their knowledge about mental health. Implementation of *Help Out a Mate* (HOAM; Liddle et al., 2019) was demonstrated to increase youth athletes' intentions to pro-vide help to other athlete friends and increase knowledge of the signs of mental illness. Mental health intervention engagement strategies in colle-giate athletes have also been evaluated in controlled trials (Donohue et al., 2004, 2016; Gulliver et al., 2012). These programs have assisted in the de-velopment of athletes' positive perspectives of mental health interventions but have not significantly improved attendance to mental health interven-tion. In response to the emergence of mental health awareness in sport programs, an international group was established (Breslin et al., 2019) to provide consensus recommendations for program designers and deliverers, policymakers, and commissioners with respect to terminology that can be operationalized when promoting mental health awareness, program design principles, and methods of evaluation.

Sport-specific mental health screening and assessment. Several extant mental health screening and assessment measures have been psychomet-rically developed for use in athlete populations. Screens help to identify athletes who are likely to benefit from mental health services. The Athlete Psychological Strain Questionnaire (APSQ) is appropriate for professional athletes (Rice et al., 2019[1]) and includes three factors (Self-regulation, Performance, External coping). Clinical cutoff scores may be used to

---

[1] This scale is included in Table 13.1 due to its model use of psychometric evaluation methodology.

determine high psychiatric distress, and scores are inversely correlated with well-being. The Student Athlete Relationships Inventory (SARI; Donohue, Miller, et al., 2007) assesses sport-specific relationship problems with teammates, family, and coaches. The SARI has demonstrated strong internal consistency and concurrent validity in high school athletes (Donohue, Miller, et al., 2007). Family scale items have been found to predict psychiatric symptoms, and psychiatric clinical cutoff scores are available (Hussey et al., 2019). The Sport Interference Checklist (SIC; Donohue, Silver, et al., 2007) assesses common interferences with sport performance in training and competition, and the extent to which athletes are motivated to pursue a sport performance professional for assistance in these areas. The SIC has been indicated to predict psychiatric symptomology in collegiate athletes, and psychiatric cutoff scores are available (Donohue et al., 2019). When assessment is desired along the continuum of mental wellness, other validated assessments should be considered, including the Sport Mental Health Continuum Short Form (SMHC; Foster & Chow, 2019) and the Sport Psychology Outcomes and Research Tool (SPORT; Hansen et al., 2019). The SMHC includes three scales specific to well-being, and the SPORT includes Athlete Wellbeing, Self-Regulation, Performance Satisfaction, and Sport-Related Distress scales. Each of these scale scores has evidenced excellent internal consistency and concurrent validity.

Sport-specific psychological interventions. These interventions have almost exclusively included components of mindfulness and cognitive behavioral therapy (CBT), and outcome study evaluations of these programs are predominately uncontrolled evaluations of athletes who have not been formally assessed for mental health disorders. While showing promise, most of these studies have been underpowered, and all of them have resulted in at least some outcomes being nonsignificant. Traditional CBT interventions include reconstruction of maladaptive thoughts to be more objective and positive, and behavioral skills training to facilitate greater positive interactions within their sports environment. Using traditional CBT, Gabana (2017) conducted an uncontrolled case trial in a female collegiate rower with major depressive disorder, and Didymus and Fletcher (2017) performed an innovative well-controlled multiple baseline study with four female hockey players who were not assessed for mental health diagnoses. The female rower was reported to evidence improvements in process measures, while the hockey players' appraisals of organizational stressors were enhanced. Internet-based CBT has been shown to decrease symptoms of depression and anxiety relative to a waitlist condition in a pilot randomized controlled trial (RCT) involving eight youth athletes who were not assessed for mental health conditions (Sekizaki et al., 2019). The *Bodies in Motion* program (Voelker et al., 2019) has been found to decrease athletes' risk for eating disorders in female collegiate athletes. This program focuses on behavioral strategies to manage sociocultural and sport-specific body image pressures, as well as promote mindful self-compassion. Utilizing quasi-experimental methodology, this program was shown to improve internalized thin appearance more so than waitlist control. Sport-specific rational emotive behavior therapy (REBT) is designed to restructure irrational beliefs to be more objective. Turner and colleagues, both in uncontrolled (Davis & Turner, in press; Turner et al., 2018) and controlled multiple baseline trials (Cunningham & Turner, 2016; Turner & Barker, 2013), have consistently demonstrated the efficacy of REBT in reducing irrational beliefs, anxiety symptoms, and factors that negatively influence sport performance in athletes who have not been assessed to evidence mental health disorders.

The Optimum Performance Program in Sports (TOPPS) is a family behavior therapy intervention that includes contingency management, goal inspiration, communication skills training, self- and environmental control, appreciation exchanges, functional analysis, job development, and financial management. The program has been evaluated in two controlled (Chow et al., 2015; Donohue, Gavrilova, Galante, Gavrilova, et al., 2018) and five uncontrolled clinical trials (Donohue et al., 2015; Galante et al., 2019; Gavrilova et al., 2017; Pitts et al., 2015; Donohue et al., in press) involving collegiate athletes and youth formally assessed for mental health disorders. Up to 8 months postbaseline, implementation of TOPPS has consistently decreased the factors of general psychiatric symptoms and depression that reportedly interfere with sport performance, and has improved relationships, particularly as mental health diagnostic severity increases. This intervention has not improved safe sexual activity and has only decreased substance use up to 4 months postbaseline, relative to traditional campus counseling in a randomized clinical trial. Lastly, mindfulness-acceptance-commitment (MAC) is focused on achieving nonjudgmental presence while performing the task at hand (Gross et al., 2016). Cognitive skills are taught utilizing psychoeducation, behavioral skills training, and mindfulness exercises. Gross et al. (2016) evaluated MAC and psychological skills training (PST) in a RCT with 1-month follow-up in 18 female collegiate athletes who were not assessed for mental health diagnosis. Results showed that MAC was more efficacious than PST in reducing substance use and hostility, and both programs demonstrated improvements in most outcome measures. Mindful sport performance enhancement (MSPE; Kaufman et al., 2009) is similar to mindfulness-based stress reduction and mindfulness-based cognitive therapy with an emphasis on sport scenarios. In an amateur baseball team ($n = 21$), Chen et al. (2018) determined that MSPE did evidence pre/post improvements and 1-month follow-up in flow state, quality of sleep, and eating disorder symptoms, but not general anxiety and depression.

Table 13.1 Five Key Readings in the Advancement of Mental Health in Athletes

Authors	Methodological Design	Key Findings
Breslin et al. (2017)	Systematic review	10 studies included from 1,216 studies retrieved: four comprising coaches or service providers, one with officials, four with athletes, and one involving a combination of coaches and athletes. A range of outcomes were used to assess indices of mental health awareness and well-being. Mental health referral was improved in six studies, while three reported an increase in knowledge about mental health disorders. Seven studies did not report effect sizes, limiting interpretation. There was substantial heterogeneity and limited validity in outcome measures of mental health knowledge and referral efficacy. Seven studies demonstrated a high risk of bias. A need for well-designed controlled intervention studies was found.
Donohue et al. (2018)	Randomized controlled clinical trial	74 collegiate athletes assessed for mental health diagnostic severity using a structured interview were randomly assigned to The Optimum Performance Program in Sports (TOPPS) or campus psychological services as usual (SAU) after baseline. Preintervention expectancy effects, demographics, and outcome measures were equivalent between interventions. Blind assessors administered measures of psychiatric symptomology, mood, factors affecting sport performance in training and competition, substance use, unsafe sex, happiness in relationships, and relationships affecting sport performance. Intervention integrity was high.

Continued

Table 13.1 *Continued*

Authors	Methodological Design	Key Findings
		Repeated-measures analyses showed participants in TOPPS demonstrated significantly better outcomes than SAU up to 8 months postrandomization on all measures except days of sex without a condom at 4 and 8 months postbaseline and substance use at 8 months postbaseline, particularly as diagnostic severity increased (i.e., no diagnosis, single diagnosis, multiple diagnosis). Attendance and consumer satisfaction were significantly higher for participants in TOPPS.
Rice et al. (2019)	Two-stage psychometric evaluation	Stage 1: 1,007 Australian elite male athletes randomly partitioned into calibration and validation samples. Exploratory factor analysis on calibration sample supported three factors (Self-Regulation, Performance, External Coping). Confirmatory factor analysis supported a similar factor model. Differential item functioning analysis indicated item equivalence relative to athletes' level of education and ethnicity. Currently injured athletes evidenced poorer Performance than injured athletes.
Turner & Barker (2013)	Multiple baselines across four youth cricketer participants	Multiple-baseline across-participants design. Rational emotive behavior therapy (REBT) was sequentially administered; participant 1 introduced to intervention in week 6 of off-season training, participant 2 in week 7, participant 3 in week 8, and participant 4 in week 10. Social desirability instructions administered prior to each data collection to limit response bias. Validated outcome measures used. REBT guided by workbook. Visual analytical techniques and Cohen's *d* showed that effects occurred for participants immediately after intervention was implemented. For irrational beliefs, participant 1 showed a 9% decrease, participant 2 showed a 34% decrease, participant 3 showed an 11% decrease, and participant 4 showed a 38% decrease from pre- to postintervention phases. For cognitive anxiety, participant 1 showed a 9% decrease, participant 2 showed a 16% decrease, participant 3 showed a 23% decrease, and participant 4 showed a 13% decrease from pre- to postintervention phase. Social validation assessed for participants, parents, and coaches after study.

Table 13.1 *Continued*

Authors	Methodological Design	Key Findings
Vella (2019)	Systematic review	Reports findings from relatively extant field of mental health within organized youth sport, including clear definitions of mental health and wellness, advantages and disadvantages of addressing youths' mental health through sport, and theoretical and empirical support for sport-based mental health intervention in youth athletes. Research recommendations are offered based on gaps in the literature, such as the need to perform longitudinal research to determine whether sport does, indeed, enhance youths' mental health, controlled intervention outcome studies, and development of methods of preventing abuse in youth sport. Practice recommendations are offered, such as need to develop policy that supports development and implementation of evidence-supported programs.

Questions to Move the Field Forward

1. Theoretical Question: Do Athletes Experience Mental Health Disorders Differently Than Nonathletes?

Epidemiological and prevalence studies comparing mental health symptomatology of demographically similar athlete and nonathlete cohorts utilizing validated diagnostic interviews have yet to occur; and extant studies that have examined prevalence of mental health symptomology utilizing retrospective reports of clinic attendance, nondiagnostic interviews, and self-report measures of symptomatology associated with mental health conditions vary considerably in methodological approach, rigor, population demographics and number, level of athletes' expertise, instrumentation, recruitment, and so on. If athletes and nonathlete peers experience mental health symptomatology similarly, including response to mental health intervention, there may be no need to establish evidence-supported mental health programming that is adapted to address sport culture. On the other hand, if athletes do evidence mental health symptomology differently than nonathlete peers, it may be necessary to alter mental health programs to address culture, activities, relationships, and other factors that are unique to sport, and perhaps justify greater mental health resources to athletes (particularly if it is reliably determined in future research that sport performance is associated with improved mental health). To answer this question, it will be necessary to develop psychometrically sound measures of mental health symptomatology that are capable of distinguishing patterns of behavior and cognition that are dysfunctional from those that are functional within the context of sport. For instance, depression scales typically include item stems that may be normal in athletes due to demanding competitions, physical training regimes, or intense scheduling (e.g., "I sleep a lot more than usual"; "I am too tired or fatigued to do a lot of things I used to do"; Beck Depression Inventory II; Beck et al., 1996). Thus, athlete responses to existing mental health assessments may lead to false symptomology rates. Assuming valid measurement, it is important that investigators conduct large-scale prevalence studies where youth and adult athletes and their nonathlete cohorts are randomly selected from larger representative populations, and that validated diagnostic measures are used to comprehensively assess all mental health conditions concurrently. Such studies ensure appropriate comparisons and should incorporate full-time elite and professional athlete populations. Given the limited access sport psychologists have typically had with professional sports organizations, such research would suggest cooperation among national and international sport psychology and sport medicine organizations and the owners/commissioners/leaders of professional sport franchises.

2. Applied Question: Is It Necessary to Adapt Evidence-Supported Mental Health Interventions That Have Been Found to Be Effective in Nonathlete Clinical Populations to Fit Sport Culture When Treating Athletes?

If there are no substantial benefits in adjusting established mental health interventions to optimally fit athletes, this would permit the larger workforce of practitioners who are not familiar with sport to be justifiably leveraged in service provision. A critical consideration in research addressing this question is consumer acceptance, which could be partially assessed by studying treatment participation rates. Thus far justification for sport-specific mental health intervention development has been limited to findings that athletes have reported relatively high rates of mental health symptomatology for particular disorders (e.g., eating disorders, anxiety disorders), perceived stigma in their pursuit of mental health intervention, and perceived stressors that are somewhat unique to sport settings. This question, however, must be answered in controlled clinical trials involving athletes, comparing interventions that have been found to ameliorate mental health disorders in nonathlete populations with sport-specific adaptations of these interventions. In this way sport-specific adaptations can be assessed for cost-effectiveness, rates of participation, and mental health symptom reduction. There needs to be a greater number of RCTs involving athletes who are formally assessed for mental health diagnoses utilizing structured interviews during baseline. Standards of clinical trial methodology in athlete populations need to improve, including assessors who are blind to experimental assignment and receive supervision that is independent of treatment providers, and assessment and control of intervention expectancy effects and outcome measure scores between participants in experimental intervention conditions at baseline. Other research practices to encourage include utilization of protocol checklists to guide intervention implementation, assessment of intervention integrity/adherence, intent to treat management of missing data, assessment of consumer satisfaction and social validation postintervention, and assessment of various interaction effects (e.g., diagnostic severity, gender). Where RCTs are difficult to implement (e.g., professional athletes), we recommend utilization of controlled multiple baseline methods across teams/participants or behaviors. Until these methods are widely adopted, the benefits of sport-specific mental health interventions will remain only promising.

Studies consistently indicate family members are reported by athletes to be critically important to their sport performance, and family-based treatments in nonathlete populations, particularly in youth, have yielded large effect sizes. Therefore, it is important to expand intervention development and evaluation of family-based approaches, and for youth athletes, within school systems. Given the likely association between sport performance and mental health, it would be prudent on both humanitarian and financial grounds if professional sport organizations and foundations allocated significant resources to the empirical development of sport-specific mental health interventions (i.e., programming as usual vs. experimental methods). Partnerships between university research teams and community stakeholders need to occur to permit cost-effective, top-notch evaluations while demonstrating commitment to the welfare of athletes.

3. Applied Question: How Can Perceptions of Mental Health Stigma in Youth Athletes Be Reduced?

While the prevalence of stigmatizing attitudes and behaviors varies among societal groups beyond sport, there is an urgent need to understand the psychology of stigma from the perspective of athletes to facilitate practical and effective support, particularly in youth. For instance, researchers have highlighted a gap in that youth perspectives of mental health are not typically examined in wellness programs. This oversight is problematic because youth have different views and interpretations of the world than adults and are often unaware of or unmotivated to pursue mental health options. Indeed, outside of the sport context, adolescents often lack medical health care knowledge specific to practitioners' expertise, role, and willingness to treat psychological problems, with many adolescents mistrusting practitioners, or perceiving them to be insensitive to their needs (Leavey et al., 2011). These attitudes to some extent have also been found in adult athletes. We believe empirical efforts are needed specific to exploring the role family has in decreasing perceived mental health stigma of athletes, including help seeking through family activities and relationships. Families impact the psychological health of the young athlete through the attitudes and beliefs of members. Theory-guided research in this area, particularly in youth, is needed. One approach that has been assumed to be effective with young athletes is the use of role models testifying to their struggles with mental health and normalizing the use of mental health services. This approach should be empirically evaluated to ascertain benefits and possible iatrogenic considerations in specific populations of youth (e.g., LGBT, ethnic minority).

4. Applied Question: Should Performance Enhancement and Mental Health Services Be Delivered to Athletes via the Same Platforms and Providers, or Should Different Professionals Work With Athletes on Performance and Mental Health Issues?

This topic has been debated in the field since the inception of applied sport psychology (Newburg, 1992). It is important that we study this issue as it involves several interrelated areas of applied sport psychology, including the proper licensure/certification of professionals working with athletes, the scope of practice for mental health/performance enhancement professionals working with athletes, the necessary education and training for those working in this area, and the expectations and satisfaction of athletes when receiving psychological services. It has been proposed that mental health–focused interventions can be the foundation of most athlete psychological interventions and will improve performance (Morgan, 1985), that unnecessary mental health interventions may be detrimental to athletic performance (Danish & Hale, 1981), and that psychotherapy can be one of many tools utilized in a holistic approach to applied sport psychology (Murphy & Murphy, 2012). Outcome research utilizing random assignment comparative trials of both approaches (mental health and performance addressed together and addressed separately) utilizing results for both performance and mental health indices is urgently needed but currently lacking. In the aforementioned Donohue, Gavrilova, Galante, Gavrilova, et al. (2018) RCT, doctoral students with no clinical practicum experience other than workshop training and ongoing supervision could implement TOPPS with demonstrated integrity while improving athletes' self-reported performance in sport and mental health. This suggests that the level of training necessary to successfully implement at least basic levels of behavioral therapies for athletes while under supervision may not be as stringent as required for independent psychological practice. It should be noted that this issue poses different implications in the United States, where the title "psychologist" is strictly regulated, versus some countries in Europe, where the term "sport psychologist" also includes sport performance professionals who are not clinical/mental health professionals (Sanchez et al., 2005). A potential model to consider in the United States is that of doctoral-level clinical/counseling psychologists working in a team setting overseeing the mental health considerations of athletes engaged in performance consulting with professionals who may have a variety of backgrounds, credentials, and training experiences. This competency-based team approach has become common, and perhaps best practice, in many areas of mental health, and research on the effectiveness, cost-effectiveness, and client satisfaction of such an approach should be a priority consideration in sport psychology research (Kaslow et al., 2012). A potential benefit of a team-based approach incorporating service provision by nondoctoral clinicians is that it could meet the rapidly increasing mental health needs of professional sports teams and organizations; universities, colleges, and schools; and national, state, and community sports organizations.

5. Applied Question: What Can Administrators in School Systems Do to Optimize Delivery of Mental Health Services for Athletes?

Division I National Collegiate Athletic Association (NCAA) universities in the United States have arguably developed the most advanced systems of mental health care for athletes, often employing clinical or counseling sport psychologists (and their supervisees) within traditional counseling centers or athletic departments. Within these systems, sport psychologists ideally work with sport performance professionals (usually at the master's level) and participate in team meetings with physicians, physical trainers, and certified experts in nutrition and strength and conditioning. Having a team of mental health professionals within one system that is directed by a licensed psychologist trained in both sport performance and mental health is an optimum milieu. Within these systems, we recommend systemic administration of validated mental health screens to identify suicide and other mental health disorders, implementation of evidence supported workshops aimed at facilitating a culture of encouragement for mental health help-seeking behavior, and implementation of mental health optimization programming that is explicitly adapted to address sport culture. These procedures establish mental health baseline scores and reduce future liability through efficient monitoring and utilization of evidence-supported treatments. Moreover, in this system athletes are more likely to comply with professional recommendations, reducing costs associated with false responding and premature termination of mental health programming. It is imperative that these protocols are implemented seamlessly from screening to treatment and formally monitored to ensure high standards in evidence-supported intervention integrity, and that the directors of these mental health teams are licensed sport psychologists with specialized training and proficiency in mental health. These directives are fundamentally possible in Division II and III NCAA universities in the United States, as well as in universities around the globe where sport clubs operate independently from universities. However, funding is required through applied clinical trial research grants, foundations, donors, and long-term governmental initiatives as reported by experts in various consensus statements and U.S. Presidential Executive Order #13824 (see the National Youth Sports Strategy). Governmental support for sport-specific mental health programming is warranted due to the strong association between societal costs, mental and physical health, and accruing evidence

supporting specialized mental health programming in athletes who participate in organized sport (which includes half of all adolescents; see Donohue,
Gavrilova, & Strong, in press). We believe it is especially important to initiate
such systems in grade schools serving children and adolescents, particularly
those in low-income communities due to their disproportionate utilization
of health care. Schools provide an excellent backdrop in which to create
sport-specific, evidence-supported mental health care systems (Vella, 2019),
such as the one outlined previously. In such systems athletes act as mental
health care models for nonathletes. Creating the aforementioned mental
health system would require a paradigm shift, as mental health professionals
in most grade schools for children and adolescents currently do very little
mental health prevention and intervention and are not focused on sport.

Conclusion

Although there has been increased interest in athletes' mental health, athletes
continue to underutilize mental health care services. To address poor service utilization, mental health awareness and engagement interventions have
been developed. Several programs have been indicated to reduce stigma associated with the pursuit of mental health care. Mental health screening tools
and mental wellness assessment measures have been psychometrically developed in college student and professional athletes, and sport-specific mental
health interventions (exclusively CBT and mindfulness based) have been
found to improve psychiatric symptomology in college athletes. However,
these programs have yet to be implemented in practice settings.

References

Beck, Steer, & Beck. (1996). Manual for the Beck Depression Inventory—II. San Antonio,
    TX: Psychological Corporation.
Breslin, G., & Leavey, G. (2019). *Mental health and well-being interventions in
    sport: Research theory and practice.* Routledge.
Breslin, G., Shannon, S., Haughey, T., Donnelly, P., & Leavey, G. (2017). A systematic re-
    view of interventions to increase awareness of mental health and well-being in athletes,
    coaches and officials. *Systematic Reviews, 6*(177), 1–15.
Breslin, G., Smith, A., Donohue, B., Donnelly, P., Shannon, S., Haughey, T. J., Vella, S. A.,
    Swann, C., Cotteril, S., Macintyre, T., Rogers, T., & Leacey, G. (2019). International con-
    sensus statement on the psychosocial and policy-related approaches to mental health
    awareness programmes in sport. *BMJ Open Sport and Exercise Medicine, 5*(1), e000585.

Chen, J.-H., Tsai, P.-H., Lin, Y.-C., Chen, C.-K., & Chen, C.-Y. (2018). Mindfulness training enhances flow state and mental health among baseball players in Taiwan. *Psychology Research and Behaviour Management, 12*, 15–21.

Chow, G., Donohue, B., Pitts, M., Schubert, K., Loughran, T., Gavrilova, Y., & Diaz, E. (2015). Utilising the Optimum Performance Programme in Sports (TOPPS) to enhance relationships, mental strength and stability, and avoidance of unsafe sexual activity and substance misuse: Results of single case-controlled trial. *Clinical Case Studies, 14*, 191–209.

Cunningham, R., & Turner, M. J. (2016). Using rational emotive behaviour therapy (REBT) with mixed martial arts (MMA) athletes to reduce irrational beliefs and increase unconditional self-acceptance. *Journal of Rational Emotive and Cognitive Behaviour Therapy, 34*(4), 289–309.

Danish, S. J., & Hale, B. D. (1981). Toward an understanding of the practice of sport psychology. *Journal of Sport Psychology, 3*, 90–99.

Davis, H., & Turner, M. J. (2020). The use of rational emotive behavior therapy (REBT) to increase the self-determined motivation and psychological well-being of triathletes. *Sport, Exercise, and Performance Psychology, 9*, 495–505. Advance online publication. https://doi.org/10.1037/spy0000191

Didymus, F. F., & Fletcher, D. (2017). Effects of a cognitive-behavioural intervention on field hockey players' appraisals of organisational stressors. *Psychology of Sport and Exercise, 30*, 173–185.

Donohue, B., Chow, G., Pitts, M., Loughran, T., Schubert, K., Gavrilova, Y., & Allen, D. N. (2015). Piloting a family-supported approach to concurrently optimise mental health and sport performance in athletes. *Clinical Case Studies, 14*, 299–323.

Donohue, B., Dickens, Y., Lancer, K., Covassin, T., Hash, A., Miller, A., & Genet, J. (2004). Improving athletes' perspectives of sport psychology consultation: A controlled evaluation of two interview methods. *Behaviour Modification, 28*, 181–193.

Donohue, B., Galante, M., Maietta, J., Lee, B., Paul, N., Perry, J. E., Corey, A., Allen, D. N. (2019). Empirical development of a screening method to assist mental health referrals in collegiate athletes. *Journal of Clinical Sport Psychology, 13*, 561–579.

Donohue, B., Gavrilova, E., & Strong, M. (2020). A sport-focused optimization approach to mental wellness for youth in low-income neighborhoods. *European Physical Education Review, 26*(3), 695–712.

Donohue, B., Gavrilova, Y., Galante, M., Burnstein, B., Aubertin, P., Gavrilova, E., Funk, A., Light, A., & Benning, S. D. (2020). Empirical development of a screening method for mental, social, and physical wellness in amateur and professional circus artists. *Psychology of Aesthetics, Creativity and the Arts, 14*, 313–324. doi:10.1037/aca0000199

Donohue, B., Gavrilova, Y., Galante, M., Gavrilova, E., Loughrana, T., Scott, J., Chow, G., Plant, C., & Allen, D. A. (2018). Controlled evaluation of an optimisation approach to mental health and sport performance. *Journal of Clinical Sport Psychology, 12*, 234–267.

Donohue, B., Miller, A., Crammer, L., Cross, C., & Covassin, T. (2007). A standardized method of assessing sport specific problems in the relationships of athletes with their coaches, teammates, family, and peers. *Journal of Sport Behavior, 30*, 375–397.

Donohue, B., O'Dowd, A., Plant, C. P., Phillips, C., Loughran, T. A., & Gavrilova, Y. (2016). Controlled evaluation of a method to assist recruitment of participants into treatment outcome research and engage student athletes into substance abuse intervention. *Journal of Clinical Sport Psychology, 10*, 272–288.

Donohue, B., Phrathep, D., Stucki, K., Kowal, I., Breslin, G., Cohen, M., White, S., Jefferson, L., White, T., Irvin, J., Reese, G., Kessler, FHP, Kieslich da Silva, A., Gabriel Santos da Silva, F., Fothergill, M., Robinson, G., Allen, H., Light, A., & Allen, D. A.

(in press). Adapting an Evidence-Supported Intervention to Optimize Mental Health and Sport Performance for Collegiate Athletes to Fit Youth from Ethnic/Racial Minority and Low-Income Neighborhoods: A National Institutes of Health Supported Stage Model Feasibility Study. *The International Journal of Psychiatry in Medicine.* doi:10.1177/00912174211006547

Donohue, B., Silver, N. C., Dickens, Y., Covassin, T., & Lancer, K. (2007). Development and psychometric evaluation of the Sport Interference Checklist. *Behaviour Modification, 31,* 937–957.

Foster, B. J., & Chow, G. M. (2019). Development of the Sport Mental Health Continuum— Short Form (Sport MHC-SF). *Journal of Clinical Sport Psychology, 13*(4), 593–608.

Gabana, N. (2017). A strengths-based cognitive behavioural approach to treating depression and building resilience in collegiate athletics: The individuation of an identical twin. *Case Studies in Sport and Exercise Psychology, 1*(1), 4–15.

Galante, M., Donohue, B., & Gavrilova, Y. (2019). The optimum performance programme in sports: A case of bulimia nervosa in a lean sport athlete. In G. Breslin & G. Leavy (Eds.), *Mental health and well-being interventions in sport: Research, theory, and practice* (pp. 9–30). Routledge.

Gavrilova, Y., Donohue, B., & Galante, M. (2017). Mental health and sport performance programming in athletes who present without pathology: A case examination supporting optimisation. *Clinical Case Studies, 16*(3), 234–253.

Gross, M., Moore, Z. E., Gardner, F. L., Wolanin, A. T., Pess, R., & Marks, D. R. (2016). An empirical examination comparing the mindfulness-acceptance-commitment approach and psychological skills training for the mental health and sport performance of female student athletes. *International Journal of Sport and Exercise Psychology, 16*(4), 431–451.

Gulliver, A., Griffiths, K. M., & Christensen, H. (2012). Barriers and facilitators to mental health help-seeking for young elite athletes: A qualitative study. *BMC Psychiatry, 12*, 1.

Hammond, T., Gialloreto, C., Kubas, H., & Davis, H. (2013). The prevalence of failure-based depression among elite athletes. *Clinical Journal of Sport Medicine, 23*, 273–277. doi:10.1097/JSM.0b013e318287b870

Hansen, A. A., Perry, J. E., Lace, J. W., Merz, Z. C., Montgomery, T. L., & Ross, M. J. (2019). Development and validation of a monitoring instrument for sport psychology practice: The Sport Psychology Outcomes and Research Tool (SPORT). *Journal of Clinical Sport Psychology, 13*(4), 543–560.

Hussey, J. E., Donohue, B., Barchard, K. A., & Allen, D. N. (2019). Family contributions to sport performance and their utility in predicting appropriate referrals to mental health optimisation programmes. *European Journal of Sport Science, 19*(7), 972–982.

Kaslow, N. J., Falender, C. A., & Grus, C. L. (2012). Valuing and practicing competency-based supervision: A transformational leadership perspective. *Training and Education in Professional Psychology, 6*(1), 47–54. https://doi.org/10.1037/a0026704

Kaufman, K. A., Glass, C. R., & Arnkoff, D. B. (2009). Evaluation of Mindful Sport Performance Enhancement (MSPE): A new approach to promote flow in athletes. *Journal of Clinical Sport Psychology, 3*(4), 334–356.

Kern, A., Heininger, W., Klueh, E., Salazar, S., Hansen, B., Meyer, T., & Eisenberg, D. (2017). Athletes connected: Results from a pilot project to address knowledge and attitudes about mental health among college student-athletes. *Journal of Clinical Sport Psychology, 11*(4), 324–336.

Leavey, G., Rothi, D., & Paul, R. (2011). Trust, autonomy and relationships: The help-seeking preferences of young people in secondary level schools in London (UK). *Journal of Adolescence, 34*(4), 685–693.

Liddle, S. K., Hurley, D., Schweickle, M., Sewann, C., & Vella, S. A. (2019). In G. Breslin & G. Leavey (Eds.), *Mental health and well-being interventions in sport: Research theory and practice*. Routledge.

Morgan, W. P. (1985). Selected psychological factors limiting performance: A mental health model. In D. H. Clarke & H. M. Eckert (Eds.), *Limits of human performance*. Human Kinetics.

Murphy, S. M., & Murphy, B. P. (2012). Preface. In S. M. Murphy (Ed.), *The Oxford handbook of sport and performance psychology* (pp. xix–xxiv). Oxford University Press.

Newburg, D. (1992). Performance enhancement - Toward a working definition. *Contemporary Thought on Performance Enhancement, 1*, 10–25.

Pitts, M., Donohue, B., Schubert, Chow, G., Lougrhan, T., & Gavrilova, Y. (2015). A systematic case examination of The Optimum Performance Programme in Sports (TOPPS) in a combative sport. *Clinical Case Studies, 14*, 178–190.

Rice, S. M., Parker, A. G., Mawren, D., Clifton, P., Harcourt, P., Lloyd, M., Kountouris, A., Smith, B., McGorry, P. D., & Purcell, R. (2019). Preliminary psychometric validation of a brief screening tool for athlete mental health among male elite athletes: The Athlete Psychological Strain Questionnaire. *International Journal of Sport and Exercise Psychology*, 1–16.

Rice, S. M., Purcell, R., Silva, S. D., Mawren, D., McGorry, P. D., & Parker, A. G. (2016). The mental health of elite athletes: A narrative systematic review. *Sports Medicine, 46*(9), 1333–1353.

Sanchez, X., Godin, P., & De Zanet, F. (2005). Who delivers sport psychology services? Examining the field reality in Europe. *Sport Psychologist, 19*, 81–92.

Schaal, K., Taet, M., Nassif, H., Thibault, V., Pichard, C., Alcotte, M., et al. (2011). Psychological balance in high level athletes: Gender-based differences and sport-specific patterns. *PLoS ONE, 6*, e19007. doi:10.1371/journal.pone.0019007

Sekizaki, R., Nemoto, T., Tsujino, N., Takano, C., Yoshida, C., Yamaguchi, T., Katagiri, N., Ono, Y., & Mizuno, M. (2019). School mental healthcare services using internet-based cognitive behavior therapy for young male athletes in Japan. *Early Intervention in Psychiatry, 13*, 79–85.

Turner, M., & Barker, J. (2013). Examining the efficacy of rational emotive behaviour therapy (REBT) on irrational beliefs and anxiety in elite youth cricketers. *Journal of Applied Sport Psychology, 25*(1), 131–147.

Turner, M. J., Ewen, D., & Barker, J. B. (2018). An idiographic single-case study examining the use of rational emotive behaviour therapy (REBT) with three amateur golfers to alleviate sport performance phobias. *Journal of Applied Sport Psychology*. Advance online publication. doi:10.1080/10413200.2018.1496186

Van Raalte, J. L., Cornelius, A. E., Andrews, S., Diehl, N. S., & Brewer, B. W. (2015). Mental health referral for student-athletes: Web-based education and training. *Journal of Clinical Sport Psychology, 9*(3), 197–212.

Vella, S. A. (2019). Mental health and organized youth sport. *Kinesiology Review, 8*, 229–236.

Voelker, D. K., Petrie, T. A., Huang, Q., & Chandran, A. (2019). Bodies in motion: An empirical evaluation of a programme to support positive body image in female collegiate athletes. *Body Image, 28*, 149–158.

14

Affective Responses to Exercise

Panteleimon Ekkekakis and Mark E. Hartman

State of the Art

Investigations into how exercise influences the way people feel were the original seed that, over the past 50 years, led to what has become the prolific scientific field of exercise psychology. The overarching conclusion from this research, as echoed in contemporary textbooks, is that "exercise makes people feel better." While there is compelling evidence that the exercise-induced "feel better" effect is indeed possible, there are also reasons to question the generalizability of this phenomenon. The main reason is the fact that few people are found to perform the minimum recommended amount of physical activity when activity is measured by mechanical devices rather than self-reports. For example, in the United States, fewer than 10% of the adult population participate in at least moderate-intensity physical activity for at least 150 minutes per week (Tucker et al., 2011). If exercise, in fact, made most people feel better, one would expect a higher level of participation.

This apparent inconsistency prompted a relaunch of research into how exercise makes people feel in the last two decades. Most early studies involved one assessment of a small sample of distinct constructs, such as state anxiety or certain components of mood (e.g., tension, depression, anger, fatigue, vigor) before the start of a session of exercise (typically performed at a "midrange" intensity, such as 60% to 70% of maximal heart rate) and one or more additional assessments after the end of the session. Especially when the participants are young, healthy, active, and physically fit college students, this methodology reliably yields postexercise scores that are more positive than the pre-exercise ones (e.g., Ensari et al., 2015; Reed & Ones, 2006). While this general methodology was used in hundreds of studies and evidently seemed uncontroversial for decades, a critical reconsideration of its various aspects uncovered possible problems (see Ekkekakis et al., 2019). Contemporary research examining affective responses to exercise and physical activity is

Panteleimon Ekkekakis and Mark E. Hartman, *Affective Responses to Exercise* In: *Sport, Exercise and Performance Psychology*. Edited by: Edson Filho and Itay Basevitch, Oxford University Press. © Oxford University Press 2021.
DOI: 10.1093/oso/9780197512494.003.0014

based on a new methodological platform, characterized by the following innovations.

First, the target construct has been identified as core affect, the primordial component of consciousness that characterizes all valenced (pleasant or unpleasant) states, including emotions and moods (Ekkekakis, 2013). The content domain of core affect is defined by two orthogonal and bipolar dimensions, namely affective valence (pleasure vs. displeasure) and perceived activation (high vs. low). Thus, major variants of core affect include such states as energy and excitement (pleasant high activation), tension and nervousness (unpleasant high activation), calmness and relaxation (pleasant low activation), and tiredness and lethargy (unpleasant low activation).

Second, because core affect is theorized to be closely tied to homeostatic regulation and the physiological condition of the body, a bout of exercise can be reasonably expected to entail dynamic changes in the dimensions of valence and activation. Therefore, rating scales of valence and activation are administered not just before and after exercise but repeatedly, before, during, and after the bout, to obtain a faithful representation of the full trajectory of the affective response over time.

Third, given the theorized link of core affect to homeostasis, studies have adopted a painstaking approach to the standardization of exercise intensity. Following guidelines from exercise physiology (Mezzani et al., 2013), the range of exercise intensity is divided into three domains, each with distinct implications for homeostasis and the ability to continue exercise. The range of *moderate intensity* extends to the lactate threshold, the highest intensity that can be maintained without an accumulation of lactate. Because the measurement of lactate requires the sampling of blood, the gas-exchange ventilatory threshold (VT) is typically used as a less invasive alternative index. Moderate-intensity exercise permits the maintenance of physiological steady state and thus entails minimal homeostatic perturbation. Importantly, most hunting, gathering, and other subsistence activities that were predominant in the daily energy budget of humans during the Pleistocene were performed within the moderate range of intensity (Raichlen et al., 2017). The domain of *heavy intensity* extends from the lactate threshold to the level of critical power, the highest level of intensity that permits the re-establishment of a physiological steady state (also coincident with the maximal lactate steady state). Because the precise determination of critical power is labor-intensive, it is often approximated by the respiratory compensation point (RCP), determined through the analysis of gas exchange data. Finally, the domain of *severe intensity* extends from critical power to the intensity associated with peak oxygen uptake (VO_2 peak). In the severe domain, even if speed or resistance remains constant, physiological parameters, such as oxygen uptake and blood lactate, rise continuously and exercise is terminated within a few minutes.

Fourth, in contemporary research, there is increased appreciation for individual differences in affective responses and the possible psychological underpinnings of such differences (Ekkekakis et al., 2005). Importantly, while individual differences in response to a given treatment often entail variations only in the degree of response (e.g., smaller or larger increases), individual differences in affective responses to the same exercise stimulus may manifest themselves as "feel better" responses in some individuals but "feel worse" responses in others. In such cases, analyses of change at the level of the group aggregate (sample mean) can produce misleading results, since an unchanged average score may conceal two divergent response patterns and may fail to accurately model the pattern of change of individual participants. Therefore, more recent studies on affective responses to exercise report changes not only in means but also in individuals and subgroups.

Using this new methodological platform, researchers have been able to decipher the complex relation between exercise intensity and affective responses (Ekkekakis et al., 2011, 2020). Specifically, within the domain of moderate intensity, most individuals report improved affective valence or continue to report positive valence. At the other end of the spectrum, in the domain of severe intensity, all or nearly all individuals report declines in affective valence. Between these two extremes, in the domain of heavy intensity, there is substantial interindividual variability, with some individuals reporting improvements and others declines in valence (Figure 14.1).

These findings paint a more nuanced picture of the relationship between exercise and affect than what was implied by "exercise makes people feel better." While the "feel better" effect is possible, it is neither automatic nor universal but rather conditional and thus less prevalent than originally thought. Five landmark studies in this line of research are summarized in Table 14.1. Next, we propose a research agenda by highlighting five high-priority questions that can propel this line of investigation forward.

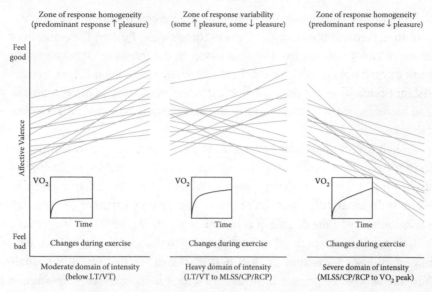

Figure 14.1. Overview of the dose-response relation between exercise intensity and affective responses. The three panels show affective valence responses of hypothetical participants during exercise performed in the moderate, heavy, and severe domains of intensity, respectively. The inserts show the pattern of oxygen uptake in the three domains of intensity. CP, critical power; LT, lactate threshold; MLSS, maximum lactate steady state; RCP, respiratory compensation point; VT, ventilatory threshold.

Table 14.1 Five Key Readings on Affective Responses to Exercise

Authors	Methodology and Design	Key Findings
Ekkekakis et al. (2008): What is the shape of the dose-response relation between exercise intensity and affective responses?	Within-subjects experiment, with three 15-minute treadmill conditions: below, at, above VT.	Running below the VT did not lower ratings on a scale of affective valence, whereas running at and above the VT did, with the decline above VT being quadratic.
Jones et al. (2018): What individual characteristics distinguish between individuals who feel worse and those who feel the same or better in response to exercise at the "heavy" range of intensity (i.e., between VT and RCP)?	Cross-sectional, correlational study. Affective responses were recorded during a graded treadmill test. Depending on changes between the VT and the RCP, participants were categorized as negative responders or neutral/positive responders.	Discriminant analysis showed that individual differences in preference for low versus high exercise intensity and sex predicted group membership in 71% of cases. Negative responders had lower preference scores and were more likely to be men.

Table 14.1 *Continued*

Authors	Methodology and Design	Key Findings
Parfitt et al. (2012): Would exercise that feels "good" result in fitness gains?	8-week randomized controlled trial, with a control and a training group. Participants in the training group were instructed to regulate their intensity to feel "good" during three 30-minute sessions per week (two supervised, one unsupervised). Control participants were instructed to continue with their normal routine.	The training group showed 23.2% improvement in the time needed to reach VT during a graded exercise test from pre- to postintervention (258.5 to 318.5 seconds), whereas the control group showed a 6.9% decline (266.7 to 248.3 seconds).
Rose & Parfitt (2008): What physiological intensity is achieved when we use a rating scale of affective valence to prescribe exercise that feels "good" or "fairly good"?	Within-subjects experiment, with eight 20-minute treadmill sessions, four with the instruction to regulate intensity to feel "good" and four with the instruction to feel "fairly good."	When instructed to exercise at an intensity that made them feel "good" or "fairly good," sedentary women intuitively selected intensities close to their ventilatory threshold and within the range the American College of Sports Medicine recommends for the enhancement and maintenance of cardiorespiratory fitness ($64 \pm 2\%$ and $68 \pm 3\%$ of maximal heart rate, respectively).
Williams et al. (2016): Is there a mediational relation connecting a prescription for self-paced exercise, affective responses, and exercise adherence?	6-month randomized controlled trial, with one group instructed to select their own pace (but not to exceed 76% of maximum heart rate) and the other group instructed to maintain intensity within the range of 64% to 76% of maximum heart rate.	Affective valence was assessed via ecological momentary assessment. Participants in the self-paced group averaged slightly higher ratings of affective valence and a higher composite score of exercise behavior (combining the duration of each session and the latency, in days, from the previous session). There was modest support for a mediational model linking self-paced exercise to exercise adherence via affective responses ($f^2 = 0.10$, where 0.02 is small, 0.15 is medium, and 0.35 is a large effect).

RCP, respiratory compensation point; VT, ventilatory threshold.

Questions to Move the Field Forward

1. Theoretical Question: What Are the Mechanistic Bases of the "Feel Better" and "Feel Worse" Effects?

Research on the psychological and neurobiological mechanisms underlying affective responses to exercise is not only of academic interest but also can serve as a valuable guide for interventions (e.g., by specifying conditions under which an intervention targeting a particular mediator may be more or less effective). Earlier mechanistic research was based on the assumption that the relation between exercise and affect was limited to the "feel better" effect. However, new evidence pointing to a complex relation necessitates an updated approach to the question of mechanisms. Mechanistic investigations should address the sources of individual differences in affective responses to an identical exercise stimulus, the dose-response relation between exercise intensity and affective responses, and the mechanistic bases of "feel worse" effects. Some of the mechanisms previously hypothesized to account for the "feel better" effect may be relevant to certain, more circumscribed, aspects of this phenomenon. For example, self-efficacy may be related to the maintenance of pleasure when the intensity of exercise presents a challenge and triggers self-doubt about one's ability to continue in the face of rising displeasure. Likewise, endorphins may be related not to feeling better per se but to the postexercise sense of relief, following a bout that was experienced as unpleasant while it lasted (Saanijoki et al., 2018).

At present, the underlying processes driving both the relatively homogeneous improvements in affect during exercise below the VT and the universal declines in affect above the RCP remain enigmatic. Below the VT (e.g., during a self-paced walk), most individuals report feeling better (especially a sense of energy), but there is no clear evidence linking this positive response to any of the mechanisms commonly discussed as explaining the "feel better" effect (e.g., there is no supporting evidence for self-efficacy, endorphins, or endocannabinoids). At the other end of the spectrum, when exercise intensity exceeds the RCP, the dominant response is affective decline, with limited individual variability. It has been proposed that this effect reflects a combination of two factors, namely the intensification of peripheral physiological symptoms related to metabolic strain and a decline in prefrontal cortical activity, which is theorized to limit the ability to cognitively regulate the rising displeasure (Ekkekakis, 2009). Declines in prefrontal cortical activity have been found to correlate with affective declines above the RCP (Tempest et al., 2014), but more research is needed. If the decrease in prefrontal activity is linked to the inability to regulate displeasure at this intensity, this finding would imply that cognitive techniques (such as attentional dissociation or cognitive reappraisal) may be of limited value for individuals exercising near the limit of their capacity.

2. Applied Question: How Can We Reliably Improve the Affective Experience of Exercise?

As noted in the introduction, a "feel better" effect associated with exercise, while possible, is conditional rather than automatic, since it appears to occur mainly within the range of moderate intensity for most individuals and within the range of heavy intensity for some. In practice, the "feel better" effect may prove to be rare. This is because the unprecedented combination of high body mass and low cardiorespiratory fitness is narrowing the range of intensity likely to be accompanied by affective improvements (and, conversely, extending the range likely leading to affective declines). The average adult in the United States today has a body mass index of 29.39 kg/m^2 (Han et al., 2019), does only 45 minutes of moderate-intensity and 19 minutes of vigorous-intensity physical activity per week (Tucker et al., 2011), and has an aerobic capacity relative to body mass that has declined by approximately one metabolic equivalent unit since the late 1960s (Lamoureux et al., 2019). In addition to numerous adverse cultural and social-psychological influences, these factors raise the probability that exercise and physical activity would reduce pleasure (Ekkekakis et al., 2018).

The affective response to exercise is a multilayered phenomenon and, as such, presents opportunities for intervention at multiple levels (Figure 14.2). While a body of evidence is being amassed on the role of certain factors (e.g., exercise intensity, audiovisual stimulation, perceived autonomy), little is known on other factors (e.g., the cultural context, the "emotional baggage" of physical education, cognitive reappraisal, the behavior of exercise leaders).

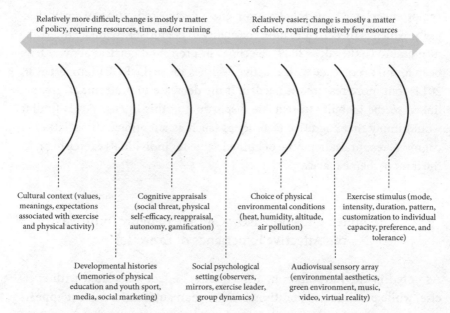

Relatively more difficult; change is mostly a matter of policy, requiring resources, time, and/or training

Relatively easier; change is mostly a matter of choice, requiring relatively few resources

Cultural context (values, meanings, expectations associated with exercise and physical activity)

Cognitive appraisals (social threat, physical self-efficacy, reappraisal, autonomy, gamification)

Choice of physical environmental conditions (heat, humidity, altitude, air pollution)

Exercise stimulus (mode, intensity, duration, pattern, customization to individual capacity, preference, and tolerance)

Developmental histories (memories of physical education and youth sport, media, social marketing)

Social psychological setting (observers, mirrors, exercise leader, group dynamics)

Audiovisual sensory array (environmental aesthetics, green environment, music, video, virtual reality)

Figure 14.2. Opportunities for interventions to improve affective responses, illustrating the multiple levels that can be targeted (from cultural and policy shifts to how exercise is implemented).

Of critical importance is the "pragmatism" of future studies; the participants and the settings to be investigated should facilitate the translation of research to practice guidelines.

3. Theoretical Question: How Do Affective Experiences Shape Memories and Affective Valuations of Exercise?

The theories used to understand, predict, and change exercise and physical activity over the past 50 years (e.g., the health belief model, the theory of planned behavior, the social-cognitive theory, the transtheoretical model) were adopted from health and social psychology. While they differ in their specifics, these theories converge on the fundamental assumption that behavior follows from cognitive appraisals (e.g., of benefits vs. barriers, self-efficacy, autonomy, relatedness). Recently, new exercise-specific theories acknowledge the role of relevant appraisals but postulate that past affective experiences associated with exercise and physical activity are also influential in shaping behavior (Brand & Ekkekakis, 2018; Conroy & Berry, 2017). A common assumption in these theoretical proposals is that repeated experiences of pleasure or displeasure during previous episodes of exercise or physical activity (e.g., in physical education, in the gym, in the rehabilitation clinic) leave a valenced "imprint" in memory (called "affective valuation" in affective-reflective theory by Brand and Ekkekakis, 2018). Subsequent activation of the stimulus-concept of "exercise" also automatically recalls the pleasure or displeasure associated with exercise, and therefore triggers the urge to either approach or avoid this behavior, respectively.

While this general idea has conceptual precedents and some empirical support in other contexts (such as addictions; Bechara & Damasio, 2005), important aspects remain unexplored. A crucial question pertains to how affective experiences of exercise and physical activity are encoded in memory. For example, would the displeasure experienced during a strenuous bout or the pleasure embedded in the sense of pride and accomplishment that is felt postexercise be more influential in how the bout is later remembered? At present, the evidence suggests that affect ratings obtained during exercise are more closely related to subsequent physical activity than those obtained postexercise (Rhodes & Kates, 2015).

As another example, in some studies, researchers have opted to represent the affective response to a bout of exercise as the overall average of ratings obtained during and after exercise, even though ratings do not remain stable over this period. Alternatively, research from the field of behavioral economics has shown that the strongest determinant of how an episode will be remembered, and whether the experience will influence subsequent behavior, is neither the average nor the total amount of pleasure reported during the episode. Instead, a "snapshot model" posits that what weighs most heavily on how an episode is remembered is the affect experienced at certain critical moments, namely the end of the episode and at the most pleasant or most unpleasant peak (Kahneman, 2000). This "peak-end rule" may also have implications for how exercise sessions are remembered (Zenko & Ekkekakis, 2019). Identifying the most consequential aspects of affective responses is a prerequisite to designing studies investigating the links between these affective responses and subsequent behavior (Figure 14.3).

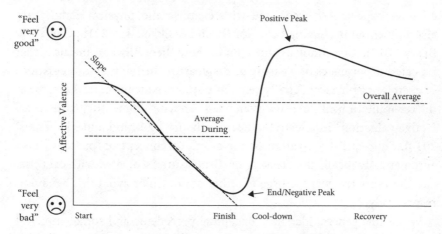

Figure 14.3. Multiple ways to operationalize the affective response to a bout of exercise, from averages (during exercise and recovery), to the slope of change, to (positive and negative) "peaks" and "end."

4. Applied Question: Can Affect-Related Messages Supplement the Focus on Health in Activity Promotion Campaigns?

The promise of disease prevention has been and continues to be the center-piece of public health campaigns to promote exercise and physical activity. This argument (i.e., be active now to reduce the risk of chronic disease, disability, and early death in the future) is based on the assumption that humans, being rational creatures, are interested in their health and will, therefore, seek, remember, and use relevant information in making behavioral decisions, such as decisions on how to allocate their discretionary time. Accordingly, it is believed that, if humans are given adequate, accurate, and compellingly presented information about the health benefits of exercise and physical activity, positive behavior change should naturally ensue. Health and exercise psychology adopted this "rationality assumption," as it was fundamentally compatible with the dominant conceptual paradigm of cognitivism.

That human behavior deviates in systematic and predictable ways from rationality was first demonstrated in studies of economic behavior and, more recently, in the context of exercise (Zenko et al., 2016). The bounded nature of human rationality is now acknowledged in medicine and public health, with authors conceding that "[providing] risk information is a weak intervention" and that "information-based approaches to changing behavior are based on partial models of human behavior" (Marteau, 2018, p. 4). The persistent failure to change the percentage of the population in industrialized countries that is regularly physically active is prompting similar acknowledgments in the field of exercise science. Perhaps most prominently, the international Lancet Physical Activity Series Working Group recognized that "the traditional public health approach based on evidence and exhortation has—to some extent—been unsuccessful so far" (Hallal et al., 2012, p. 254). The diplomatic qualifiers "to some extent" and "so far" notwithstanding, this statement is a paradigm-shifting concession that the modus operandi of the past 50 years was misguided.

While a successor paradigm will probably take a while to emerge, promoting exercise and physical activity on the basis of immediate rewards, such as pleasure, enjoyment, and a sense of fulfillment, appears as the most conceptually defensible candidate. According to Shrank and Choudhry (2012), "perhaps we need to find a way to make doing the right thing 'feel good' to patients" (p. 264). This could be accomplished if we could somehow establish a "very basic, subconscious connection between happy feelings and certain behavior" (p. 265). However, at present, comparative evaluations of the current approach based on appeals to rationality (i.e., promising future health benefits) and an approach emphasizing immediate affective rewards are still lacking (Figure 14.4).

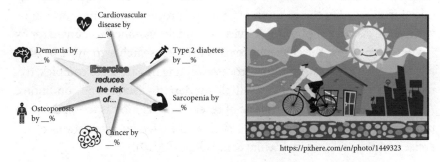

https://pxhere.com/en/photo/1449323

Figure 14.4. Alternative ways to promote exercise and physical activity. The left panel is an example of typical appeals to rationality (i.e., promise of future health benefits using specific numerical information). The right panel is aimed, through repetition, to establish a connection between physical activity and pleasure, without words or numbers.

5. Theoretical Question: How Do Affective and Reflective Processes Interact in Shaping Exercise Behavior?

Emerging theories of exercise and physical activity behavior (Brand & Ekkekakis, 2018; Conroy & Berry, 2017) postulate that these behaviors result from the interaction of two categories of processes, one (called "Type 1") with past affective experiences at its core and another (called "Type 2") with reflective cognition at its core. Predictions when the two categories are concordant are straightforward (i.e., avoidance of exercise when negative reflective evaluations co-occur with negative past affective experiences). The situation is more complex when the two are discordant (e.g., when one believes that exercise will benefit health but is burdened by negative affective experiences).

The interactions between the affective and reflective processes probably cannot be reduced to deriving the algebraic sum of two opposing vectors. The affective-reflective theory (Brand & Ekkekakis, 2018) postulates that the availability of self-control resources may act as a moderator, allowing reflective processes to impose willful plans in the presence of negative urges associated with affective processes (e.g., a person determined to implement a New Year's resolution after years of efforts halted by pain, exhaustion, or embarrassment). On the other hand, when self-control resources are diminished (e.g., under conditions of stress, cognitive load, time pressure), affective processes seize control of behavior. Similar complex interactions are posited by dual-process models proposed in other contexts, such as food choice (e.g., Shiv et al., 2005; Wirz et al., 2018). Within exercise psychology, early studies investigating dual-process models have mostly dealt with the question of whether the addition of "Type 1" processes accounts for unique variance in exercise or physical activity beyond the variance accounted for by "Type 2" processes. The challenge for this line of research is to move beyond models of these two categories of processes acting in parallel to complex, dynamic models that incorporate multiple moderating factors and conditions. A prerequisite to bringing this type of research to fruition is to improve the measurement of "Type 1" processes, such as the affective associations of exercise and physical activity (Zenko & Ekkekakis, 2019).

Conclusion

Over the past two decades, the study of affective responses to exercise has made considerable advances from the days of reiterating the "exercise makes people feel better" mantra. The overhaul of the methodological platform has enabled researchers to delineate the shape of the dose-response relation between exercise intensity and affect. In turn, this has opened the door to investigations and theoretical models that attempt to link the affective experiences of exercise to subsequent behavior. This line of research has the potential to reshape not only exercise psychology (by proposing theoretical models that offer an expanded view of the mechanisms underlying exercise and physical activity behavior) but also exercise science in general (by changing the principles that underlie exercise prescriptions and physical activity recommendations). Certainly, considerable work remains. Hopefully, the questions we have identified here will inspire a new generation of investigators to become involved.

References

Bechara, A., & Damasio, A. R. (2005). The somatic marker hypothesis: A neural theory of economic decision. *Games and Economic Behavior, 52*(2), 336–372. https://doi.org/10.1016/j.geb.2004.06.010

Brand, R., & Ekkekakis, P. (2018). Affective–reflective theory of physical inactivity and exercise: Foundations and preliminary evidence. *German Journal of Exercise and Sport Research, 48*(1), 48–58. https://doi.org/10.1007/s12662-017-0477-9

Conroy, D. E., & Berry, T. R. (2017). Automatic affective evaluations of physical activity. *Exercise and Sport Sciences Reviews, 45*(4), 230–237. https://doi.org/10.1249/JES.0000000000000120

Ekkekakis, P. (2009). Illuminating the black box: Investigating prefrontal cortical hemodynamics during exercise with near-infrared spectroscopy. *Journal of Sport and Exercise Psychology, 31*(4), 505–553. https://doi.org/10.1123/jsep.31.4.505

Ekkekakis, P. (2013). *The measurement of affect, mood, and emotion: A guide for health-behavioral research.* Cambridge University Press.

Ekkekakis, P., Hall, E. E., & Petruzzello, S. J. (2005). Variation and homogeneity in affective responses to physical activity of varying intensities: An alternative perspective on dose-response based on evolutionary considerations. *Journal of Sports Sciences, 23*(5), 477–500. https://doi.org/10.1080/02640410400021492

Ekkekakis, P., Hall, E. E., & Petruzzello, S. J. (2008). The relationship between exercise intensity and affective responses demystified: To crack the 40-year-old nut, replace the 40-year-old nutcracker! *Annals of Behavioral Medicine, 35*(2), 136–149. https://doi.org/10.1007/s12160-008-9025-z

Ekkekakis, P., Hartman, M. E., & Ladwig, M. A. (2020). Affective responses to exercise. In G. Tenenbaum & R. C. Eklund (Eds.), *Handbook of sport psychology* (4th ed., pp. 233–253). Wiley. https://doi.org/10.1002/9781119568124.ch12

Ekkekakis, P., Ladwig, M. A., & Hartman, M. E. (2019). Physical activity and the "feel-good" effect: Challenges in researching the pleasure and displeasure people feel when they exercise. In S. R. Bird (Ed.), *Research methods in physical activity and health* (pp. 210–229). Routledge. https://doi.org/10.4324/9781315158501-20

Ekkekakis, P., Parfitt, G., & Petruzzello, S. J. (2011). The pleasure and displeasure people feel when they exercise at different intensities: Decennial update and progress towards a tripartite rationale for exercise intensity prescription. *Sports Medicine, 41*(8), 641–671. https://doi.org/10.2165/11590680-000000000-00000

Ekkekakis, P., Zenko, Z., & Werstein, K. M. (2018). Exercise in obesity from the perspective of hedonic theory: A call for sweeping change in professional practice norms. In S. Razon & M. L. Sachs (Eds.), *Applied exercise psychology: The challenging journey from motivation to adherence* (pp. 289–315). Routledge. https://doi.org/10.4324/9780203795422-23

Ensari, I., Greenlee, T. A., Motl, R. W., & Petruzzello, S. J. (2015). Meta-analysis of acute exercise effects on state anxiety: An update of randomized controlled trials over the past 25 years. *Depression and Anxiety, 32*(8), 624–634. https://doi.org/10.1002/da.22370

Hallal, P. C., Andersen, L. B., Bull, F. C., Guthold, R., Haskell, W., & Ekelund, U. (2012). Global physical activity levels: Surveillance progress, pitfalls, and prospects. *Lancet, 380*(9838), 247–257. https://doi.org/10.1016/S0140-6736(12)60646-1

Han, L., You, D., Zeng, F., Feng, X., Astell-Burt, T., Duan, S., & Qi, L. (2019). Trends in self-perceived weight status, weight loss attempts, and weight loss strategies among adults in the United States, 1999–2016. *JAMA Network Open, 2*(11), e1915219. https://doi.org/10.1001/jamanetworkopen.2019.15219

Jones, L., Hutchinson, J. C., & Mullin, E. M. (2018). In the zone: An exploration of personal characteristics underlying affective responses to heavy exercise. *Journal of Sport and Exercise Psychology, 40*(5), 249–258. https://doi.org/10.1123/jsep.2017-0360

Kahneman, D. (2000). Evaluation by moments: Past and future. In D. Kahneman & A. Tversky (Eds.), *Choices, values, and frames* (pp. 693–708). Cambridge University Press. https://doi.org/10.1017/CBO9780511803475.039

Lamoureux, N. R., Fitzgerald, J. S., Norton, K. I., Sabato, T., Tremblay, M. S., & Tomkinson, G. R. (2019). Temporal trends in the cardiorespiratory fitness of 2,525,827 adults between 1967 and 2016: A systematic review. *Sports Medicine, 49*(1), 41–55. https://doi.org/10.1007/s40279-018-1017-y

Marteau, T. M. (2018). Changing minds about changing behavior. *Lancet, 391*(10116), 116–117. https://doi.org/10.1016/S0140-6736(17)33324-X

Mezzani, A., Hamm, L. F., Jones, A. M., McBride, P. E., Moholdt, T., Stone, J. A., Urhausen, A., Williams, M. A., European Association for Cardiovascular Prevention and Rehabilitation, American Association of Cardiovascular and Pulmonary Rehabilitation, & Canadian Association of Cardiac Rehabilitation. (2013). Aerobic exercise intensity assessment and prescription in cardiac rehabilitation: A joint position statement of the European Association for Cardiovascular Prevention and Rehabilitation, the American Association of Cardiovascular and Pulmonary Rehabilitation and the Canadian Association of Cardiac Rehabilitation. *European Journal of Preventive Cardiology, 20*(3), 442–467. https://doi.org/10.1177/2047487312460484

Parfitt, G., Alrumh, A., & Rowlands, A. V. (2012). Affect-regulated exercise intensity: Does training at an intensity that feels "good" improve physical health? *Journal of Science and Medicine in Sport, 15*(6), 548–553. https://doi.org/10.1016/j.jsams.2012.01.005

Raichlen, D. A., Pontzer, H., Harris, J. A., Mabulla, A. Z., Marlowe, F. W., Josh Snodgrass, J., Eick, G., Colette Berbesque, J., Sancilio, A., & Wood, B. M. (2017). Physical activity patterns and biomarkers of cardiovascular disease risk in hunter-gatherers. *American*

Journal of Human Biology, *29*(2), 10.1002/ajhb.22919. https://doi.org/10.1002/ajhb.22919

Reed, J., & Ones, D. S. (2006). The effect of acute aerobic exercise on positive activated affect: A meta-analysis. *Psychology of Sport and Exercise*, *7*(5), 477–514. https://doi.org/10.1016/j.psychsport.2005.11.003

Rhodes, R. E., & Kates, A. (2015). Can the affective response to exercise predict future motives and physical activity behavior? A systematic review of published evidence. *Annals of Behavioral Medicine*, *49*(5), 715–731. https://doi.org/10.1007/s12160-015-9704-5

Rose, E. A., & Parfitt, G. (2008). Can the Feeling Scale be used to regulate exercise intensity? *Medicine and Science in Sports and Exercise*, *40*(10), 1852–1860. https://doi.org/10.1249/MSS.0b013e31817a8aea

Saanijoki, T., Tuominen, L., Tuulari, J. J., Nummenmaa, L., Arponen, E., Kalliokoski, K., & Hirvonen, J. (2018). Opioid release after high-intensity interval training in healthy human subjects. *Neuropsychopharmacology*, *43*(2), 246–254. https://doi.org/10.1038/npp.2017.148

Shiv, B., Fedorikhin, A., & Nowlis, S. M. (2005). Interplay of the heart and the mind in decision-making. In S. Ratneshwar & D. G. Mick (Eds.), *Inside consumption: Consumer motives, goals, and desires* (pp. 166–184). Routledge. https://doi.org/10.4324/9780203481295-15

Shrank, W. H., & Choudhry, N. K. (2012). Therapy: Affect and affirmations — A "basic" approach to promote adherence. *Nature Reviews Cardiology*, *9*(5), 263–265. https://doi.org/10.1038/nrcardio.2012.35

Tempest, G. D., Eston, R. G., & Parfitt, G. (2014). Prefrontal cortex haemodynamics and affective responses during exercise: A multi-channel near infrared spectroscopy study. *PLoS ONE*, *9*(5), e95924. https://doi.org/10.1371/journal.pone.0095924

Tucker, J. M., Welk, G. J., & Beyler, N. K. (2011). Physical activity in U.S. adults: Compliance with the physical activity guidelines for Americans. *American Journal of Preventive Medicine*, *40*(4), 454–461. https://doi.org/10.1016/j.amepre.2010.12.016

Williams, D. M., Dunsiger, S., Emerson, J. A., Gwaltney, C. J., Monti, P. M., & Miranda, R., Jr. (2016). Self-paced exercise, affective response, and exercise adherence: A preliminary investigation using ecological momentary assessment. *Journal of Sport and Exercise Psychology*, *38*(3), 282–291. https://doi.org/10.1123/jsep.2015-0232

Wirz, L., Bogdanov, M., & Schwabe, L. (2018). Habits under stress: Mechanistic insights across different types of learning. *Current Opinion in Behavioral Sciences*, *20*, 9–16. https://doi.org/10.1016/j.cobeha.2017.08.009

Zenko, Z., & Ekkekakis, P. (2019). Internal consistency and validity of measures of automatic exercise associations. *Psychology of Sport and Exercise*, *43*, 4–15. https://doi.org/10.1016/j.psychsport.2018.12.005

Zenko, Z., Ekkekakis, P., & Kavetsos, G. (2016). Changing minds: Bounded rationality and heuristic processes in exercise-related judgments and choices. *Sport, Exercise, and Performance Psychology*, *5*(4), 337–351. https://doi.org/10.1037/spy0000069

15

Health Behavior and Exercise Adherence

Selen Razon and Michael Sachs

State of the Art

Behavioral compliance or adherence is a fundamental problem in health care settings in general (Osei-Frimpong, 2017) and within exercise settings in particular (Picha & Howell, 2018). The discipline of exercise psychology is concerned with the biopsychosocial bases of exercise behavior (Razon & Sachs, 2018). The purpose of this chapter is first to review the literature related to theories and research concerning the discipline of exercise psychology. Next, we identify five major unanswered questions within the discipline. These questions revolve around the most commonly studied and least well-understood aspects of exercise behavior and the problem of sustaining adherence to exercise behavior. Specifically, we examine main topic areas related to the antecedents, determinants, consequences, individual differences, and measurement in exercise behavior and exercise adherence. The importance of effectively answering these questions will be discussed in light of the knowledge that low levels of physical activity (PA) are a global concern (Condello et al., 2017) and physical inactivity remains the greatest public health problem of the 21st century (Piggin & Bairner, 2016).

First, regarding the literature in exercise psychology, antecedents (i.e., what precedes) of exercise behavior have been equated to multiple contributors operating at different levels of influence. As such, it is conceptualized that exercise behavior is influenced by social (e.g., social support), biological (e.g., genetic makeup), demographic (e.g., age, education levels, socioeconomic status [SES]), and psychological (e.g., motivational) factors (Teixeira et al., 2012). Particularly relevant to the field of exercise psychology, research on exercise motivation from the perspective of self-determination theory (SDT; Deci & Ryan, 2000) has bourgeoned in recent years. Briefly, SDT postulates that two types of motivation, intrinsic and

Selen Razon and Michael Sachs, *Health Behavior and Exercise Adherence* In: *Sport, Exercise and Performance Psychology*. Edited by: Edson Filho and Itay Basevitch, Oxford University Press. © Oxford University Press 2021. DOI: 10.1093/oso/9780197512494.003.0015 extrinsic, regulate individuals' behaviors. To that end, *intrinsic motivation* governs activities that one does because of their inherent rewards. When intrinsically motivated, the individual feels a sense of enjoyment, excitement, and mastery (Deci & Ryan, 2010). For instance, one can exercise for the associated feelings of enjoyment or for the challenge of participating in an exercise when they are intrinsically motivated. In contrast to intrinsic motivation, *extrinsic motivation* governs activities that are done for instrumental gains, or to achieve some outcome that is separated from the activity itself. For example, one can exercise to earn a tangible or social reward or to avoid disapproval of others when they are extrinsically motivated (Teixeira et al., 2012). Additionally, SDT has introduced the notion of *basic psychological needs*. Specifically, SDT argues that individuals possess three basic psychological needs: (a) a need for autonomy (i.e., feelings of self-sufficiency vs. being controlled), (b) a need for competence (i.e., perception of mastery over a task), and (c) a need for relatedness (i.e., perceptions of personal connection with others). All of these needs are considered essential for the development of intrinsic motivation. As seen in Table 15.1, research has shown consistent support that a sense of autonomy and competence, along with intrinsic and extrinsic motivation, distinctly contributes to initial exercise behavior as well as its long-term sustenance (Teixeira et al., 2012).

Next, with regard to major determinants (i.e., most decisive life factors) of exercise behavior and its long-term adherence, researchers have investigated the role of a large array of lifestyle determinants across several age groups. As seen in Table 15.1, findings suggest that while previous history of activity is positively associated with exercise behavior, other factors such as screen use, smoking, language difficulties, gestation, childrearing, and lack of time are negatively associated with it (Condello et al., 2017).

Of the psychological consequences of exercise behavior, research has mainly revolved around the consequences of exercise on mood states and cognitive functioning. To that end, with regard to anxiety disorders, which are the most prevalent mental disorder (World Health Organization [WHO], 2017), exercise is considered an evidence-based alternative for improving anxiety symptoms among individuals suffering from anxiety disorders (Stubbs et al., 2017; see Table 15.1). With regard to its cognitive effects, research findings indicate that especially at higher intensities (VO_{2max}), acute bouts of exercise result in positive effects on long-term memory consolidation; hence, high-intensity exercise is recommended for preventing cognitive impairments in older adults (Labban & Etnier, 2018). A recent review has also summarized experimental evidence demonstrating the positive effects of exercise on cognitive function (Etnier et al., 2019). These advances are important because, with one new dementia diagnosis every 3 seconds, cognitive decline in the elderly is a key public health concern worldwide (WHO, 2017).

Another important component of this literature pertains to the linkage between exercise behavior research and individual differences. To that end, an underpinning theory is that individuals may feel greater motivation to engage in exercise depending on their personality traits (see Table 15.1). Consequently, drawing upon the classic "Big Five" or the five-factor model (McCrae & John, 1992), personality traits including extraversion (e.g., talkative, assertive, energetic), openness to experience (e.g., intellectual, creative), and conscientiousness (e.g., orderly, responsible, dependable) have been associated with high levels of exercise behavior (Allen et al., 2017).

Last but not least, within the field of exercise psychology, psychometrically sound measures are key for the establishment of effective inferences and the advancement of additional inquiries. It is important to note that sport and exercise psychology is a theoretical and applied discipline at the intersection of psychology and kinesiology/exercise science. As such, measurements used by scientists and applied practitioners are diverse and are either physiological (e.g., heart rate, heart rate variability, power output, galvanic skin response) or psychological in nature (e.g., questionnaires, interviews, observations). Subsequently, perhaps due to its unique position of drawing upon distinct fields, measurement and overall scientific rigor within the field have at times come under scrutiny. For instance, a recent critical review concerning the measurement of exercise behavior and its contributing factors revealed that a large number of published works have failed to follow appropriate measurement and reporting guidelines (Zenko & Ekkekakis, 2019). Ultimately, the authors have advanced recommendations to facilitate better practices in the field (see Table 15.1).

Table 15.1 Five Key Readings in Exercise Psychology

Authors	Methodological Design	Key Findings
Allen et al. (2017)	A sample of 10,227 adults completed self-report measures of physical activity and personality in 2006 (Time 1), 2010 (Time 2), and 2014 (Time 3).	Conscientiousness and openness to experience predicted increases in exercise behavior. Findings indicated that personality is important in considering exercise behavior.
Condello et al. (2017)	Systematic review of 17 empirical studies published from January 2004 to April 2016. A systematic literature review and meta-analysis of observational studies that investigated the behavioral determinants of exercise behavior were conducted.	In preschoolers and children, screen use was negatively associated with overall exercise behavior; the higher the screen use in preschoolers and children, the less physically active they were. In children and adolescents, previous history of exercise was positively associated with overall exercise behavior. In adolescents, current physical education classes and school sports were positively associated with overall exercise behavior. In adults, baseline exercise levels were positively associated with overall exercise behavior. Language difficulties were negatively associated with overall exercise behavior. In older adults, smoking was negatively associated with overall exercise behavior. Across all ages, transitioning into an institution (i.e., middle school, high school, college), gestation, childrearing, and lack of time were negatively associated with overall exercise behavior.
Stubbs et al. (2017)	Meta-analysis of articles published up to December 2015. Altogether, six randomized control trials including 262 adults were analyzed.	Exercise significantly decreased anxiety symptoms in experimental groups with respect to control. Exercise is effective in improving anxiety symptoms in people with a current anxiety disorder diagnosis.

Continued

Table 15.1 *Continued*

Authors	Methodological Design	Key Findings
Teixeira et al. (2012)	Systematic review of 66 empirical studies published until June 2011, including experimental, cross-sectional, and prospective studies that have measured the link between exercise motivation and short-term and long-term exercise behavior.	Perceptions of autonomy predict initial exercise participation and long-term exercise adherence across a range of samples and settings. Well-internalized extrinsic motivations, such as personally valuing certain *outcomes* of exercise (e.g., becoming healthier), are particularly important for initial adoption of exercise. Intrinsic motivation (i.e., valuing the actual *experience* of exercise) is particularly important for long-term adherence to exercise.
Zenko & Ekkekakis (2019)	Critical review of 37 studies in which automatic associations (i.e., implicit attitudes) to sedentary behavior, physical activity, and/or exercise were measured.	Of the 37 studies, 27 (73%) did not include a justification for the measure chosen. Additional problems included the nonreporting of psychometric information (e.g., validity, internal consistency, test-retest reliability) and the lack of standardized procedures. The authors emphasized the need to select measures based on theory, psychometric validity, and reliability, as well as the importance of using standardized measurement protocols.

Questions to Move the Field Forward

1. Applied Question: What Is the Potential of Exercise-Related Technologies and Technology-Supported Exercise Programs to Instill Motivation and Adherence for Long-Term Exercise Behavior?

In light of the information that motivation is a primary antecedent of health behavior change (Suarez & Spaccarotella, 2019), this is the first important question to be addressed in future research. Recently, the use of technologies for exercise has seen a substantial increase (Razon, Wallace, et al., 2019). Today, commercially available wearable physical activity tracking devices and exergaming remain practical tools designed to improve exercise habits (Filho et al., 2018; Filho & Tenenbaum, 2018). To that end, the new generation of activity trackers features properties of both pedometers and accelerometers. They also provide individuals with an easy and affordable way to monitor activity and energy expenditure (Dominick et al., 2016). Similarly to wearable physical activity tracking devices, exergames are technologies that aim to increase individuals' physical activity by requiring them to be physically active in the course of game playing. Therefore, exergames or exergame programs come with gaming qualities (e.g., use of exercise equipment; tailoring to individual's fitness level) that differ from casual video games and aim to promote exercise behavior (Vazquez et al., 2018). However, the evidence with regard to the effectiveness of these technologies to generate/support the motivation needed for long-term exercise behavior change or exercise adherence is mixed at best (Suarez & Spaccarotella, 2019).

From a practical standpoint, it is important to explain whether these technologies instill motivation for long-term exercise behavior. Specifically, evidence-based practice requires decision-making through careful use of the best available evidence gathered from numerous sources to improve the prospect of a positive outcome (Barends et al., 2017). Thus, practitioners who are expected to follow evidence-based practice guidelines are in need of additional evidence regarding the effectiveness of these new tools for long-term behavior change. Furthermore, previous research indicates that the uninformed use of these technologies in exercise interventions may not only preclude individuals from meeting their exercise goals but also result in amotivation and reduced self-efficacy with regard to their exercise behavior (Kerner & Goodyear, 2017).

While these technologies are promoted as ways to motivate people to be active, there is a scarcity of research data about the effectiveness of these approaches to influence exercise motivation for true behavior change (Kerner & Goodyear, 2017). Therefore, consistent with the most recent calls for additional research on the topic (Gell et al., 2020), further large sample size investigations, including individual qualitative approaches for gathering real-person experiences that assess the motivational component of multiple technologies, would best help address the question (Farnell & Barkley, 2017). While doing this, it would also be important to further consider how these technologies impact other perceptions such as self-esteem and self-confidence (Kerner & Goodyear, 2017), all of which exert indirect effects on motivation and behavior change (Bruning & Kauffman, 2016).

2. Applied Question: What Are the Best Strategies to Help Individuals Exercise Initially and Then Exercise Regularly?

The second question for exercise psychology addresses advancing practical applications. This question relates to the determinants of exercise behavior. As previously outlined, amid multiple lifestyle factors (e.g., screen time, previous levels of activity, and smoking) that influence exercise behavior and exercise adherence, can we develop effective and time-efficient strategies to increase exercise behavior? In fact, as recently proposed by the American College of Sports Medicine (ACSM), there is a need to help exercise and health professionals provide practical, innovative, and effective recommendations to individuals who struggle to find ways to exercise (Cohen & Sachs, 2021; Ferguson-Stegall & Robb, 2019).

This is important to address because exercise is a fundamental human need and physical activity interventions typically fail (Guest et al., 2020). In fact, with the ever-increasing prospects of more people becoming sedentary, finding ways to integrate exercise into one's daily life can present substantial challenges. This is perhaps not surprising considering that the percentage of adults getting adequate amounts of exercise remains quite low. Particularly in the United States, recent reviews have reported that only about 20% of adults engage in the recommended amounts of exercise (Clarke et al., 2017). Furthermore, this percentage is known to decrease with age, with about 13% of those 65 years or older engaging in the recommended amounts of physical activity (Clarke et al., 2017).

From a scientist-practitioner standpoint, the best way to address this question is to design practical exercise interventions and test the short- and long-term effectiveness of these interventions in increasing exercise behavior and exercise adherence in sedentary individuals. To that end, consistent with some recent promptings (Ferguson-Stegall & Robb, 2019), practical interventions could focus on setting more realistic goals and helping individuals build less intimidating but workable exercise plans. For instance, for individuals who are busy at work, approaches such as breaking exercise into short bouts and using active workstations, including under-the-desk ellipticals, standing desks, treadmill desks, or even bicycle desks, can facilitate light exercise during the workday—these can all be tested. Similarly, to make time at home more active, interventions to help include exercise into downtime, as well as into a number of household chores, should be tested. These practical interventions to increase active time at home can be diverse, such as taking brisk walks, doing push-ups or squats for every 30 minutes of screen time, holding wall-sits while doing laundry, and having activity challenges and competitions between household members (Cohen & Sachs, 2021). Finally, as an alternative to more traditional forms of exercise, the effectiveness of engaging in and maintaining nontraditional but (to some potentially) more enjoyable forms of exercise such as yoga, active commuting, and active recreation, including age-group sports and partner/social dancing, should be examined.

3. Applied Question: What Are the Preferred Exercise Types That Lead to the Optimal Dose-Response Relationship Between Exercise Practice and Biopsychosocial Effects?

This question addresses the consequences of exercise behavior, in view of practical considerations encompassing the nature of the dose-response relationship. Dose-response relationship can be defined as the relationship between the frequency, intensity, time, and type of exercise and its desired biopsychosocial effects (Lox et al., 2016). Specifically, there is now considerable evidence that exercise exerts positive effects on mood states (Stubbs et al., 2017) and cognition (Labban & Etnier, 2018). Nevertheless, data are still lacking to confirm what type of exercise, as well as its regularity and intensity and duration, are needed to achieve desired outcomes on mental health and cognitive functioning (Chen et al., 2018).

This is important to address because issues such as mood disorders and cognitive decline are prevalent (McIntyre & Carvalho, 2016). Nearly 10% of adults experience a mood disorder in any given year in the United States (National Institute of Mental Health [NIMH], 2017), and almost half of them experience severe symptoms. The prevalence of cognitive decline is 11.1%, or one in nine adults in the United States (Centers for Disease Control and Prevention [CDC], 2019). Cognitive decline costs close to $300 billion per year (Cuyler, 2019). Further complicating the matter, the pharmacological therapy that is typically prescribed for these conditions is associated with multiple negative side effects (Fink et al., 2018). Consequently, exercise therapy that is low in cost and with minimal to no negative side effects could become a viable alternative to conventional therapies. Nevertheless, to best help individuals achieve the psychological benefits associated with exercise, there is a need for clearer guidelines drawn from well-defined dose-response relationships.

Consistent with our previous recommendations, from an evidence-based practice standpoint, additional research is needed to help address this question. Specifically, there is a need for further rigorous studies to test the effectiveness of exercise either as a main or adjunct treatment to mood disorders and cognitive decline. To that end, while keeping in mind that, most likely, a balance between aerobic and anaerobic exercise would provide the most health benefits, research is still needed to determine the most effective type, duration, frequency, and intensity of exercise for individuals with these conditions. Studies should also test personalized exercise strategies, since it is possible that different individuals will benefit more from specific types and duration of exercise and, thus, advancing recommendations based upon one's clinical features and individual responses could boost treatment efficacy in these conditions. Prospective studies with follow-up, including a large number of participants, are essential to clarify the effects of particular exercise prescriptions specifically with regard to clinical populations (Teixeira et al., 2012).

4. Applied Question: How to Prescribe the Best Exercise "Training" According to Personal Characteristics?

With regard to individual characteristics and the influences they exert on exercise behavior, another key practical question is how to best combine the numerous individual variables each person presents and provide people with prescriptions that will maximize their exercise participation and adherence. Individual characteristics include, but are not limited to, gender, age, SES, educational level, religion, race/ethnicity, relationship status, employment status, comorbidities, children, past experience with/adherence to exercise, and perhaps even personality traits such as introversion, extroversion, neuroticism, openness to experience, and contentiousness. Subsequently, there is a considerable challenge to synthesize all of this information into one meaningful prescription that will work for people in both acute and chronic terms. Ideally, research would allow us to advance more refined algorithms that would enable plugging in data on these various factors to establish an exercise prescription for a given individual. However, it is unlikely we will see this in the near future.

Nevertheless, this is still an important question to address because these differences can affect perceived barriers and motivations for participation and adherence (Cohen & Sachs, 2021; Razon & Sachs, 2018). Furthermore, given the low adherence rates to exercise even in highly structured clinical re-habilitation settings (Jansons et al., 2017), there may be a need to reconsider the priorities that guide the conventional ways to prescribe exercise and how much of the individual and their uniqueness to consider. Perhaps the idea of an advanced individualized exercise prescription could be best understood in light of recent approaches in medicine. Individualized precision medicine that is gaining popularity (Klein & Foroud, 2017) considers one's unique ge-netic makeup and genetic expression as well as their map of hormones prior to prescribing therapies (Moyer et al., 2019). Similarly to precision medicine, more advanced personalized exercise prescriptions can consider a number of factors such as individuals' genotype, phenotype, current training status, and nutritional intake (Swinton et al., 2018).

Furthermore, clinicians and practitioners may assume a more active role in administering a concise demographic intake initially and following up with prompts related to the person's preferences, history of exercise adher-ence, and current circumstances related to work, family, children, child care, financial resources, etc., and attempt to maximize the effectiveness of exer-cise recommendations. To that end, rather than overcomplicating matters, one could even simply inquire about what the person likes in terms of phys-ical activity because, in exercise as well, individuals stick with what they like to do. Additionally, focusing on the term *physical activity*, especially physical activities that are fun for the individual, may likely serve as the basic/critical element to increase exercise participation and adherence. Such an approach would also prevent practitioners from getting "in trouble" by focusing too much on the terms *exercise* and *sport*, which may be negatively value laden for some individuals (Ciaccio & Sachs, 2018). In summary, drawing upon this question/need, with exercise being a volitional activity for most indi-viduals (Ryan & Deci, 2017), practitioners would maximize effectiveness for increasing exercise behavior by recommending activities that people enjoy but that also align with their unique characteristics.

5. Methodological Question: What Are the Best Methods to Conduct Applied Research in the Exercise and Physical Activity Domain?

The last question that needs to be addressed is a methodological one. To that end, it is important to note that, to bridge the research-practice gap, the field of sport and exercise psychology typically conducts applied research (Keegan et al., 2017). Applied research aims to solve specific, practical problems affecting an individual or a group (e.g., does mental imagery improve exercise performance?). Basic research, on the other hand, is a systematic methodology that aims to further the understanding of fundamental aspects of a phenomenon and of observable facts (e.g., which neural pathways are involved in mental imagery during exercise?) (Thomas et al., 2015). This said, experimental research commonly favors controlled environments with carefully manipulated variables and well-designed conditions that relate to the phenomena under consideration. Nevertheless, the world of applied research can be complex and rather disorganized, since it involves real-life situations, with uncontrolled and weakly defined variables. As a result, with applied paradigms, researchers often witness variables that behave in ways that challenge the basic assumptions of research (Keegan et al., 2017). In light of this information, an imminent question to address is how to conduct high-quality and rigorous applied research in the field.

To reiterate, this is an important question to address because applied researchers may need to operate within a messy environment with limited control. Nevertheless, research that is messy and with limited scientific rigor is reckless (Hofseth, 2018). To that end, problems of rigor are not new to the field of sport and exercise psychology. A number of recent inquiries have called upon the ever-increasing need to improve rigor within the field (Razon, Lebeau, et al., 2019; Smith & McGannon, 2018). Consequently, it is only through increased rigor and high-quality research that we could (a) improve applied practices to deliver positive outcomes, (b) enrich training of applied practitioners, (c) enhance the field's liability and transparency and, ultimately, (d) increase the credibility of the field as a whole (Keegan et al., 2017).

The best way to address this question is by following recent recommendations for increasing rigor in research coming from the field. For instance, in qualitative frameworks, recent recommendations (McGannon et al., 2019) for increasing rigor have strongly suggested that researchers in the field should (a) acknowledge that exploring one's experiences can be done through more than just interviews and that the field needs to go beyond individual interviews and use additional qualitative research methods, such as focus groups, narrative inquiry, and case studies; (b) go beyond interrater reliability and member checking by considering other rigor methods (e.g., social reliability, critical friends, peer review, intercoder guidelines, member reflections, synthesized and dialogic member checking); and (c) ensure that epistemologies also align with contemporary forms of rigor and trustworthiness with regard to the notion of epistemological coherence. Lastly, consistent with the general recommendations for strengthening the practice of scientific research in exercise and sport sciences (Halperin et al., 2018), quantitative research in the field would benefit from (a) increased validity of used measures, (b) more longitudinal designs, (c) further replication of previous findings, and (d) higher reporting of trivial and/or nonsignificant results.

Conclusion

Although the psychology of exercise must be considered to gain a greater understanding of the human experience of exercise, including response to exercise and associated outcomes, investigation and application of this knowledge are still in a bourgeoning stage. From a broader perspective, while there is a general understanding in terms of how the psychological and biological interact to influence each other over the course of exercise, there are still many questions we have to address. We are confident that through the habit of scientific inquiry and an evidence-based mindset, researchers and practitioners will come to address these questions and help advance the understanding of the psychology of exercise.

References

Allen, M. S., Magee, C. A., Vella, S. A., & Laborde, S. (2017). Bidirectional associations between personality and physical activity in adulthood. *Health Psychology, 36*, 332–336. https://doi.org/10.1037/hea0000371

Barends, E., Villanueva, J., Rousseau, D. M., Briner, R. B., Jepsen, D. M., Houghton, E., & Ten Have, S. (2017). Managerial attitudes and perceived barriers regarding evidence-based practice: An international survey. *PloS ONE, 12*(10), e0184594. doi:10–1371/journal.pone.0184594

Bruning, R., & Kauffman, D. (2016). Self-efficacy beliefs and motivation in writing development. In C. MacArthur, S. Graham, & J. Fitzgerald (Eds.), *Handbook of writing research* (pp. 160–173). The Guilford Press.

Centers for Disease Control and Prevention (CDC). (2019). Subjective cognitive decline: A public health issue. https://www.cdc.gov/aging/data/subjective-cognitive-decline-brief.html

Chen, F. T., Etnier, J. L., Wu, C. H., Cho, Y. M., Hung, T. M., & Chang, Y. K. (2018). Dose-response relationship between exercise duration and executive function in older adults. *Journal of Clinical Medicine, 7*, 279. https://doi.org/10.3390/jcm7090279

Ciaccio, J. B., & Sachs, M. L. (2018). A rose by any other name . . . . In S. Razon & M. L. Sachs (Eds.), *Applied exercise psychology: the challenging journey from motivation to adherence* (pp. 15–19). Routledge.

Clarke, T. C., Norris, T., & Schiller, J. S. (2017). Early release of selected estimates based on data from the 2016 National Health Interview Survey. *National Center for Health Statistics.* http://www.bobmorrison.org/wp-content/uploads/2017/01/cdc-report-on-uninsured-and-other-population-stats.pdf

Cohen, B., & Sachs, M. L. (2021). *Excusercise: Inexcusable excuses for not exercising.* Excusercise Publications.

Condello, G., Puggina, A., Aleksovska, K., Buck, C., Burns, C., Cardon, G., Carlin, A., Simon, C., Ciarapica, D., Coppinger, T., Cortis, C., D'Haese, S., De Craemer, M., Di Blasio, A., Hansen, S., Iacoviello, L., Issartel, J., Izzicupo, P., Jaeschke, L., . . . Boccia, S. (2017). Behavioral determinants of physical activity across the life course: A "determinants of diet and physical activity" (DEDIPAC) umbrella systematic literature review. *International Journal of Behavioral Nutrition and Physical Activity, 14,* 58. https://doi.org–10.1186/s12966-017-0510-2

Cuyler, R. (2019). Estimating the direct and indirect costs of dementia. Care, planning, lifestyle research. https://braincheck.com/blog/costs-of-dementia

Deci, E. L., & Ryan, R. M. (2000). The "what" and "why" of goal pursuits: Human needs and the self-determination of behavior. *Psychological Inquiry, 11,* 227–268. https://doi.org/10.1207/S15327965PLI1104_01

Deci, E. L., & Ryan, R. M. (2010). Intrinsic motivation. In I. B. Weiner & W. E. Craighead (Eds.), *The Corsini encyclopedia of psychology* (pp. 1–2). John Wiley & Sons.

Dominick, G. M., Winfree, K. N., Pohlig, R. T., & Papas, M. A. (2016). Physical activity assessment between consumer-and research-grade accelerometers: A comparative study in free-living conditions. *JMIR mHealth and uHealth, 4,* e110. doi:10.2196/mhealth.6281

Etnier, J. L., Drollette, E. S., & Slutsky, A. B. (2019). Physical activity and cognition: A narrative review of the evidence for older adults. *Psychology of Sport and Exercise, 42,* 156–166. https://doi.org/10.1016/j.psychsport.2018.12.006

Farnell, G., & Barkley, J. (2017). The effect of a wearable physical activity monitor (Fitbit One) on physical activity behavior in women: A pilot study. *Journal of Human Sport and Exercise, 12,* 1230–1237. doi:10.14198/jhse.2017.124.09

Ferguson-Stegall, L., & Robb, J. D. (2019). Effective strategies to increase physical activity in the working years. *ACSM's Health and Fitness Journal, 23,* 26–33. doi:10.1249/FIT.0000000000000508

Filho, E., di Fronso, S., Robazza, C., & Bertollo, M. (2018). Exergaming. In S. Razon & M. L. Sachs (Eds.), *Applied exercise psychology: The challenging journey from motivation to adherence* (pp. 122–134). Routledge.

Filho, E., & Tenenbaum, G. (2018). Advanced technological trends in exercise psychology. In S. Razon & M. L. Sachs (Eds.), *Applied exercise psychology: The challenging journey from motivation to adherence* (pp. 111–121). Routledge.

Fink, H. A., Jutkowitz, E., McCarten, J. R., Hemmy, L. S., Butler, M., Davila, H., Ratner, E., Calvert, C., Barclay, T. R., Brasure, M., Nelson, V. A., & Kane, R. L. (2018). Physical activity interventions to prevent cognitive decline, mild cognitive impairment, and clinical Alzheimer-type dementia: A systematic review. *Annals of Internal Medicine, 168,* 30–38. doi:10.7326/M17-1528

Gell, N. M., Grover, K. W., Savard, L., & Dittus, K. (2020). Outcomes of a text message, Fitbit, and coaching intervention on physical activity maintenance among cancer survivors: A randomized control pilot trial. *Journal of Cancer Survivorship, 14*, 80–88. https://doi.org/10.1007/s11764-019-00831-4

Guest, C., Guest, D. D., & Smith-Coggins, R. (2020). How to care for the basics: Sleep, nutrition, exercise, and health. In L. W. Roberts (Ed.), *Roberts academic medicine handbook* (pp. 571–580). Springer.

Halperin, I., Vigotsky, A. D., Foster, C., & Pyne, D. B. (2018). Strengthening the practice of exercise and sport-science research. *International Journal of Sports Physiology and Performance, 13*, 127–134.

Hofseth, L. J. (2018). Getting rigorous with scientific rigor. *Carcinogenesis, 39*, 21–25. https://doi.org/10.1093/carcin/bgx085

Jansons, P. S., Haines, T. P., & O'Brien, L. (2017). Interventions to achieve ongoing exercise adherence for adults with chronic health conditions who have completed a supervised exercise program: Systematic review and meta-analysis. *Clinical Rehabilitation, 31*, 465–477. https://doi.org/10.1177/0269215516653995

Kerner, C., & Goodyear, V. A. (2017). The motivational impact of wearable healthy lifestyle technologies: A self-determination perspective on Fitbits with adolescents. *American Journal of Health Education, 48*, 287–297. https://doi.org/10.1080/19325037.2017.1343161

Klein, C. J., & Foroud, T. M. (2017). Neurology individualized medicine: When to use next-generation sequencing panels. *Mayo Clinic Proceedings, 92*, 292–305. https://doi.org/10.1016/j.mayocp.2016.09.008

Labban, J. D., & Etnier, J. L. (2018). The effect of acute exercise on encoding and consolidation of long-term memory. *Journal of Sport and Exercise Psychology, 40*, 336–342. https://doi.org/10.1123/jsep.2018-0072

Lox, C. L., Ginis, K. A. M., & Petruzzello, S. J. (2016). *The psychology of exercise: Integrating theory and practice*. Routledge.

Keegan, R. J., Cotteril, S., Woolway, T., Appaneal, R., & Hutter, V. (2017). Strategies for bridging the research-practice "gap" in sport and exercise psychology. *Revista de Psicología del Deporte, 26*, 75–80.

McCrae, R. R., & John, O. P. (1992). An introduction to the five-factor model and its applications. *Journal of Personality, 60*, 175–215. https://doi.org/10.1111/j.1467-6494.1992.tb00970.x

McGannon, K. R., Smith, B., Kendellen, K., & Gonsalves, C. A. (2019). Qualitative research in six sport and exercise psychology journals between 2010 and 2017: An updated and expanded review of trends and interpretations. *International Journal of Sport and Exercise Psychology, 17*, 1–21. https://doi.org/10.1080/1612197X.2019.1655779

McIntyre, R. S., & Carvalho, A. F. (2016). Mood disorders and general medical comorbidities: Shared biology and novel therapeutic targets. *Current Molecular Medicine, 16*, 104–105.

Moyer, A. M., Matey, E. T., & Miller, V. M. (2019). Individualized medicine: Sex, hormones, genetics, and adverse drug reactions. *Pharmacology Research & Perspectives, 7*, e00541.

National Institute of Mental Health (NIMH). (2017). Any mood disorders. https://www.nimh.nih.gov/health/statistics/any-mood-disorder.shtml

Osei-Frimpong, K. (2017). Patient participatory behaviors in healthcare service delivery: Self- determination theory (SDT) perspective. *Journal of Service Theory and Practice, 27*, 453–474. https://doi.org/10.1108/JSTP-02-2016-0038

Picha, K. J., & Howell, D. M. (2018). A model to increase rehabilitation adherence to home exercise programs in patients with varying levels of self-efficacy. *Musculoskeletal Care, 16*, 233–237. https://doi.org/10.1002/msc.1194

Piggin, J., & Bairner, A. (2016). The global physical inactivity pandemic: An analysis of knowledge production. *Sport, Education and Society, 21*, 131–147. https://doi.org/10.1080/13573322.2014.882301

Razon, S., Lebeau, J. C., Basevitch, I., Foster, B., Akpan, A., Mason, J., Boiangin, N., & Tenenbaum, G. (2019). Effects of acute exercise on executive functioning: Testing the moderators. *International Journal of Sport and Exercise Psychology, 17*, 303–320. https://doi.org/10.1080/1612197X.2017.1349821

Razon, S., & Sachs, M. L. (Eds.). (2018). *Applied exercise psychology: The challenging journey from motivation to adherence*. Routledge.

Razon, S., Wallace, A., Ballesteros, J., Koontz, N., Judge, L. W., & Montoye, A. H. (2019). Perceptions of physical activity tracking devices: A survey analysis. *Physical Educator, 76*, 258–284. doi:10.18666/TPE-2019-V76-I1-8470

Ryan, R. M., & Deci, E. L. (2017). *Self-determination theory: Basic psychological needs in motivation, development, and wellness*. Guilford Press.

Smith, B., & McGannon, K. R. (2018). Developing rigor in qualitative research: Problems and opportunities within sport and exercise psychology. *International Review of Sport and Exercise Psychology, 11*, 101–121. https://doi.org/10.1080/1750984X.2017.1317357

Stubbs, B., Vancampfort, D., Rosenbaum, S., Firth, J., Cosco, T., Veronese, N., Salum, G. A., & Schuch, F. B. (2017). An examination of the anxiolytic effects of exercise for people with anxiety and stress-related disorders: A meta-analysis. *Psychiatry Research, 249*, 102–108. https://doi.org/10.1016/j.psychres.2016.12.020

Suarez, E., & Spaccarotella, K. (2019). Effects of Fitbit use on physical activity in cardiac rehabilitation patients. *Graduate Journal of Sport, Exercise & Physical Education Research, 10*, 26–36.

Swinton, P. A., Hemingway, B. S., Saunders, B., Gualano, B., & Dolan, E. (2018). A statistical framework to interpret individual response to intervention: Paving the way for personalized nutrition and exercise prescription. *Frontiers in Nutrition, 5*, 41.

Teixeira, P. J., Carraça, E. V., Markland, D., Silva, M. N., & Ryan, R. M. (2012). Exercise, physical activity, and self-determination theory: A systematic review. *International Journal of Behavioral Nutrition and Physical Activity, 9*, 78. https://doi.org/10.1186/1479-5868-9-78

Thomas, J. R., Nelson, J. K., & Silverman, S. J. (2015). *Research methods in physical activity* (5th ed.). Human Kinetics.

Vazquez, F. L., Otero, P., García-Casal, J. A., Blanco, V., Torres, A. J., & Arrojo, M. (2018). Efficacy of video game-based interventions for active aging. A systematic literature review and meta-analysis. *PloS ONE, 13*(12), e0208192. doi:10.1371/journal.pone.0208192

World Health Organization. (2017). Global action plan on the public health response to dementia: 2017–2025. https://apps.who.int/gb/ebwha/pdf_files/EB140/B140_28-en.pdf?ua=1

Zenko, Z., & Ekkekakis, P. (2019). Critical review of measurement practices in the study of automatic associations of sedentary behavior, physical activity, and exercise. *Journal of Sport and Exercise Psychology, 41*, 271–288. https://doi.org/10.1123/jsep.2017-0349

16

Mindfulness in Exercise Psychology

Sarah Ullrich-French and Anne E. Cox

State of the Art

Mindfulness is a popular construct currently applied in a wide variety of contexts to support health behaviors and general well-being. Empirical evidence supports many health benefits of mindful movement (e.g., yoga, tai chi) and is beginning to support the role that mindfulness may play in exercise motivational processes and behavior (Cox, Ullrich-French, & Austin, 2020). As such, mindfulness is emerging as a potential pathway to positive exercise experiences. Mindfulness is increasingly used as a strategy to support sport performance, and this also represents an important area of research (e.g., Noetel et al., 2019) but falls outside the scope of this chapter. This chapter addresses current research on mindfulness within the context of exercise.

When defining mindfulness, there is general consensus on two key aspects (Bishop et al., 2004; Kabat-Zinn, 2003). The first reflects attention to and awareness of the present moment. Awareness reflects consciousness of both internal and external stimuli. Internal awareness can include the breath, thoughts, emotions, or muscular engagement while moving. Perceiving one's environment via sensory input reflects external awareness. Within awareness, one may focus or concentrate on one particular stimulus or allow many stimuli to pass in and out of awareness. The second key element is an attitude of openness, receptivity, curiosity, nonjudgment, and acceptance. Awareness and attention that are nonreactive and accepting create an optimal state of vividness and clarity that allows for optimal psychological functioning (Brown & Ryan, 2003).

Mindfulness can be considered as a generalized trait or as a state. Trait mindfulness reflects a tendency or disposition toward being mindful across a range of daily activities and over time. State mindfulness reflects the degree of mindfulness in a specific situation. Thus, there are interindividual

Sarah Ullrich-French and Anne E. Cox, *Mindfulness in Exercise Psychology* In: *Sport, Exercise and Performance Psychology*. Edited by: Edson Filho and Itay Basevitch, Oxford University Press. © Oxford University Press 2021.
DOI: 10.1093/oso/9780197512494.003.0016

differences in trait mindfulness and intraindividual differences in state mind-fulness across situations or over time. Trait and state mindfulness have been distinguished empirically by differential prediction of well-being outcomes (Brown & Ryan, 2003) and motivation variables in the context of physical ac-tivity (Cox, Ullrich-French, & Austin, 2020).

The majority of mindfulness research in the context of exercise has exam-ined the role of trait mindfulness. Overall, this research has demonstrated consistent associations between trait mindfulness and exercise-related cognitions and emotions (see Schneider et al., 2019). For example, higher trait mindfulness is linked to higher autonomous forms of motivation (Kang et al., 2017; Ruffault et al., 2016) and satisfaction with physical activity (Tsafou et al., 2016, 2017). The relationship between trait mindfulness and exercise behavior has been less consistent (Kang et al., 2017; Kangasniemi et al., 2015) but has shown small effects with self-reported physical activity (Tsafou et al., 2017) and physical activity maintenance (Ulmer et al., 2010).

Mindfulness within the context of exercise may hold more relevance to exercise-related experiences compared to trait mindfulness due to being more proximal to the outcomes of interest, such as exercise-related affect, cognitions, and motives. Because state mindfulness varies across activi-ties (Brown & Ryan, 2003), Tsafou et al. (2016) created the Mindfulness in Physical Activity Scale ("When I am doing physical activity, I am aware of what I am doing"). Mindfulness contextualized to physical activity was mod-erately and positively related to physical activity, while trait mindfulness was not (Tsafou et al., 2016). In a follow-up study, mindfulness contextualized to physical activity was found to mediate the relationship between trait mind-fulness and physical activity (Tsafou et al., 2017). In both studies, contextual mindfulness was positively associated with satisfaction with physical ac-tivity. However, there is no evidence supporting the psychometric properties of the contextualized measure nor other examples of exercise-contextualized assessments of mindfulness.

The degree to which individuals are mindful while engaging in a specific physical activity is a more precise window into exercise experiences than either trait or contextualized mindfulness. Using two items to assess state mindfulness, Yang and Conroy (2018) found that within-person affective experiences assessed through ecological momentary assessment varied as a function of state mindfulness, specifically that lower negative affect was re-ported while moving and being more mindful than while sitting or reporting less mindfulness. However, these results were based on two items from a general measure of state mindfulness not designed for exercise. To address the need for measurement designed for the physical activity context, the State Mindfulness Scale for Physical Activity (SMS-PA; Cox, Ullrich-French, & French, 2016) was developed. The SMS-PA, based on Tanay and Bernstein's (2013) State Mindfulness Scale, originally assessed mental (e.g., thoughts, emotions) and physical (e.g., physical sensations) targets of mindfulness. The SMS-PA expanded the number of items capturing awareness of bodily movement and sensation to increase salience to physical activity. The SMS-PA can be used as a single score or as two subscales reflecting mindfulness of the mind and mindfulness of the body. Findings are most consistent for the state mindfulness of the body scale, including robust associations with higher intrinsic motivation for physical activity, psychological need satisfaction, and body appreciation and lower body appearance concerns (Cox, Ullrich-French, & French, 2016; Cox, Ullrich-French, Cole, & D'Hondt-Taylor, 2016; Cox, Ullrich-French, & Austin, 2020). The SMS-PA has also been shown to successfully discriminate mindfulness conditions as a manipulation check in experimental studies (Cox, Ullrich-French, Tylka, et al., 2020; Cox, Ullrich-French, Hargreaves, & McMahon, 2020). Given the infancy of this work, it is clear that the ability to adequately assess a hierarchy of trait, contextual, and state mindfulness will be helpful for furthering this research (Yang & Conroy, in press).

There has been inconsistent and often no use of theory in mindfulness-based research relative to physical activity or exercise. However, mindfulness aligns well with several popular theories that are used to explain motivation and positive exercise experiences, including self-determination theory (SDT) and dual-process models. Articulation for how mindfulness can facilitate autonomous motivation was introduced over 40 years ago by Deci and Ryan (1980), who described how characteristics of mindfulness disrupt maladaptive automatic and reactive patterns and allow an individual to make decisions aligned with values, needs, and interests that support psychological needs for competence and autonomy. Empirical tests of specific SDT theoretical propositions are limited. Dual-process models (e.g., Brand & Ekkakakis, 2018) addresses the distinction between explicit (cognitive) and implicit (affective) processes and suggest that implicit processes will dominate when sufficient self-regulation is lacking. Evidence supports significant predictive capability of implicit processes (e.g., pleasure experienced during an activity) leading to increasing emphasis on understanding the quality of the physical activity experience and strategies for maximizing pleasure during exercise.

Dual-process models provide a framework for better understanding how state and trait mindfulness support positive affective experiences during exercise.

Mindful movement is a deliberate practice of fully experiencing physical activity through "whole practice," where one objectively self-observes core elements of physical movement, breathing, feelings, and thoughts (Asztalos et al., 2012). Combining mindfulness with movement is found in activities such as yoga, tai chi, qigong, and Feldenkrais. One of the most popular forms of mindful movement is yoga (Clarke et al., 2018), where intentional cues often direct nonjudgmental attention to the physical and psychological experience, thereby supporting emotional regulation and distress tolerance. Strong evidence supports positive outcomes of yoga that encompass both physical and psychological wellness (Chu et al., 2016; Cox, Ullrich-French, Tylka, Cook-Cottone, & Neumark-Sztainer, 2020; Cox, Ullrich-French, Cole, & D'Hondt-Taylor, 2016; Klatte et al., 2016) even over and above mindful practice without movement (Hunt et al., 2018).

The positive associations between mindfulness and exercise-related variables as well as the positive outcomes of mindful movement have led to a wide variety of mindfulness-based interventions. There is robust support for the effectiveness of incorporating mindfulness into acceptance-based interventions (e.g., mindfulness-based stress reduction [MBSR], acceptance and commitment theory [ACT], and self-compassion) to positively influence exercise behavior (Meyer et al., 2018; Palmeira et al., 2017). However, there are wide inconsistencies in intervention duration, session length, delivery, content, and follow-up. In a recent systematic review of the role of mindfulness in physical activity, 40 studies were included, 19 were cross-sectional, and only one received a quality rating as "strong" (Schneider et al., 2019). The review revealed more consistent effects of mindfulness on psychological outcomes (e.g., satisfaction, motivation, affect) than on physical activity behaviors (Schneider et al., 2019). Mindfulness and physical activity behavior may be indirectly associated with and mediated by other psychological or physiological factors. More rigorous methodology and application of theory will be needed to establish reliable effects of mindfulness interventions and understanding of mechanisms of influence.

There is growing interest in mindfulness, including in exercise contexts. The research evidence is supportive of the use of mindfulness as a strategy to enhance exercise-related outcomes as well as mindful movement to play a key role in enhancing mindfulness skills and positive well-being (see

Table 16.1 Five Key Readings in Mindfulness Related to Exercise Psychology

Authors	Methodological Design	Key Findings
Cox et al. (2020)	Longitudinal cohort design (16-week yoga class)	Increases in state mindfulness predict increases in autonomous motivation directly and indirectly through psychological need satisfaction.
Hunt et al. (2018)	Randomized control; five treatment groups with active and inactive control groups	All active treatments resulted in decreased anxiety compared to inactive control. Both yoga alone and combined with mindfulness training led to the most adaptive responses to a stress challenge.
Ruffault et al. (2016)	Cross-sectional study	Trait mindfulness moderates (strengthens) the positive relationship between intrinsic motivation for exercise and self-report physical activity.
Schneider et al. (2019)	Systematic review	Mindfulness-based interventions (MBIs) do not conclusively lead to increased physical activity behavior. Future MBIs should be physical activity specific and target psychological factors that sustain physical activity using rigorous longitudinal and experimental designs.
Yang & Conroy (2018)	Smartphone-based 14-day experience sampling design across life contexts	Lower momentary negative affect was reported while moving and being more mindful than when sitting or being less mindful.

Ullrich-French & Cox, 2020, for a review). Table 16.1 identifies five key readings; however, there is much to learn about mindfulness in exercise and we pose some key questions to move our understanding forward.

Questions to Move the Field Forward

1. Theoretical Question: What Are the Processes by Which State and Trait Mindfulness Support Physical Activity Behavior?

Although a number of studies have now shown that state and trait mindfulness associate positively with exercise-related cognitions, motivation, and behavior, they are often lacking a clear theoretical foundation or deeper exploration of the processes explaining the connection. It is critical to understand different processes because they will inform appropriate mindfulness interventions that are aimed at supporting positive exercise experiences. For example, this knowledge will help answer the question of whether time is best spent cultivating general mindfulness skills that will enhance dispositional mindfulness or creating contexts that facilitate state mindfulness during exercise. The pathways by which trait and state mindfulness support exercise behavior may be independent, overlap to some degree, or interact with one another. Investigating these pathways will require studies grounded in theory that systematically build upon each other.

Dual-mode models, monitor and acceptance theory (MAT), and SDT are but a few frameworks with which to begin these investigations. For example, bringing attention to present-moment exercise experiences may help individuals gain awareness of the naturally pleasant sensations of exercising, supporting the implicit processes in dual-mode models. Consistent with MAT (Lindsay & Creswell, 2017), the acceptance part of state mindfulness may also help lower affective reactivity, allowing individuals to be more accepting of unpleasant physical or mental experiences while exercising. Heightened attention coupled with lower reactivity may then afford individuals the mental space and clarity to make decisions during their exercise session that best support their feelings of competence and autonomy, critical antecedents of intrinsic motivation according to SDT. These theoretical perspectives provide a springboard from which to conduct future examinations of how state mindfulness during exercise supports positive exercise experiences and behavior.

Trait mindfulness, on the other hand, may facilitate exercise behavior for the very simple reason that it leads to more frequent state mindfulness while exercising, demonstrating overlapping. There is some evidence for this relationship in the general psychology literature and in the context of physical activity (Cox et al., 2020). On the other hand, although trait mindfulness may increase the experience of state mindfulness during exercise, one can experience state mindfulness even in the absence of strong trait mindfulness, demonstrating independent pathways. In addition, state mindfulness may have differential effects for those higher or lower in trait mindfulness, reflecting an interaction effect. There may also be unique pathways connecting trait mindfulness to exercise behavior and experiences. For example, greater mindfulness in everyday life may increase one's awareness of the desire to exercise and the clarity with which to meet one's physical needs in this way and make the decision to exercise. Trait mindfulness may also associate with the types of goals that facilitate exercise behavior (e.g., more internalized goals). Finally, we need to examine how trait mindfulness impacts state mindfulness during exercise and how being mindful during exercise impacts trait mindfulness over time. Conducting theoretically grounded studies that are intentional about investigating state or trait mindfulness or both will better illuminate the processes by which mindfulness facilitates positive exercise experiences.

2. Theoretical Question: What Are the Key Moderators of Mindfulness?

We know that mindfulness is a complex, multidimensional construct. We also know that constructs do not exist in a vacuum, but exist alongside a host of other psychological, social, physical, and contextual factors. While research consistently reports on adaptive associations and effects of mindfulness on psychological factors related to physical activity, there are examples of null and mixed findings, particularly for behavioral outcomes, that suggest there are confounding or moderating factors to consider alongside mindfulness. It is imperative to consider who may benefit more or less from mindfulness intervention. Neuroticism (Norris et al., 2018) and distress tolerance (Hsin Hsu et al., 2013) have been found to moderate the effects of mindfulness interventions and support the need for more exploration of moderators of mindfulness in the context of exercise. Moderators can be used to explain how exposure to mindfulness may not lead to the same benefits for all. Studies have begun to explore mediators to explain the effects of mindfulness on physical activity, such as satisfaction and stress (Tsafou et al., 2017). However, exploration of potential moderators of the effect of mindfulness on exercise outcomes is lacking.

One potential moderating variable pertains to the experience of the person relative to physical activity broadly or the specific activity being examined. For example, those with more experience with yoga or meditation report higher state mindfulness during exercise (e.g., Cox, Ullrich-French, & French, 2016). Furthermore, those who participate in more physical activity report higher state mindfulness compared to those who do none to occasional activity (Ullrich-French et al., 2017). Whether there are only differences in level of mindfulness or whether mindfulness may associate differently with outcomes has yet to be explored in an exercise context. One assumption requiring testing is that more experience being physically active and more experience practicing a particular skill should lead to better body awareness and insight and may thus set the stage for stronger effects of mindfulness. Some evidence suggests trait mindfulness could be a moderator of the relationship between intrinsic motivation and physical activity behavior (Ruffault et al., 2016). However, we have not found being higher in trait mindfulness to be a necessary component for achieving the motivational benefits of being mindful during exercise (Cox et al., 2020). Research specifically testing whether trait mindfulness moderates the effects of a mindfulness intervention is needed. Drawing from research in other contexts (e.g., Norris et al., 2018; Hsin Hsu et al., 2013), there likely are inter- and intraindividual differences that may moderate the effects of mindfulness on exercise.

To more fully understand the unique role of mindfulness in physical activity, we need to consider what the primary moderating variables are that may dampen or magnify the impact of mindfulness. Consideration of such factors is important to more reliably understand the role of mindfulness and to better design interventions and practical applications of mindfulness. To accomplish this, several types of studies will be necessary. First, descriptive work that explores a wide range of potential moderators will need to take place to provide foundational descriptive evidence for which moderators to explore more deeply. Next, well-planned rigorous experimental studies with strong measurement will be needed that properly assess the relevant aspects of mindfulness as well as the moderator. Such research will need adequate power to detect moderation and capture adequate variability in both mindfulness and the respective moderator.

3. Methodological Question: What Considerations Need to Be Taken When Designing Studies to Test the Role of Mindfulness During Exercise?

Despite quickly expanding research on mindfulness in exercise, there are relatively few rigorous study designs (Schneider et al., 2019). For example, an increasing number of studies are employing experimental designs to test the effect of state mindfulness during exercise on a variety of outcomes. In doing so, there are a number of study design elements that need to be carefully considered because they impact the conclusions we can draw from such studies and ultimately impact both theory and practice. There are no clear-cut answers for the best experimental design; however, carefully considering *why, what, who, where, when, and how* questions will help researchers make the most informed decisions.

A good starting place is considering *why* state mindfulness would have an impact on the dependent variable of interest. This requires a conceptual or theoretical rationale. Perhaps aligned with MAT, greater state mindfulness during exercise is hypothesized to support more positive affective responses because it will reduce affective reactivity. The why will then lead to *what* to focus on. Given the multifaceted nature of mindfulness and the infinite number of mindfulness practices available, one must carefully consider *what* aspects of mindfulness they wish to induce in their experiment: awareness, attention, acceptance, or all three. Next, *where* should those qualities of mindfulness be directed? The mind, the body, the environment, or all three? In this example, it would be critical to include acceptance in a mindfulness manipulation since it is theorized to reduce affective reactivity according to MAT. The *why* and the *what* answers will guide the researcher to the specific type of mindfulness manipulation or intervention (*how and when*) they wish to test.

Another important *what* question is what the mindfulness intervention or manipulation will be compared to. Within-person and between-person designs offer flexibility for comparison. Using a quasi-experimental design in a more naturalistic setting may require hunting for a good comparison group, whereas true experimental designs will use a more traditional control or active control group. For example, if you are manipulating mindfulness to test if it enhances affect during exercise, then you may choose to compare it to an exercise condition that is somewhat neutral (e.g., listening to a podcast) or one that is known to support positive affect (e.g., listening to music). To test if moving while mindful is a superior strategy for decreasing anxiety compared to a seated mindfulness practice, the control group may be a seated form of mindfulness rather than a second exercise condition.

The next question is *who* the participants are. It is important to consider that participants' experiences while exercising will be influenced by a host of factors not related to mindfulness such as their fitness level, physical activity history, and tolerance for exertion. Participant response to a mindfulness manipulation will also be shaped by their levels of trait mindfulness and experience engaging in both static and movement-based mindfulness practices. Whether and how to control for these factors of course depend on the research question, but they should be considered nonetheless. Final considerations include *where* an experiment should take place (e.g., lab or naturalistic setting) and *how/when* mindfulness should be experimentally induced (e.g., providing instructions at the beginning or listening to an audio mindfulness script). Every decision involves a tradeoff, but systematically working through these questions will lead to a well-informed study design.

4. Methodological Question: How Do You Assess Mindfulness During Exercise?

The multifaceted nature of mindfulness gives rise to a wide variety of mindfulness measures. However, to meaningfully move our understanding and application of mindfulness during exercise forward, more thought needs to be given to appropriate assessment. Most measures are self-report, and the vast majority assess trait mindfulness. The wide variety of trait measures that capture different aspects of mindfulness lead to difficulty in making comparisons across studies. The importance of capturing specific aspects of mindfulness depends on the research goals, but most often researchers rely on a total score and fail to attend to the differences between global mindfulness and specific aspects of mindfulness. Additionally, evidence suggests that state and contextualized mindfulness are more salient to exercise-related outcomes. As noted by Yang and Conroy (2019), there is a need to capture a hierarchy of mindfulness to account for the global (trait), contextual, and specific situational (state) levels of mindfulness.

Moving toward the goal of capturing a broader hierarchy of mindfulness means more work needs to be done in the exercise context. There are only a few examples of research assessing mindfulness at the context (Tsafou et al., 2016, 2017) or state level during physical activity (SMS-PA; Cox, Ullrich-French, & French, 2016). In addition, these contextualized and state measure of mindfulness for physical activity do not adequately capture the two key elements of mindfulness. The SMS-PA captures attention and awareness but lacks adequate representation of the nonjudgment and acceptance qualities of attention, which may be especially important to capture as they are proposed to be critical explanatory mechanisms for positive outcomes of mindfulness according to MAT (Lindsay & Cresswell, 2017).

Researchers should consider moving beyond using self-report instruments to assess state mindfulness in particular. Self-reports have inherent limitations, including that such assessments require consciousness of complex and nuanced mindfulness processes. More objective tools of neuroimaging can provide new insight into the mechanisms of mindfulness and complement self-report measures. As application of these technologies increases, there is growing understanding of the neural mechanisms underlying mindfulness (see Tang et al., 2015). For example, the use of functional magnetic resonance imaging (fMRI) and electroencephalography (EEG) have revealed the brain regions that are activated while being mindful and even shown differences in gray matter for those who practice mindful meditation (e.g., Desbordes et al., 2012). Despite being useful for testing neuroplasticity following mindfulness interventions, these techniques have limited ability to capture mindfulness while moving in complex real-world exercise or physical activity contexts and are not an accessible option for many researchers. Triangulated assessment from more subjective self-report and more objective neuroimaging instruments at the trait, context, and state levels will provide a more complete picture of mindfulness and physical activity.

To test the mechanisms of mindfulness, adequate measurement is needed that addresses the appropriate level, the triangulation of forms of assessments, as well as capturing the critical elements of both monitoring (awareness) and acceptance (nonjudgment). The ability to empirically distinguish the qualities and degree of mindfulness within the context of movement will be critical in gaining more fine-grained testing of the mechanisms of mindfulness during exercise. This information will assist development of the most effective interventions fostering strategies to increase mindfulness skills.

5. Applied Question: What Forms of Physical Activity Are Suited (or Not) to Mindfulness Interventions?

Some forms of physical activity or settings may be more conducive to being mindful while moving. Mindful movement practices including yoga, tai chi, and Pilates actively incorporate mindfulness within the physical practice. For example, the instructor may direct participants to notice their breath and physical sensations. Another type of movement that may be particularly

234 HEALTH AND WELL-BEING

well suited to incorporating mindfulness is walking. Walking has been used in studies testing the effects of mindful exercise (Cox, Ullrich-French, Hargreaves, & McMahon, 2020; Yang & Conroy, 2018) and is a primary vehicle for practicing mindfulness in various programs (e.g., MBSR). Walking is appealing because it is accessible, inexpensive, and flexible and affords the opportunity to easily apply guided mindfulness practices to a well-practiced movement (e.g., directing attention to the sensations of the engagement of muscles). It is clear that various forms of mindful movement and walking offer ideal contexts within which to practice mindfulness; however, we know far less about many other popular forms of exercise. This is where the work lies.

Many forms of mindful movement are lower intensity activities. What is not clear is what happens at higher intensities of exercise, such as exercise at or above the ventilatory threshold (VT). This is a critical question because exercise above the VT is almost universally unpleasant and results in negative affective experiences (Brand & Ekkekakis, 2018). We do not yet know whether drawing attention, even with acceptance and nonjudgment, to the inevitably uncomfortable interoceptive cues (e.g., muscle pain, perspiration, increased heart rate and respiration) will have a positive or negative impact on affective experiences and in turn long-term behavioral choices.

Likewise, the mode of activity is an important consideration for the application of mindfulness. Because limited modes of physical activity have been examined, it will be necessary to test and compare different activity modes and contexts. The constrained action hypothesis suggests that internal focus of attention interferes with automatic processes of motor control (McNevin et al., 2003). We do not know how being mindful during physical activity, particularly focusing internally, will impact different types of motor behaviors. There may be some types of physical activity or exercise that are not conducive to mindfulness strategies. Additionally, at early stages of learning, mindfulness may not facilitate safe or appropriate motor skill execution. However, walking and perhaps other well-practiced motor skills such as running or biking may provide an ideal mind-body movement pair. It is necessary to focus attention on the appropriate cues needed to safely execute some exercises, especially when learning new and/or complex motor coordination patterns (e.g., safe weightlifting technique). While attention and awareness may facilitate such tasks, it is unknown how mindful qualities of openness and curiosity play a role in performance or motor skill execution.

Research that tests different intensity levels, modes of exercise, and stages of learning is needed to better understand the most appropriate ways to incorporate mindfulness into physical activity and exercise. Another unexplored area is to what degree an exerciser's goals align with mindful practice. There may be contexts that are not appropriate for incorporating mindfulness. Determination of appropriate application of mindfulness across physical activities cannot be made until there is adequate replication across different types of exercise and exercisers.

Conclusion

The potential for applying mindfulness in the exercise context for enhancing positive outcomes is clear, but there is a lot of work yet to be done. Gaps in our knowledge include what modes of exercise, for whom, and how is mindfulness best applied to exercise. Employing rigorous study designs, applying the appropriate level and mode of assessment, and identifying moderators will increase the precision of conclusions made, particularly for identifying mechanisms for the effects of mindfulness and the application of effective interventions. The questions identified previously serve as a starting place and demonstrate the breadth of theoretical, methodological, and applied issues that have yet to be systematically pursued.

References

Asztalos, M., Wijndaele, K., De Bourdeaudhuij, I., Philippaerts, R., Matton, L., Duvigneaud, N., & Cardon, G. (2012). Sport participation and stress among women and men. *Psychology of Sport and Exercise, 13*, 466–483.

Bishop, S. R., Lau, M., Shapiro, S., Carlson, L., Anderson, N. D., Carmody, J., & Devins, G. (2004). Mindfulness: A proposed operational definition. *Clinical Psychology: Science and Practice, 11*, 230–241.

Brand, R., & Ekkekakis, P. (2018). Affective–reflective theory of physical inactivity and exercise. *German Journal of Exercise and Sport Research, 48*, 48–58.

Brown, K. W., & Ryan, R. M. (2003). The benefits of being present: Mindfulness and its role in psychological well-being. *Journal of Personality and Social Psychology, 84*, 822–848.

Chu, P., Gotink, R. A., Yeh, G. Y., Goldie, S. J., & Hunink, M. M. (2016). The effectiveness of yoga in modifying risk factors for cardiovascular disease and metabolic syndrome: A systematic review and meta-analysis of randomized controlled trials. *European Journal of Preventive Cardiology, 23*, 291–307.

Clarke, T. C., Barnes, P. M., Black, L. I., Stussman, B. J., & Nahin, R. L. (2018). *Use of yoga, meditation, and chiropractors among US adults aged 18 and over*. US Department of Health and Human Services, Centers for Disease Control and Prevention, National Center for Health Statistics.

Cox, A. E., Ullrich-French, S., & Austin, B. (2020). Testing the role of state mindfulness in facilitating autonomous physical activity motivation. *Mindfulness, 11*, 1018–1027.

Cox, A., Ullrich-French, S., Cole, A., & D'Hondt-Taylor, M. (2016). The role of mindfulness during yoga in predicting self-objectification and reasons for exercise. *Psychology of Sport and Exercise, 22*, 321–327. https://doi.org/10.1016/j.psychsport.2015.10.001

Cox, A., Ullrich-French, S., & French, B. (2016). Validity evidence for state mindfulness scale scores in a physical activity context. *Measurement in Physical Education and Exercise Science, 20*, 38–49. https://doi.org/10.1080/1091367X.2015.1089404

Cox, A. E., Ullrich-French, S., Hargreaves, E., & McMahon, A. (2020). The effects of mindfulness and music on affective responses to self-paced treadmill walking. *Sport, Exercise, and Performance, Psychology, 9*, 571–584. https://doi.org/10.1037/spy0000192

Cox, A. E., Ullrich-French, S., Tylka, T., Cook-Cottone, C., & Neumark-Sztainer, D. (2020). Examining the effects of mindfulness based yoga instruction on positive embodiment and affective responses. *Journal of Eating Disorders, 28*, 458–475.

Deci, E. L., & Ryan, R. M. (1980). The empirical exploration of intrinsic motivational processes. In L. Berkowitz (Ed.), *Advances in experimental social psychology* (Vol. 13, pp. 39–80). Academic Press.

Desbordes, G., Negi, L. T., Pace, T. W., Wallace, B. A., Raison, C. L., & Schwartz, E. L. (2012). Effects of mindful-attention and compassion meditation training on amygdala response to emotional stimuli in an ordinary, non-meditative state. *Frontiers in Human Neuroscience, 6*, 292. doi:10.3389/fnhum.2012.00292

Hsin Hsu, S., Collins, S. E., & Marlatt, G. A. (2013). Examining psychometric properties of distress tolerance and its moderation of mindfulness-based relapse prevention effects on alcohol and other drug use outcomes. *Addictive Behaviors, 38*, 1852–1858. https://doi.org/10.1016/j.addbeh.2012.11.002

Hunt, M., Al-Braiki, F., Dailey, S., Russell, R., & Simon, K. (2018). Mindfulness training, yoga, or both? Dismantling the active components of a mindfulness-based stress reduction intervention. *Mindfulness, 9*, 512–520. doi:10.1007/s12671-017-0793-z

Kabat-Zinn, J. (2003). Mindfulness-based interventions in context: Past, present, and future. *Clinical Psychology: Science and Practice, 10*, 144–156.

Kang, Y., O'Donnell, M. B., Strecher, V. J., & Falk, E. B. (2017). Dispositional mindfulness predicts adaptive affective responses to health messages and increased exercise motivation. *Mindfulness, 8*, 387–397.

Kangasniemi, A. M., Lappalainen, R., Kankaanpää, A., Tolvanen, A., & Tammelin, T. (2015). Towards a physically more active lifestyle based on one's own values: The results of a randomized controlled trial among physically inactive adults. *BMC Public Health, 15*, 260.

Klatte, R., Pabst, S., Beelmann, A., & Rosendahl, J. (2016). The efficacy of body-oriented yoga in mental disorders: A systematic review and meta-analysis. *Deutsches Ärzteblatt International, 113*(12), 195.

Lindsay, E. K., & Creswell, J. D. (2017). Mechanisms of mindfulness training: Monitor and acceptance theory (MAT). *Clinical Psychology Review, 51*, 48–59.

McNevin, N., Shea, C., & Wulf, G. (2003). Increasing the distance of an external focus of attention enhances learning. *Psychological Research, 67*, 22–29.

Meyer, J. D., Torres, E. R., Grabow, M. L., Zgierska, A. E., Teng, H. Y., Coe, C. L., & Barrett, B. P. (2018). Benefits of 8-wk mindfulness-based stress reduction or aerobic training on seasonal declines in physical activity. *Medicine and Science in Sports and Exercise, 50,* 1850.

Noetel, M., Ciarrochi, J., Van Zanden, B., & Lonsdale, C. (2019). Mindfulness and acceptance approaches to sporting performance enhancement: A systematic review. *International Review of Sport and Exercise Psychology, 12*(1), 139–175. https://doi.org/10.1080/1750984X.2017.1387803

Norris, C. J., Creem, D., Hendler, R., & Kober, H. (2018). Brief mindfulness meditation improves attention in novices: Evidence from ERPs and moderation by neuroticism. *Frontiers in Human Neuroscience, 12,* Article 315. https://doi.org/10.3389/fnhum.2018.00315

Palmeira, L., Pinto-Gouveia, J., & Cunha, M. (2017). Exploring the efficacy of an acceptance, mindfulness and compassionate-based group intervention for women struggling with their weight (Kg-Free): A randomized controlled trial. *Appetite, 112,* 107–116.

Ruffault, A., Bernier, M., Juge, N., & Fournier, J. F. (2016). Mindfulness may moderate the relationship between intrinsic motivation and physical activity: A cross-sectional study. *Mindfulness, 7,* 445–452. doi:10.1007/s12671-015-0467-7

Schneider, J., Malinowski, P., Watson, P. M., & Lattimore, P. (2019). The role of mindfulness in physical activity: A systematic review. *Obesity Reviews, 20,* 448–463. doi/abs/10.1111/obr.12795

Tanay, G., & Bernstein, A. (2013). State mindfulness scale (SMS): Development and initial validation. *Psychological Assessment, 25,* 1286–1299. doi: 10.1037/a0034044

Tang, Y.-Y., Hölzel, B. K., & Posner, M. I. (2015). The neuroscience of mindfulness meditation. *Nature Reviews Neuroscience, 16,* 213–225.

Tsafou, K. E., De Ridder, D. T., van Ee, R., & Lacroix, J. P. (2016). Mindfulness and satisfaction in physical activity: A cross-sectional study in the Dutch population. *Journal of Health Psychology, 21,* 1817–1827.

Tsafou, K. E., Lacroix, J. P., Van Ee, R., Vinkers, C. D., & De Ridder, D. T. (2017). The relation of trait and state mindfulness with satisfaction and physical activity: A cross-sectional study in 305 Dutch participants. *Journal of Health Psychology, 22,* 1221–1232.

Ullrich-French, S., & Cox, A. E. (2020). Mindfulness and exercise. In D. Hackfort & R. J. Schinke (Eds.), *Routledge international encyclopedia of sport and exercise psychology, Vol. 1: Theoretical and methodological concepts* (pp. 303–321). London https://doi.org/10.4324/9781315187228

Ullrich-French, S., González Hernández, J., & Hildago Montesinos, M. D. (2017). Validity evidence for the adaptation of the state mindfulness scale for physical activity (SMS-PA) in Spanish youth. *Psicothema, 29,* 119–125. https://doi.org/10.7334/psicothema2016.204

Ulmer, C. S., Stetson, B. A., & Salmon, P. G. (2010). Mindfulness and acceptance are associated with exercise maintenance in YMCA exercisers. *Behaviour Research and Therapy, 48,* 805–809.

Yang, C. H., & Conroy, D. E. (2018). Momentary negative affect is lower during mindful movement than while sitting: An experience sampling study. *Psychology of Sport and Exercise, 37,* 109–116.

Yang, C., & Conroy, D. E. (2019). Mindfulness and physical activity: A systematic review and hierarchical model of mindfulness. *International Journal of Sport and Exercise Psychology.* https://doi.org/10.1080/1612197X.2019.1611901

17

Exercise and Aging

Michel Audiffren and Nathalie André

State of the Art

Cognitive performance generally declines with aging, but a high interindividual variability can be observed in the population, with some individuals declining more quickly than others (Hertzog et al., 2009). Genetic and lifestyle factors explain a large part of this interindividual variability. Lifestyle factors include physical activity (PA) and food habits. For instance, epidemiological studies show that practicing PA regularly reduces the risk of dementia, cognitive impairment, and cognitive decline with aging (e.g., Rockwood & Middleton, 2007). However, maintaining a new healthy habit for a long period, such as the regular practice of physical activity, requires higher cognitive functions, such as executive functions (Hall & Fong, 2015). This chapter focuses on the bidirectional relationship between chronic exercise (i.e., planned, structured, and repeated bouts of PA) and cognitive health in the elderly. In this introductory section, we first describe the causal link between chronic exercise and cognitive performance in older adults. Then, we discuss the causal link between the efficiency of high-level cognitive functions, such as executive functions (e.g., planning), and adherence to exercise. In the second section, we present five major questions related to this topic that need to be addressed to advance the field forward.

The causal relationship between exercise and cognitive aging has been extensively studied during the last 50 years. Randomized controlled trials (RCTs) are the only valid protocols allowing to establish this causal link. Recent meta-analyses of RCTs revealed that there is a small to moderate positive effect of chronic exercise on cognition in older adults (e.g., Sanders et al., 2019). Arthur Kramer and his team were the first to propose that this positive effect of chronic exercise is selective rather than general; that is, brain regions mostly affected by the deleterious effect of aging benefit mostly from chronic exercise (e.g., Colcombe et al., 2003). In a well-known meta-analysis

Michel Audiffren and Nathalie André, *Exercise and Aging* In: *Sport, Exercise and Performance Psychology.*
Edited by: Edson Filho and Itay Basevitch, Oxford University Press. © Oxford University Press 2021.
DOI: 10.1093/oso/9780197512494.003.0017

on chronic exercise and cognitive performance in older adults (Colcombe & Kramer, 2003), results indicated that the effect size is larger for executive functions (e.g., inhibitory control, cognitive flexibility) than for other cognitive functions (e.g., speed of information processing, visuospatial processes).

Executive functions (EFs) can be conceived as an umbrella of high-level top-down cognitive functions requiring effortful control and the activation of a large frontoparietal network. Core EFs include maintenance and updating of relevant information in working memory; controlled inhibition of prepotent impulses, intrusive thoughts, awkward emotions, or automatic motor responses; and mental set shifting, also known as cognitive flexibility. Other high-level cognitive functions such as volition, planning, sustained attention, and self-regulation have also been considered intrinsically linked to EFs. Executive functions play an important role in daily living, allowing individuals to mentally shift through ideas, to reason before acting, to cope with novel and unexpected challenges, to resist temptations, and to stay focused on a specific goal (Diamond, 2013). In the domain of sport and exercise, EFs seem to be crucial for the process of successful pacing regulation (Hyland-Monks et al., 2018).

Today, the efficacy and effectiveness of exercise programs aimed to slow down cognitive aging and improve EFs have been largely supported. The current questions in debate concern the type of exercise and program that lead to the largest effect size and the explanatory mechanisms that underpin these positive effects. In RCT studies demonstrating a causal link between chronic exercise and cognition, researchers generally compare cognitive performances before the beginning and after the end of the exercise program in a treatment and a control group. The control group generally participates in light-intensity exercises, such as stretching exercises, balance exercises, toning exercises, or a combination of all or part of these different categories of exercise. These exercises generally induce null or small positive effects when comparing cognitive performances of the control group before and after the program. By contrast, several types of exercise programs led to a moderate to large improvement of cognitive functions in the treatment group. The meta-analysis of Colcombe and Kramer (2003) suggests that programs combining aerobic exercise (e.g., jogging, Nordic walking, cycling) and resistance exercises and lasting more than 6 months give the largest positive effects. In addition, coordination exercises seem to have a beneficial effect on cognitive functions but through different mechanisms depending on the intervention, such as the training of EFs (Voelcker-Rehage et al., 2011).

Different mechanisms have been proposed to explain these positive effects of chronic exercise on cognitive aging. The *cardiovascular hypothesis* (Tarumi & Zhang, 2015) suggests that cardiovascular adaptations to endurance exercise ameliorate brain oxygenation and consequently brain functions through attenuation of age-related arterial stiffness and/or endothelial dysfunction. The *neurotrophic hypothesis* (Cotman & Berchtold, 2002) proposes that voluntary exercise can increase brain levels of several neurotrophic factors, such as the brain-derived neurotrophic factor (BDNF), leading to a stimulation of neurogenesis and angiogenesis, an increased resistance to brain insult, and an improvement of learning and cognitive performance. The *inflammatory hypothesis* (Petersen & Pedersen, 2005) assumes that the production and releasing of cytokines, such as interleukin-10 (IL-10), during skeletal muscle fiber contractions induces a protective and anti-inflammatory effect against chronic diseases associated with brain tissue inflammation. The *effort hypothesis* (Audiffren & André, 2019) propounds that regular practice of effortful exercises initiates a virtuous circle linking PA and effortful control in a bidirectional way. On the one hand, chronic exercise leads to an improvement of EFs and effortful control. On the other hand, gains in EFs and effortful control effectiveness lead to a reciprocal facilitation of the maintenance of PA over time. It is important to note that these four mechanisms are thought to occur synergistically rather than antagonistically.

As mentioned earlier, EFs play a crucial role in self-regulating exercise pace. In addition, they play a determinant role in adherence to exercise. For instance, it can be hypothesized that aging people who have a high efficacy in planning (i.e., the ability to plan actions until their completion) and in remembering planned actions just before they have to be completed (i.e., prospective memory) will have a higher efficacy in maintaining a healthy behavior, such as regularly practicing physical activity. In the same way, it can be hypothesized that older adults who have a performant-controlled inhibition (i.e., the ability to stop or repress prepotent impulses, unwanted and intrusive thoughts, embarrassing emotions, or automatic responses) will have a higher capacity to resist the desire to stop exercise when the feeling of discomfort, pain, or fatigue is too high. McAuley and his coworkers (2011) conducted the first study that showed a causal link between efficacy of EFs and adherence to exercise in older adults. More precisely, they have shown significant indirect effects of executive function on adherence via self-efficacy. More recently, Best, Nagamatsu, and Liu-Ambrose (2014) showed that the gain in EFs induced by an exercise program predicts the adherence to PA during the 1-year follow-up period in an elderly population. Table 17.1 summarizes five key studies that contributed greatly to the advancement of the field and posited the positive effect of chronic exercise on cognitive aging as evidence based. In the following section, we will present five major questions that need to be addressed in the future to advance theory and methodology in the field and improve future interventions targeting older adults.

Table 17.1   Five Key Readings in Exercise and Cognitive Aging

Authors	Methodological Design	Key Findings
Best et al. (2014)	Intervention study Latent growth curve analysis	The higher the gain in executive functions following a 12-month resistance exercise training in the elderly, the higher the adherence to a subsequent exercise routine over a 1-year period
Colcombe et al. (2003)	Cross-sectional study Structural MRI	Cortical areas negatively affected by aging are positively impacted by exercise.
Colcombe et al. (2006)	Intervention study Structural MRI	A program of 6 months of aerobic exercises in older adults led to significant increases in gray and white matter volume of the anterior cingulate cortex and the superior temporal gyrus, two key structures involved in effortful control.
Colcombe & Kramer (2003)	Meta-analysis	The effect size of the positive effect of chronic exercise on cognitive functions is larger for executive functions compared to other cognitive functions in aging people.
Erickson et al. (2011)	Intervention study Structural MRI	A program of 12 months of aerobic exercise increased hippocampal volume of the elderly by 2%.

Questions to Move the Field Forward

While research in the area of exercise psychology has made significant advances in the comprehension of the bidirectional relationship between exercise and cognition, certain questions remain unanswered. In this section, we present five of these unanswered major questions.

1. Theoretical and Applied Question: What Is the Specific Contribution of Each Explanatory Mechanism to the Link Between Exercise and Cognition?

The first question relates to theoretical and practical issues and concerns the real contribution of the four main plausible mechanisms presented earlier in this chapter to the positive effect of chronic exercise on cognitive aging. We previously explained that each of these four mechanisms (i.e., neurotrophic hypothesis, inflammatory hypothesis, effort hypothesis, and cardiovascular hypothesis) could contribute synergistically to the benefits of exercise on cognitive functions. Nevertheless, some questions remain unanswered: Does one of these mechanisms induce larger effects than the others? Are the effects of these four mechanisms additive or overadditive? Answering these two questions could help researchers and trainers to optimize exercise programs aiming to enhance cognition. In this perspective, if one of the four mechanisms explains a large part of variance of the gain in cognitive performance (e.g., 70%), preference should be given to the type of exercise mostly soliciting this mechanism. For instance, if the inflammatory hypothesis explains the largest part of variance of the phenomenon, it could be interesting to focus on exercises leading to a higher releasing of myokines. By contrast, if the neurotrophic mechanism interacts positively with the effort mechanism, it could be judicious to conceive exercise programs that simultaneously stimulate releasing of neurotrophic factors and effortful control in order to magnify the effects of chronic exercise on cognition.

The best way to address this question would be to conduct a series of intervention studies satisfying three criteria. First, each intervention study should allow to compare several types of exercise programs (e.g., aerobic, resistance, and coordination exercises, and different combinations of these three types of exercise). Second, the principal outcome related to cognitive health (e.g., a battery of cognitive tasks tapping EFs and effortful control) and mediating variables reflecting a specific mechanism should be assessed before and after the end of the intervention program. For instance, the plasmatic concentration of IL-10 cytokines could be viewed as a mediator of the relation between exercise and cognition regarding the inflammatory hypothesis. In the same way, the serum level of BDNF could be used as a mediator with regard to the neurotrophic hypothesis and the maximal oxygen uptake during incremental exercise (VO_{2max}) as a mediator concerning the cardiovascular hypothesis. Finally, considering the effort hypothesis, the connectivity within the salience network underpinning effortful control could be conceived as a mediator of the linkage between exercise and cognition. Third, results of these intervention studies should be analyzed through structural equation modeling, allowing to determine the weight of each plausible mechanism in the causal relationship between exercise and cognition.

2. Theoretical and Applied Question: How Do Individual Characteristics Help to Address Theoretical and Practical Issues?

The second question relates to theoretical and practical issues and concerns the moderating effect of individual characteristics on the magnitude of the effect of chronic exercise on cognitive aging. Relevant participant characteristics include polymorphism genotypes, neurological status, chronological age, and gender. Individual characteristics moderating the effects of chronic exercise on high-level cognitive functions, such as EFs and declarative memory, are particularly relevant for two main reasons.

First, the interaction between a moderating variable, such as the neurological status, and an intervening variable, such as the type of exercise program, on cognitive functions has theoretical value. The observation of such an interaction would suggest that the brain mechanism negatively affected by the neurological problem shares commonalities with the neurophysiological mechanism positively impacted by chronic exercise (i.e., when two factors interact); as such, it could be inferred that these two factors influence the same mechanism. However, this inference could be made if, and only if, there is no ceiling or floor effect; that is, the combination of both effects does not reach an upper or lower limit.

Second, identifying the older population groups that are more sensitive to the positive effect of chronic exercise on cognition also presents a practical interest. This information can help public policies to ameliorate prevention programs aiming to improve the well-being and the cognitive health of older adults by targeting more subtly specific populations (e.g., frail elderly). However, it is important to use a pertinent protocol to observe the expected interaction.

The majority of the studies that examined interaction effects between a moderating variable associated with an individual characteristic and the effect of chronic exercise on cognitive aging used cross-sectional or longitudinal studies. The main problem of these protocols is that they do not allow to evidence the causal relationship between exercise and cognition. Consequently, results can be interpreted in two ways: a group of older adults presenting a specific characteristic (e.g., valine homozygous for the BDNF gene) can be either more sensitive to the effects of chronic exercise on cognitive functions, more capable to practice physical exercises regularly, or both. In addition, the "State of the Art" section presents some arguments suggesting that the two relationships exist. Only RCT intervention studies can demonstrate the direction of the causal link, even in specific populations. Consequently, we need more intervention studies examining interactions between a specific individual characteristic (e.g., postmenopausal women with and without hormone treatment) and a specific exercise program (e.g., stretching vs. aerobic exercises) to identify the mechanism explaining the interaction and to delineate the subpopulations more positively impacted by the chronic effect of exercise.

3. Methodological Question: How Best to Examine the Intention-Exercise Relationship?

The third question relates to methodological issues and concerns the weak predictive power of health models regarding behavioral change in older adults. The reflection around this question is definitely an epistemological concern and criticizes the use of global conceptual models, such as the theory of planned behavior (Ajzen, 1991). Such models refer to a structured sequential scheme that serves as either a causal chain of determinants or a sequential chain of states for a given human behavior.

Global conceptual models of behavioral change poorly predict change in older adults for two main reasons. First, the expected behavior is generally a new behavior, which has to dislodge or supersede competing customary behaviors, change habits, remove impediments, and accommodate to life context, all elements that are strongly rooted in older adults. Second and closely related to the first reason, almost all the conceptual models used in health and social sciences are banked on intention, while no published experimental demonstration can be found that intention is first among all possible determinants of behavior.

Some insightful debates have been held on the legitimacy of global conceptual models in health and social psychology (e.g., Schwarzer, 2014) by questioning their usefulness for the understanding of human behavior and their effectiveness for predicting and controlling behavior change. In fact, the validity of a global conceptual model is seldom examined through the validity of its individual components, the psychometric soundness of its observed variables, or the appropriateness of statistical tools used for validation. The proposed approaches, such as expanding the model (e.g., Kosma, 2014; Park et al., 2017) or using auxiliary assumptions (i.e., assumptions that link the theory to an actual observation; see Trafimow & Earp, 2016), are not always suitable to models based on behavior change because of the inherent irrationality of certain behaviors and their low reproducibility. It would be more appropriate and heuristic to use observation-based predictive conceptual models, rather than prescriptive/descriptive models, as the experimental evidence of the latter is quite problematic (André & Laurencelle, 2020). Indeed, researchers usually use confirmatory approaches, whose goal is to methodologically reconcile the initial hypothesized model with the emerging (best-fit) statistical model. This upward reconciliation is fostered by the supporters of confirmatory statistical techniques (confirmatory factor analysis, structural equation modelling) and authorized by their leniency for imperfect models. This approach leads to confirm the original model to the detriment of actual observed differences, which might nevertheless contain important information. For this reason, scholars should elaborate competing models and bank on their predictive validity.

The intention-behavior relationship could be the first to be experimentally examined to verify the role of intention in behavior change when the past behavior is determined mainly by routine behaviors (e.g., van Bree et al., 2013). Moreover, there is a need to identify determinants negatively related to behavior change such as resistances to change or past failures.

4. Theoretical Question: How to Clarify the Role of High-Level Cognitive Functions in the Behavior Change Process?

The fourth question relates to theoretical issues and concerns the crucial role of high-level cognitive functions in maintenance of exercise in elderly. As mentioned earlier, changing behavior is complex because it relies on high-level cognitive functions (e.g., EFs), which decline with aging. More and more research is showing that high-level cognitive functions, such as controlled inhibition for physical activity (e.g., Best et al., 2014) or prospective memory in medication prescription (e.g., Insel et al., 2016), predict the maintenance of a new behavior. However, the relationship between high-level cognitive functions and maintenance of exercise remains underexplored. Consequently, there is a need to answer the following question: does the improvement of EFs, effortful control, and prospective memory through training help aging people to maintain durably a new behavior, such as exercising regularly?

The best way to address this question is to examine the complexity of the behavior that needs to be changed and maintained. It is frequently mentioned that the higher the complexity of the targeted behavior, the lower the likelihood of successful behavioral change (e.g., Rothman, 2000). However, what is a complex behavior? For instance, is smoking cessation more complex than starting to exercise? We assume here that it is not the complexity of the target behavior itself that must be questioned but rather the nature of the cognitive change involved. A new perspective on the study of behavior change is considered here by distinguishing behaviors that primarily target stopping an unhealthy behavior (e.g., smoking, drug abuse, alcohol consumption, video game playing, gambling, sex addiction, or binge eating) from those that primarily focus on starting a new healthy behavior (exercising, following a medication treatment, self-examination, diet regimen, or condom use).

It is reasonable to assume that stopping a behavior requires the use of the controlled inhibition function many times a day to resist the desire to express this specific behavior, which requires effortful control. In another respect, a sedentary senior who would like to start a new behavior, such as practicing physical activity several times a week, would also have to exert an inhibitory control over the desire to stop exercising when the feeling of discomfort or fatigue is too high. However, the individual certainly exerts this inhibitory control less frequently than when stopping a strong habit (Audiffren & André, 2015). In addition, someone who wants to start a new behavior must plan this new activity and remember to begin at the appropriate time (prospective memory), two higher cognitive functions directly related to self-regulation and EFs. A first interesting approach would be to examine whether the two categories of behavioral change (i.e., stopping a habit or starting a new behavior) require the same executive components and in which percentage of involvement. A second interesting approach would be to understand how a substitution behavior (e.g., a pleasant healthy behavior with a low perceived cost, such as jogging at the preferred speed) could help stop an unhealthy behavior, such as smoking, in order to help maintenance.

5. Theoretical and Applied Question: How Best to Examine the Complete Virtuous Circle Linking Exercise and Cognition?

The fifth and last question focuses on examining the bidirectional causal relationship between exercise and cognition (i.e., the complete virtuous circle) in a single protocol. As discussed in the previous sections, practicing physical exercise regularly improves memory and EFs. Symmetrically, improvement of EFs and prospective memory facilitates adherence to exercise programs. To our knowledge, only one intervention-based study (Best et al., 2014; see Table 17.1) examined the complete virtuous circle linking exercise and cognition. However, a theory needs more support to be substantiated. Consequently, there is a need for more intervention studies in the area, including a follow-up period of at least 12 months to test the hypothesis of the virtuous circle.

The validity of the virtuous circle has a very important practical purpose regarding the efficacy and effectiveness of physical exercise–based rehabilitation programs for vulnerable populations with physical deconditioning such as patients with low back pain and fragile older adults. It would be interesting to test the efficacy and effectiveness of intervention programs using physical exercises, cognitive exercises, and a combination of both types of exercise. These programs could be conceived to induce gains in EFs and prospective memory and to examine if these gains increase physical activity maintenance in the 12 months postintervention. Two categories of cognitive exercises could be used separately or in combination: (a) strategy-based exercises that train people to learn strategies to better store information in episodic and prospective memory, leading to improved organization of their activities, and focus of attention, and (b) process-based exercises that train people to perform cognitive tasks repeatedly, selectively tapping EFs and prospective memory.

Another important question concerns the transferability of cognitive function gains to other domains of behavior change (e.g., changes in food habits toward healthy eating), with the hypothesis that varying exercise types (e.g., physical and cognitive, strategy based and process based) within a training program would facilitate such far-transfer effects, which need to be examined in such intervention studies.

Conclusion

The positive effect of chronic exercise on cognitive aging is no more debated in the scientific and medical literature. It can be viewed as a far-transfer effect of exercise on cognitive functions, and more particularly on executive control. What needs to be improved in the future is the understanding of the synergistic effects of the different mechanisms leading to these positive effects in order to propose more effective exercise programs and magnify their effects at the behavioral level. In addition, it seems crucial to identify moderators of this causal relationship in order to tailor these exercise programs to individual characteristics. Finally, theory-driven behavioral change techniques based on cognitive processes must be elaborated to increase compliance and adherence of the older participants to the exercise programs.

References

Ajzen, I. (1991). The theory of planned behavior. *Organizational Behavior and Human Decision Processes, 50*(2), 179–211.

André, N., & Laurencelle, L. (2020). Where do the conceptual models for behaviour change come from, and how are they used? A critical and constructive appraisal. *Quantitative Methods for Psychology, 16*(1), 1–8.

Audiffren, M., & André, N. (2015). The strength model of self-control revisited: Linking acute and chronic effects of exercise on executive functions. *Journal of Sport and Health Science, 4*, 30–46.

Audiffren, M., & André, N. (2019). The exercise-cognition relationship: A virtuous circle. *Journal of Sport and Health Science, 8*, 339–347.

Best, J. R., Nagamatsu, L. S., & Liu-Ambrose, T. (2014). Improvements to executive function during exercise training predict maintenance of physical activity over the following year. *Frontiers in Human Neurosciences, 8*(353), 1–9.

Colcombe, S. J., Erickson, K. I., Raz, N., Webb, A. G., Cohen, N. J., McAuley, E., & Kramer, A. F. (2003). Aerobic fitness reduces brain tissue loss in aging humans. *Journal of Gerontology: Medical Sciences, 58A*(2), 176–180.

Colcombe, S. J., Erickson, K. I., Scalf, P. E., Kim, J. S., Prakash, R., McAuley, E., Elavsky, S., Marquez, D. X., Hu, L., & Kramer, A. F. (2006). Aerobic exercise training increases brain volume in aging humans. *Journal of Gerontology: Medical Sciences, 61A*(11), 1166–1170.

Colcombe, S., & Kramer, A. F. (2003). Fitness effects on the cognitive function of older adults: A meta-analytic study. *Psychological Science, 14*(2), 125–130.

Cotman, C. W., & Berchtold, N. C. (2002). Exercise: A behavioral intervention to enhance brain health and plasticity. *Trends in Neurosciences, 25*(6), 295–301.

Diamond, A. (2013). Executive functions. *Annual Review of Psychology, 64*, 135–168.

Erickson, K. I., Voss, M. W., Prakash, R. S., Basak, C., Szabo, A., Chaddock, L., Kim, J. S., Heo, S., Alves, H., White, S. M., Wojcicki, T. R., Mailey, E., Vieira, V. J., Martin, S.

A., Pence, B. D., Woods, J. A., McAuley, E., & Kramer, A. F. (2011). Exercise training increases size of hippocampus and improves memory. *Proceedings of the National Academy of Sciences, 108*(7), 3017–3022.

Hall, P. A., & Fong, G. T. (2015). Temporal self-regulation theory: A neurobiologically informed model for physical activity behavior. *Frontiers in Human Neuroscience, 9*, 117.

Hertzog, C., Kramer, A. F., Wilson, R. S., & Lindenberger, U. (2009). Enrichment effects on adult cognitive development: Can the functional capacity of older adults be preserved and enhanced? *Psychological Sciences in the Public Interest, 9*(1), 1–65.

Hyland-Monks, R., Cronin, L., McNaughton, L., & Marchant, D. (2018). The role of executive function in the self-regulation of endurance performance: A critical review. *Progress in Brain Research, 240*, 353–370.

Insel, K. C., Einstein, G. O., Morrow, D. G., Koerner, K. M., & Hepworth, J. T. (2016). Multifaceted prospective memory intervention to improve medication adherence. *Journal of the American Geriatrics Society, 64*, 561–568.

Kosma, M. (2014). An expanded framework to determine physical activity and falls risks among diverse older adults. *Research on Aging, 36*(1), 95–114.

McAuley, E., Mullen, S. P., Szabo, A. N., White, S. M., Wójcicki, T. R., Mailey, E. L., Gothe, N. P., Olson, E. A., Voss, M., Erickson, K., Prakash, R., & Kramer, A. F. (2011). Self-regulatory processes and exercise adherence in older adults: Executive function and self-efficacy effects. *American Journal of Preventive Medicine, 41*(3), 284–290.

Park, J. Y., Chiu, W., & Won, D. (2017). Sustainability of exercise behavior in seniors: An application of the extended theory of planned behavior. *Journal of Physical Education and Sport, 17*(1), 342–347.

Petersen, A. M. W., & Pedersen, B. K. (2005). The anti-inflammatory effect of exercise. *Journal of Applied Physiology, 98*, 1154–1162.

Rockwood, K., & Middleton, L. (2007). Physical activity and the maintenance of cognitive function. *Alzheimer's & Dementia, 3*, S38–S44.

Rothman, A. J. (2000). Toward a theory-based analysis of behavioural maintenance. *Health Psychology, 19*, 64–69.

Sanders, L. M. J., Hortobagyi, T., la Bastide-van Gemert, S., van der Zee, E. A., & van Heuvelen, M. J. G. (2019). Dose-response relationship between exercise and cognitive function in older adults with and without cognitive impairment: A systematic review and meta-analysis. *PloS ONE, 14*(1), e0210036.

Schwarzer, R. (2014). Life and death of health behavior theories. *Health Psychology Review, 8*, 53–56.

Tarumi, T., & Zhang, R. (2015). The role of exercise-induced cardiovascular adaptation in brain health. *Exercise and Sport Sciences Reviews, 43*(4), 181–189.

Trafimow, D., & Earp, B. D. (2016). Badly specified theories are not responsible for the replication crisis in social psychology: Comment on Klein. *Theory and Psychology, 26*, 540–548.

van Bree, R. J. H., van Stralen, M. M., Bolman, C., Mudde, A. N., de Vries, H., & Lechner, L. (2013). Habit as moderator of the intention–physical activity relationship in older adults: A longitudinal study. *Psychology and Health, 28*(5), 514–532.

Voelcker-Rehage, C., Godde, B., & Staudinger, U. M. (2011). Cardiovascular and coordination training differentially improve cognitive performance and neural processing in older adults. *Frontiers in Human Neuroscience, 5*, 26.

18

Youth Sport

Daniel Gould and Michael Mignano

A better understanding of sport for children and youth is a topic of paramount importance in the field of sport psychology for a number of reasons. First, millions of children are involved in sport worldwide (Tremblay et al., 2014). Second, it has been demonstrated that sport participation has a number of important physical, social, and psychological consequences for children and youth (e.g., Eime et al., 2013). Many of these consequences have been shown to be beneficial (e.g., improved health, learned life skills such as emotional regulation, and teamwork). However, other outcomes of youth sport have been shown to be negative (e.g., physical injury, stress, and burnout). Third, children participate in sport during important developmental periods of their lives where being physically active can influence long-term physical and mental health and development. Fourth, society sees sport as an important avenue for both achievement and the development of young people.

Given the importance of sport participation for children, it is not surprising that sport psychology researchers have been interested in the topic since the late 1970s (Smith et al., 1979). Interest in the area has grown over the years with studies conducted on a variety of topics such as motivation for participation, moral development, sport parenting, and effective coaching. We now have entire books (e.g., Knight et al., 2017) and special issues of journals like *Kinesiology Review* (e.g., Smith & Gould, 2019) devoted to the subject. A growing and devoted group of researchers around the world also focus their agendas on youth sport issues.

While we have learned much about sport psychology for young athletes, more questions remain unanswered than have been answered. Therefore, this chapter focuses on what is unknown about sport psychology research concentrated on youth sports. That is, what are key questions for the field moving forward and what are the best ways to address those questions? We will begin by first summarizing five exemplary research studies that have

Daniel Gould and Michael Mignano, *Youth Sport* In: *Sport, Exercise and Performance Psychology.*
Edited by: Edson Filho and Itay Basevitch, Oxford University Press. © Oxford University Press 2021.
DOI: 10.1093/oso/9780197512494.003.0018

appeared in the youth sport literature and identifying what made them so impactful. Then, five key questions facing the field moving forward are addressed. In doing so, we will discuss why each question is important and the most effective ways to study that question.

State of the Art

Based on our knowledge of the youth sports research, five key studies have been identified that capture the state of the art of youth sport psychological research. The design and key findings of these exemplary studies are summarized in Table 18.1.

The first study is Smith, Smoll, and Curtis's (1979) investigation of youth sport coaches, which was one of the first intervention studies conducted in the area. This seminal work has also spawned several extensions and replications (e.g., Smith et al., 2007) as well as practical publications and programs.

The second study is one of the first author's and his colleagues (Gould et al., 1996) and was part of a series of mixed-method studies designed to examine burnout in young athletes. We chose the second qualitative study in the series and included it because this work was one of the few studies to date that actually identified burned-out young athletes, as opposed to assessing burnout in active participants.

The third study is Vella, Cliff, and Okely's (2014) longitudinal quantitative analysis of youth sport motivation and dropout using a national data set in Australia. It is one of the few studies to distinguish between sport dropout and sport transfers and was guided by a comprehensive socioecological model.

Visek and colleagues' (2015) mixed-method study examining how fun is defined in youth sport is the fourth study identified. We liked its comprehensive nature and focus on developing a fun integration theory.

Finally, Weiss, Bolter, and Kipp's (2016) mixed-method evaluation of the First Tee life skills–based golf program was included. It is an example of a well-conducted evaluation of a youth sport program.

An examination of these five studies revealed that they were guided by theory or focused on theory development, were methodologically sound, and asked questions of practical importance. These studies often included mixed methods using the appropriate method for the question being posed and reflect how quantitative and qualitative methods can augment one another, providing unique information.

Table 18.1 Five Key Readings in the State of the Youth Sport Literature

Authors	Methodological Design	Key Findings
Gould et al. (1996)	Qualitative; second phase of a study that conducted interviews of 10 highly burned-out junior elite tennis players; used an integrated working model of burnout and semistructured interview approach; Profile and Hierarchical Content Analysis	Better understanding of burnout to help prevent and provide strategies for tennis players and junior athletes. The researchers showed and labeled categories based on the hierarchical content analysis, including signs, symptoms, and characteristics of burnout; factors leading to burnout; and advice for preventing future burnout.
Smith et al. (1979)	Experimental; coach effectiveness training intervention with 34 male Little League coaches; experimental coach group was exposed to a preseason training program utilizing empirically derived effective guidelines and compared to control coaches in the same leagues who did not experience such training	Trained coaches showed more positive behaviors and were viewed more favorably than the control (untrained) coaches group. Young athletes who played for trained coaches showed significant increases in self-esteem and higher levels of intrateam attraction, despite no differences in won-lost records. Seminal research in understanding youth sport coaches' use of encouragement, punishment, and technical methods of instruction.
Vella et al. (2014)	Quantitative; data set from the Kindergarten (K) cohort of the Longitudinal Study of Australian Children (LSAC), an examination of the social, environmental, and economic impacts on development and well-being; 4,042 child participants of a nationally representative sample; measured sports participation with social-ecological predictors	Found seven socioecological predictors of sports participation in organized sports and four predictors of burnout. Study distinguished between complete sport dropout and sport transfers. Overall, girls, children of lower socioeconomic backgrounds, and children who receive low parental support were found to encounter the highest risks of low sport participation and high sport dropout rates.

Table 18.1 *Continued*

Authors	Methodological Design	Key Findings
Visek et al. (2015)	Mixed methods; concept mapping and structured group data collection; youth soccer athletes (n = 142), parents (n = 57), and coaches (n = 37) were interviewed using brainstorming, sorting, and rating activities related to fun in sports	The fun integration theory was developed from this study using the framework of fun using a novel mixed-methods assessment of participants in sport (FUN MAPS). Overall, 81 fun-determinants were found and categorized into 11 themes such as positive team dynamics, trying hard, positive coaching, learning, and improving.
Weiss et al. (2016)	Mixed methods; program evaluation of First Tee, a national youth life skills organization; two-part study; Study 1's purpose was to compare First Tee with other organized activities on life skills transfer and developmental outcomes. Study 2's purpose was to assess life skills transfer across 3 years; further validity of the Life Skills Transfer Survey.	Studies added to the positive youth development framework and evaluated the impact of a youth sport life skills organization to determine program efficacy; significantly contributed to the existing knowledge base by using essential research design features such as a comparison group, statistical analysis, longitudinal phase, and validity of a life skills transfer measure.

Questions to Move the Field Forward

1. Applied Question: How Can the Professionalization of Youth Sports Be Curbed?

The professionalization of youth sport is a worldview that occurs when youth sport coaches and parents adopt, often implicitly, an elite entertainment model of sport that places heavy emphasis on competitive success, early sport specialization, intensive training, and the pursuit of extrinsic rewards like receiving trophies and earning rankings (Gould, 2009). The professionalized model of youth sport can be contrasted with a more holistic child-focused view that places primary emphasis on fostering the physical, psychological, and social development of the child. The goals of holistic youth sports should be for every child to have a positive experience, engage in healthy physical activity, learn social skills and values, and have fun (Committee on Sports Medicine and Fitness & Committee on School Health, 2001).

Addressing the professionalization of youth sports via applied interventions is important because it is thought to lead to a range of problematic behaviors. These include coaches focusing most of their attention only on the most skilled children, coaches and parents yelling at children for not performing well, increased early sports specialization, intense year-round training, parental pressure on children to win or achieve results, and the berating of officials and various unethical behaviors (e.g., violating rules, use of performance-enhancing drugs).

Given that professionalization of youth sport is a sociocultural issue, it must be addressed at that level. Some organizations in the United States, for example, such as the Positive Coaching Alliance and Aspen Foundation Project Play, have been trying to shift the narrative away from this model to a more child-centered holistic approach through nationwide social messaging, engaging stakeholders, and bringing media attention to the issue. In addition, national sport governing bodies such as USA Hockey and the United States Tennis Association have reorganized their youth sport programs to better align with a holistic child development versus a professionalized model. This has involved such initiatives as modifying the rules and teachings of the games at the entry levels so that they are more developmentally appropriate and eliminating rankings and national competitions. While these initiatives are laudable and encouraging, few, if any, efforts have been made to evaluate their effectiveness. Evaluation research is needed to determine if these efforts are effective in achieving their goals and what specific elements of the programs are effective. It is also important to note that there is an entirely separate body of evaluation research theories, methods, and knowledge that exists. Thus, investigators interested in assessing if efforts to shift youth sport stakeholders from professionalized to more holistic views should use this body of evaluation scientific knowledge and methods to guide their research efforts (e.g., Patton, 2014). Moreover, programs designed to shift the youth sport narrative could be designed, implemented, and evaluated by using existing research dissemination and communication models, like diffusion theory, which explains how new ideas and technology spread through a social system (Dearing & Kerr, 2012). Specifically, these models suggest that targeting persuasive information toward key influencers in specific social settings (e.g., respected and influential youth sport coaches) is more effective than mass appeals.

2. Theoretical and Methodological Question: Does Youth Sport Participation Influence Short- and Long-Term Physical Activity and Health-Enhancing Behaviors?

With the growth and expansion of technology around the world and increasingly sedentary lifestyles, physical inactivity and obesity levels have risen in children and youth. For example, in the United States, only one in four children aged 6 to 15 years meets minimum physical activity guidelines (Dentro et al., 2014). This is important because a lack of physical activity is associated with a variety of health problems in both children and adults (Pfeiffer & Wierenga, 2019). Moreover, sport participation is assumed to be a major vehicle for combatting physical inactivity in young people. However, this assumption has rarely been tested, and there is some evidence that children who play sports do not meet minimal physical activity guidelines (Leek et al., 2011). Not only are children less physically active because of factors like the decline of unstructured or free play, but also many young people lack fundamental physical literacy skills like jumping, throwing, and skipping that serve as the building blocks of movement throughout their lives (Tremblay et al., 2018).

Given current high rates of physical inactivity in young people, an important question related to applied interventions, theory, and methodological development is to examine how youth sport participation influences short- and long-term physical activity and health-enhancing behaviors in children and youth. Specifically, what role does sport participation play in helping children reach minimum physical activity guidelines, become adults who remain physically active, and engage in positive health-oriented behaviors? Identifying mechanisms to explain why some individuals engage in physical activity while others do not is an additional topic of importance.

Relative to the short-term effects of the role sport can play in meeting physical activity requirements, observational or accelerometer studies that assess the amounts of time young athletes spend being physically active in practices and games are needed. These are important because some studies have shown that children, especially in entry-level sport programs, are not meeting minimal physical activity requirements (Leek et al., 2011), despite the fact that many of these programs have enhanced physical activity as a goal. Randomized intervention protocols like the one described by Guagliano and colleagues (2012) provide an excellent example for conducting future studies examining whether training youth coaches influences the amount of physical activity their athletes experience during practices and games.

In terms of the study of long-term physical activity effects, after reviewing the literature, Pfeiffer and Wierenga (2019) identified two key methodological approaches. These included retrospective recall and longitudinal studies. Longitudinal studies have been more common in the literature and consist of short-term studies that look across short periods of time like the 4 years of high school (e.g., Pfeiffer et al., 2006) and long-term studies that track sport participants anywhere from 9 to 40 years (e.g., Kjønniksen et al., 2009). Reviewers have concluded that most of these studies found a positive relationship between youth sport participation and future physical activity levels. However, effect sizes were small (Trost et al., 2002).

Moving forward in this area, Pfeiffer and Wierenga (2019) offered several recommendations for researchers to examine. First, relationships may differ across geographic regions and cultural contexts (e.g., European sport club system vs. U.S. school-based sport system). Second, questions specific to the type, intensity, and frequency of youth sport involvement (vs. general physical activity levels) should be added to existing large-scale national physical activity and health surveillance studies. Third, more short-term longitudinal studies should be conducted so that dose-response relationships can be examined to determine if relationships are stronger across different periods of life. Finally, examining how the relationship between sport participation and physical activity participation might vary across different life transitions is critical (e.g., middle to high school, high school to college, college to post–college graduation). Researchers should also begin to assess potential factors that might influence the youth sport participation and adult physical activity relationship like type of sport played (e.g., golf vs. wrestling), the participant's level of sport engagement, motivation for participation (e.g., intrinsic vs. extrinsic), and quality of coaching. Cluster analytic studies that compare those who go on to stay physically active versus those who do not could be very useful. With the increase in anterior cruciate ligament and other serious injuries in young athletes and the correlation between having these injuries and the early onset of arthritis (Lohmander et al., 2004), understanding how youth sport injury history influences future physical activity involvement is important.

To date, the focus in this area of research has been on predicting how youth sport participation relates to future physical activity participation. However, researchers should begin to look at other health-enhancing outcomes by examining the relationship between youth sport participation and adult nutritional patterns and weight management. Finally, more emphasis needs to be placed on deriving explanations for why youth sport participation is related to later physical activity participation. For example, do young athletes develop habits of being physically active? Do they develop an intrinsic love for physical activity and moving, or are messages of living a healthy lifestyle internalized? There is a need to pursue theoretical explanations for these relationships.

3. Theoretical and Methodological Question: How Does Youth Sport Participation Influence the Mental Health and Well-Being of Children and Youth?

Mental health issues such as depression, anxiety, and substance abuse are on the rise in children and youth (Bor et al., 2014; Twenge et al., 2018), with the rates of anxiety disorders being highest among youth aged 15 to 19 years when compared to all age groups (World Health Organization, 2017). It has also been reported that over half of all mental issues have an onset before the age of 14 years (Kessler et al., 2005). Clearly, facilitating mental health in young people must be a global priority as both the financial and moral costs of not doing so are enormous.

With sport being such a pervasive and important childhood activity and mental health issues increasing in children and youth, the role that sport can play in facilitating the mental health of young people is a critical theory and methodology development question needing study. This is an especially important question in light of findings showing that sport participation has the potential to be both facilitative (e.g., higher self-esteem, lower anxiety, increased resilience, fewer mental health problems) and debilitative (e.g., increased stress and burnout, harassment, and maltreatment) when it comes to children's mental health (Vella, 2019).

Many types of studies are needed in this area. First, because the evidence linking youth sport participation to both facilitative and debilitative mental health has typically been cross-sectional and noncausal, research needs to address causality. This might involve comparisons of sport versus nonsport participants longitudinally while controlling for other factors like socioeconomic status and participation in other youth activities. Vella (2019) has also indicated that identifying mediating and moderating factors influencing the youth sport participation–mental health link is important. Such factors as program dosage, type of sport, engagement level of the participants, and participant characteristics should be considered. Finally, more intervention development and evaluation studies are needed like those conducted by Vella and colleagues (2018) to assess the effectiveness of the Ahead of the Game (https://aheadofthegame.org.au, 2019) program, an intervention designed to both improve mental health knowledge and prevent or reduce the impact of mental health problems in adolescents through community sport clubs.

4. Theoretical and Applied Question: What Does Effective Coaching Look Like for Children of Different Ages and in Different Sport Contexts?

It has been repeatedly demonstrated that coaches and coaching behaviors have important influences on a range of outcomes including young athletes' motivation, continued participation, stress, anxiety levels, and burnout (e.g., see Gould, 2016). While researchers have certainly learned a great deal about effective youth sport coaching, they have not looked at this question developmentally and considered the sport context. There is a need to examine what effective coaching looks like for children of different ages and in different sport contexts. This question has important theoretical and applied implications and will need varied methods to be answered.

It is important for future researchers to examine this topic because developmental psychologists have found that children of various ages are not alike, but rather differ in many important cognitive, emotional, and social ways. For example, important stages of child development have been identified such as early (ages 1 to 8 years) and late childhood (ages 9 to 11) as well as early (ages 12 to 14), middle (ages 15 to 17), and late stages of adolescence (ages 18 to 21; see Eccles, 1999; Sanders, 2013). While researchers have conducted studies on children of various ages, few investigations have systematically looked at how effective coaching practices might be similar and/or different depending on the age and development level of the young athletes involved.

Horn (2019), in reviewing the literature specifically on coaches' feedback patterns and young athletes' psychosocial well-being, suggested that researchers should examine how to best provide young athletes with coaching feedback during critical transitions such as from elementary to middle school and from high school to college. She recommended that coaching feedback differences accompanying athlete transitions from recreation to competitive sport programs be examined. Furthermore, Horn (2019) stressed the need for researchers not only to examine how coaches' feedback patterns differ across critical development and sport environment transitions but also to make efforts to better understand why coaches behave the way they do, as well as how variables such as emotional intelligence or assumptions related to Dweck's (2006) theory of implicit abilities influence their coaching.

This research topic is best approached using multiple methods. Observational studies using existing coaching assessment instruments would be useful in identifying how coaches behave in varying contexts with children of different ages. Traditional surveys that assess perceptions of their coaches' styles and behaviors could be administered to large groups of young athletes of different ages and from varied contexts to identify more versus less effective and/or preferred coaching styles. Of course, this might be difficult to do with children younger than 8 years of age, where different methods might be employed. Finally, case studies of exemplary coaches of children of varying ages and in varying contexts could be employed, and these might involve observations and in-depth interviews.

5. Theoretical Question: When, Under What Conditions, and How Are Life Skills Developed in Youth Sports and Do These Life Skills Transfer Beyond Sport?

A topic of considerable interest to both sport psychology and youth development researchers that has theory development, methodological, and applied implications is determining if, when, how, and under what conditions life skills are developed in young athletes. Life skills have been defined as "those internal personal assets, characteristics and skills such as goal setting, emotional control, self-esteem, and hard work ethic that can be facilitated or developed in sport and are transferred for use in non-sport settings" (Gould & Carson, 2008, p. 60). Life skills can be developed through sport participation, although most researchers have concluded that they typically are not an automatic by-product of participation, but are best developed when explicitly fostered by coaches (Turnnidge et al., 2014). Life skills are also more likely to be developed when a caring sport climate is created and when participants are highly engaged in their sport (Gould et al., 2012).

While much has been learned about life skills development through sport, more needs to be known. These include the conditions under which they are developed and if and how those life skills developed through sports transfer beyond sport to other areas of young people's lives. This is an important issue to study because developing life skills can not only help young athletes have more enjoyable sport experiences but also provide opportunities to learn characteristics and skills that can help them be more effective and civically engaged adults. However, while it is often assumed that life skills learned in sport transfer to other domains, this is not always the case (Martinek et al., 2001). More needs to be known about if and when transfer occurs, what factors cause life skills transfer, and the reasons transfer takes place. Pierce, Gould, and Camiré (2016) developed a comprehensive model outlining how transfer might occur as well as predicting relationships between key variables.

There are several avenues for future research related to life skills transfer and positive youth development through sport. Scholars need to not only investigate how life skills are developed in sport but also examine if they do indeed transfer to nonsport settings (e.g., school, home, work). This could be done in several ways. First, retrospective interviews could be conducted with former athletes relative to the life skills they felt they developed in sport and later transferred to nonsport settings. The advantage of this approach is that the person would have time to actually implement any life skills learned in sport to other aspects of their life. A second approach would be to conduct longitudinal studies that track life skills developed in sport over time including one's postathletic career to determine what skills transferred beyond sport. It would be especially interesting to compare the sport participants to children who take part in other nonsport activities as well as to children who did not take part in sport or extracurricular activities. This would help determine what unique contributions sport might make to life skills development and transfer. Studies are also needed to test some of the proposed relationships that Pierce and his colleagues (2016) forwarded in their life skills model. For example, are life skills more likely to transfer when the sport context they are learned in is similar to the conditions in the transfer context? Do life skills transfer more often when sport coaches emphasize doing so and reinforce such transfer? Finally, do the concepts of near transfer (transferring between very similar contexts) versus far transfer (transferring to different contexts) help explain life skills transfer?

Conclusion

Helping children gain the many physical, psychological, and social benefits of sport participation is one of the most important areas of research in the field of sport and exercise psychology. Youth sport offers a unique opportunity to positively influence millions of children across the globe. To do this, however, researchers must ask questions that will have major impact and use the most appropriate and advanced methods for addressing those questions. We hope this chapter will help both current and future youth sport researchers to do so.

References

Bor, W., Dean, A. J., Najman, J., & Hayatbakhsh, R. (2014). Are child and adolescent mental health problems increasing in the 21st century? A systematic review. *Australian and New Zealand Journal of Psychiatry, 48*, 606–616.

Committee on Sports Medicine and Fitness & Committee on School Health. (2001). Organized sports for children and preadolescents. *Pediatrics, 107*(6), 1459–1462.

Dearing, J. W., & Kerr, K. F. (2012). Historical roots of dissemination and implementation science. In R. C. Brownson, G. A. Colditz, & E. K. Proctor (Eds.), *Dissemination and implementation research in health: Translating science to practice* (pp. 55–71). Oxford University Press.

Dentro, K. N., Beals, K., Crouter, S. E., Eisenmann, J. C., McKenzie, T. L., Pate, R. R., Saelens, B. E., Sisson, S. B., Spruijt-Matz, D., Southern, M. S., Katzmarzyk, P. T. (2014). Results from the United States' 2014 report card on physical activity for children and youth. *Journal of Physical Activity and Health, 11*(s1), S105–S112.

Dweck, C. S. (2006). *Mindset: The new psychology of success*. Random House.

Eccles, J. S. (1999). The development of children ages 6 to 14. *Future of Children, 9*(2), 30–44.

Eime, R. M., Young, J. A., Harvey, J., Charity, M. J., & Payne, W. R. (2013). A systematic review of the psychological and social benefits of participation in sport for children and adolescents: Informing development of a conceptual model of health through sport. *International Journal of Behavioral Nutrition and Physical Activity, 10*(1), 98–112.

Gould, D. (2009). The professionalization of youth sports: It's time to act! *Clinical Journal of Sports Medicine, 19*(1), 81–82.

Gould, D. (2016). Quality coaching counts. *Phi Delta Kappan, 97*(8), 13–28.

Gould, D., & Carson, S. (2008). Life skills development through sport: Current stands and future directions. *International Review of Sport and Exercise Psychology, 1*(1), 58–78.

Gould, D., Flett, M. R., & Lauer, L. (2012). The relationship between psychological development and the sports climate experienced by underserved youth. *Psychology of Sport & Exercise, 13*(1), 80–87.

Gould, D., Tuffey, S., Udry, E., & Loehr, J. (1996). Burnout in competitive junior tennis players: II. Qualitative analysis. *Sport Psychologist, 10*(4), 341–366.

Guagliano, J. M., Lonsdale, C., Kolt, G. S., & Rosnekrantz, R. R. (2012). Increasing girls' physical activity during an organised youth sport basketball program: A randomised controlled trial protocol. *BMC Public Health, 14*, 383.

Horn, T. S. (2019). Examining the impact of coaches' feedback patterns on the psychosocial well-being of youth sport athletes. *Kinesiology Review, 8*, 244–251.

Kessler, R. C., Berglund, P., Demler, O., Jin, R., Merikangas, K. R., & Walters, E. E. (2005). Lifetime prevalence and age-of-onset distributions of DSM-IV disorders in the National Comorbidity Survey Replication. *Archives of General Psychiatry, 62*(6), 593–602.

Kjønniksen, L., Anderssen, N., & Wold, B. (2009). Organized youth sport as a predictor of physical activity in adulthood. *Scandinavian Journal of Medicine & Science in Sports, 19*(5), 646–654.

Knight, C. J., Harwood, C. G., & Gould, D. (Eds.). (2017). *Sport psychology for young athletes*. Routledge.

Leek, D., Carlson, J. A., Cain, K. L., Henrichon, S., Rosenberg, D., Patrick, K., & Sallis, J. F. (2011). Physical activity during youth sports practices. *Archives of Pediatrics & Adolescent Medicine, 165*(4), 294–299.

Lohmander, L. S., Östenberg, A., Englund, M., & Roos, H. (2004). High prevalence of knee osteoarthritis, pain, and functional limitations in female soccer players twelve years after anterior cruciate ligament injury. *Arthritis & Rheumatism: Official Journal of the American College of Rheumatology, 50*(10), 3145–3152.

Martinek, T., Schilling, T., & Johnson, D. (2001). Transferring personal and social responsibility of underserved youth to the classroom. *Urban Review, 33*(1), 29–45.

Patton, M. Q. (2014). *Qualitative research and evaluation methods* (4th ed.). Sage.

Pfeiffer, K. A., Dowda, M., Dishman, R. K., McIver, K. L., Sirard, J. R., Ward, D. S., & Pate, R. R. (2006). Sport participation and physical activity in adolescent females across a four-year period. *Journal of Adolescent Health, 39*(4), 523–529.

Pfeiffer, K. A., & Wierenga, M. J. (2019). Sport for all: Promoting physical activity through youth sports. *Kinesiology Review, 8*, 204–210.

Pierce, S., Gould, D., & Camiré, M. (2016). Definition and model of life skills transfer. *International Review of Sport and Exercise Psychology, 10*(1), 186–211.

Sanders, R. A. (2013). Adolescent psychosocial, social, and cognitive development. *Pediatric Review American Academy of Pediatrics, 34*(8), 354–358.

Smith, A. L., & Gould, D. (2019). Contemporary youth sport: Critical issues and future directions. Special Issue. *Kinesiology Review, 8*(3).

Smith, R. E., Smoll, F. L., & Cumming, S. P. (2007). Effects of a motivational climate intervention for coaches on young athletes' sport performance anxiety. *Journal of Sport and Exercise Psychology, 29*, 39–59.

Smith, R. E., Smoll, F. L., & Curtis, B. (1979). Coach effectiveness training: A cognitive-behavioral approach to enhancing relationship skills in youth sport coaches. *Journal of Sport and Exercise Psychology, 1*(1), 59–75.

Tremblay, M. S., Gray, C. E., Akinroye, K., Harrington, D. M., Katzmarzyk, P. T., Lambert, E.V., . . . Prista, A. (2014). Physical activity of children: A global matrix of grades comparing 15 countries. *Journal of Physical Activity and Health, 11*(s1), S113–S125.

Tremblay, M. S., Longmuir, P. E., Barnes, J. D., Belanger, K., Anderson, K. D., Bruner, B., . . . Kolen, A. M. (2018). Physical literacy levels of Canadian children aged 8–12 years: Descriptive and normative results from the RBC Learn to Play–CAPL project. *BMC Public Health, 18*(2), 1036.

Trost, S. G., Owen, N., Bauman, A. E., Sallis, J. F., & Brown, W. (2002). Correlates of adults' participation in physical activity: Review and update. *Medicine & Science in Sports & Exercise, 34*(12), 1996–2001.

Turnnidge, J., Côté, J., & Hancock, D. J. (2014). Positive youth development from sport to life: Explicit or implicit transfer? *Quest, 66,* 203–217. doi:10.1080/00336297.2013.867275

Twenge, J. M., Joiner, T. E., Rogers, M. L., & Martin, G. N. (2018). Increases in depressive symptoms, suicide-related outcomes, and suicide rates among US adolescents after 2010 and links to increased new media screen time. *Clinical Psychological Science, 6*(1), 3–17.

Vella, S. A. (2019). Mental health and organized youth sports. *Kinesiology Review, 8,* 229–236.

Vella, S. A., Cliff, D. P., & Okely, A. D. (2014). Socio-ecological predictors of participation and dropout in organized sports during childhood. *International Journal of Behavioral Nutrition and Physical Activity, 11,* 62. http://dx.doi.org/10.1186/1479-5868-11-62

Vella, S. A., Swann, C., Batterham, M., Boydell, K. M., Eckermann, S., Fogarty, A., . . . Noetel, M. (2018). Ahead of the game protocol: A multi-component, community sport-based program targeting prevention, promotion and early intervention for mental health among adolescent males. *BMC Public Health, 18*(1), 390–401.

Visek, A. J., Achrati, S. M., Mannix, H., McDonnell, K., Harris, B. S., & DiPietro, L. (2015). The fun integration theory: Toward sustaining children and adolescents sport participation. *Journal of Physical Activity & Health, 12,* 424–433. http://dx.doi.org/10.1123/jpah.2013-0180

Weiss, M. R., Bolter, N. D., & Kipp, L. E. (2016). Evaluation of The First Tee in promoting positive youth development: Group comparisons and longitudinal trends. *Research Quarterly for Exercise and Sport, 87*(3), 271–283.

World Health Organization. (2017). *Depression and other common mental disorders: Global health estimates.* WHO reference number: WHO/MSD/MER/2017.2.

19

Career Transitions and Change

Roy David Samuel

Over the last decade, the athlete's career transition literature has shifted from a deterministic (or linear) to a probabilistic (nonlinear) perspective. Athletes' careers can be perceived as a roller coaster ride, shaped by transitions, change-events, appraisals, decision-making, coping, and environmental influences. Transitions are turning phases in athletes' career development, associated with a set of specific demands. They can be classified as normative, nonnormative, and quasi-normative. Change-events are distinct events or longitudinal processes that disrupt the athletic engagement status quo and create emotional and cognitive imbalance and initiate a demand for change (Stambulova & Samuel, 2020).

Athletes can enjoy a fruitful and meaningful career as long as they positively adapt to the various transitional periods and changes encountered, potentially creating multiple career pathways. Furthermore, research has expanded to additional sport performers, such as e-sport and extreme sports athletes, coaches, and referees. Finally, the lives of sport performers have considerably changed in the past decade as a result of the globalization process, social media, and migration, requiring career researchers to modify existing conceptualizations. This chapter, therefore, provides a critical examination of the recent developments in the career transition and change literature, mainly focusing on critical questions to be asked and a prospective view of this field.

State of the Art

Several key conceptual and research developments have been integrated in the past decade in the sport career literature (for an overview see Stambulova et al., 2020): (a) a within-career transition and change perspective (Drew et al., 2019; Samuel, Stambulova, & Ashkenazi, 2020; Samuel & Tenenbaum, 2011a; Stambulova, 2016), (b) a dual-career perspective (Stambulova & Wylleman,

Roy David Samuel, *Career Transitions and Change* In: *Sport, Exercise and Performance Psychology.*
Edited by: Edson Filho and Itay Basevitch, Oxford University Press. © Oxford University Press 2021.
DOI: 10.1093/oso/9780197512494.003.0019

2019), and (c) the cultural praxis of athletes' careers (Ryba et al., 2018; Ryba et al., 2016). In addition, research attention is still given to examining adaptation to athletic retirement (Park et al., 2013) as well as to the effectiveness of career transition support/intervention programs (Samuel, 2013; Stambulova, 2016; Pummell & Lavallee, 2019). Finally, there are a few research attempts focused on the career transitions of additional sport performers, such as soccer referees (Samuel et al., 2017) and coaches (Knight et al., 2015; Samuel, Basevitch, et al., 2020). Table 19.1 presents five highlighted publications within these areas of research. Largely, these readings suggest that various types of transitions and change-events shape athletes' careers, with multiple factors potentially affecting athletes' adaptation. Furthermore, a nonlinear and highly dynamic transitional experience is evident.

Change-events. Proposing a dynamic and probabilistic view of the athlete's career, Samuel and Tenenbaum (2011a) presented the scheme of change for sport psychology practice (SCSPP). The novelty of this framework is in emphasizing athletes' cognitive appraisals and decision-making in response to a wide range of *change-events* (Stambulova et al., 2020). This perspective suggests that both "positive" and "negative" types of change-events can lead to change: instability in athletes' careers and mindset, which deserve adequate consideration. Several studies provided support for the basic tenets of the SCSPP (Knowles & Lorimer, 2014; Samuel & Tenenbaum, 2011b, 2013; Samuel et al., 2016). For example, a recent cross-national study concerning the modifications of regulations and refereeing in competitive judo since 2013 indicated that these modifications were perceived rather negatively by athletes and coaches. Participants' decision-making mostly involved consulting with others and making a conscious decision to change, mainly focusing on adjusting tactical skills. The participants' motivation decreased following these modifications. Finally, there were cross-cultural differences in how participants responded to this change-event, emphasizing the importance of context in change-event studies (Samuel, Basevitch, et al., 2020).

Recently, the SCSPP was integrated with the athletic career transition model (see Stambulova, 2016) to explain complex, multiphase transitions, such as the cultural transition of the Israeli men's U18 national handball team that migrated to Germany for a full season to train and compete in a high-level environment (Samuel, Stambulova, et al., 2020). This integrated career change and transition framework (ICCT) portrays an interplay among perceived transition demands, resources, and barriers in the transition appraisals, decision-making, and coping, and provides a probabilistic view on transition pathways (Samuel, Stambulova, et al., 2020).

Junior-to-senior transition. The junior-to-senior transition (JST) is the most researched within-career transition in sport (Drew et al., 2019). It might last from several months to a few years and is considered a highly challenging period in athletes' careers, involving increases in competition intensity, season duration, level of opponents, and intensified on- and off-court demands. As a result, only 20% to 30% of athletes manage to adapt, while most athletes either drop out or move to a recreational level of sport/exercise (Stambulova & Samuel, 2020). Recent JST research is focused on the role of the environment in nurturing athletes' development. For example, Henriksen et al. (2014) presented a case study of a golf team in a sport academy in Denmark with limited success in effective JST. This struggling environment was characterized by a lack of supportive training groups and role models, little understanding from the nonsport environment, no integration of efforts among different parts of the environment, and an incoherent organizational culture.

In addition, Pehrson et al., (2017) validated an empirical model called "phases in the JST of Swedish ice hockey players" among professional coaches and players. This model proposes four phases—preparation, orientation, adaptation, and stabilization—containing specific demands, barriers, resources, coping strategies, and outcomes. This study confirmed the longitudinal nature of the JST and the idea of moving back and forth between phases (i.e., nonlinear individual JST trajectories).

Nonnormative and quasi-normative transitions. In addition to the JST, other types of transitions also received research attention. Nonnormative transitions (e.g., injuries, deselection; Blakelock et al., 2016; Ivarsson et al., 2018; McEwen et al., 2018) are less predictable and are risky in terms of a crisis outcome (Stambulova & Samuel, 2020). For example, Blakelock et al. found that elite adolescent English soccer players (aged 15 to 18) who were released (i.e., 23% of the players) from their clubs experienced meaningful psychological distress at relatively high rates, both 1 week and 3 weeks following deselection. Additionally, quasi-normative transitions are predictable for a particular category of athletes (Stambulova & Samuel, 2020), such as Olympic athletes who transition to Olympic training centers (Poczwardowski et al., 2014) or participate in the Olympic Games (Schinke et al., 2015).

Other sport performers. A few studies have also examined career changes of additional sport performers, such as soccer referees and coaches. For example, Samuel et al. (2017) found that Israeli soccer referees experienced a highly dynamic career, comprising multiple types of transitions and change-events. The most significant ones were *receiving an international badge, changing to the assistant referee group, a transition to a higher league,* and *a transition to a lower league.* Knight et al. (2015) initially interviewed Canadian coaches regarding the work-environment factors that influence coach transitions. Four higher order themes describing reasons coaches transitioned between positions were identified: (a) interpersonal considerations, (b) work demands, (c) career concerns, and (d) positive coaching experiences. In a subsequent study, they (Knight et al., 2015) identified two overarching themes depicting reasons (i.e., "push" and "pull") for transitions: seeking opportunities to be more successful and leaving a negative or challenging work environment.

Table 19.1 Five Key Readings in the Area of Transitions and Change in the Sport Career

Authors	Methodological Design	Key Findings
Drew et al. (2019)	A meta-study of qualitative studies on the JST; a total of 27 qualitative studies were included ($n = 261$)	Four overarching themes were identified: individual factors, external factors, cultural factors, and intervention strategies. The JST is a complex and dynamic process occurring over varying time periods underpinned by multiple factors. Synthesizing the findings, the individual, external, cultural model of the JST was presented, with three underpinning features: transition preconditions, transition variables, and transition outcomes.
Park et al. (2013)	A systematic review of studies on the transition out of sport; 126 qualitative (44%), quantitative (44%), and mixed-model (12%) studies were reported ($n = 13,511$)	15 variables associated with the quality of end-of-career transitions were identified: athletic identity, demographic issues, the voluntariness of retirement decision, injuries/health problems, career/personal development, sport career achievement, educational status, financial status, self-perception, control of life, relationship with a coach, disengagement/dropout, time passed after retirement, life changes, and balance of life. Athletic identity, injuries/health problems, and a conflict with a coach were associated with negative adjustment.

Continued

Table 19.1 *Continued*

Authors	Methodological Design	Key Findings
Ryba et al. (2016)	15 professional athletes with transnational experience; a life story method was used in a two-step interview process; thematic, structural, and performative data analyses were applied	The cultural transition process was constituted in social practices and shifting modes of participation within and between sport/work and other contexts. The experiences of the athletic transition rather than transition to a new society dominated participants' stories, with a belief in the universal language of sport in all cultures. The three-phase cultural transition model is suggested. It represents the developmental tasks throughout the transition phases and underlying psychological mechanisms facilitating cultural adaptation.
Samuel & Tenenbaum (2011b)	A cross-sectional and retrospective design; 338 athletes representing five professional levels and various sports; measures: change-event experiences, athletic identity	Athletes experience multiple types of change-events in their careers, with different profiles of perception, emotional reaction, and coping. Athletic identity correlates positively with the perceived significance of the change-event
Schinke et al. (2015)	The Canadian Olympic boxing team members' meta-transitions through the Olympic quadrennial period are discussed	Six meta-transitions within the Olympic cycle 2013–2016 are identified: (a) entering the National Team Program, (b) entering major international tournaments, (c) Olympic qualification, (d) focused preparation for the Olympics, (e) to the Olympic podium, and (f) to the post-Games. Each meta-transition is described in terms of its demands, resources, barriers, coping process/strategies, possible pathways, and outcomes relevant to athletes' preparation, performance, and development.

JST, junior-to-senior transition.

Questions to Move the Field Forward

In this section, five critical questions are formulated, suggesting areas of thought and study to advance this field. Each question is initially stated, then the importance of addressing that question is explained, and then the best ways to address the question are specified. The initial four questions are mostly conceptual-methodological, whereas the final one presents applied challenges.

1. Theoretical Question: What Is the Interplay Between Career Development and Career Transitions?

Currently, there are two parallel lines of research in the athlete's career area. The career development (CD) research, typically conceptualized using the holistic athletic career model (Wyllemanet al., 2013), suggests a predetermined career route from childhood to retirement, with structured normative transitions (Stambulova et al., 2020). The career transition (CT) research, typically conceptualized by the athletic career transition model (Stambulova, 2016) and the SCSPP (Samuel & Tenenbaum, 2011a), proposes a highly dynamic view, with various transitions and change-events being perceived as driving forces in shaping career pathways (Stambulova & Samuel, 2020). Research indicates a highly complex athlete-environment interaction, manifested in both developmental processes (e.g., Henriksen et al., 2014, Samuel, Stambulova, et al., 2020; Schinke et al., 2015) and transitional experiences (e.g., Poczwardowski et al., 2014; Ryba et al., 2016; Samuel & Tenenbaum, 2011b; Samuel et al., 2015, 2016). Thus, an integrated perspective for the study of an athlete's career is suggested to advance the field.

An integrated development-transition framework should be developed and tested, identifying the potential pathways athletes might experience as a result of within-career transitions. Furthermore, the range of factors that might influence athletes' adaptation to various transitions and the effects on their development need to be explored. Special consideration should be given to the athlete-environment interactions, acknowledging that there is no "perfect" environment for athletes' development. In addition, much of the research to date applied retrospective designs, which might lead to bias in athletes' narratives when describing decision-making processes and adaptation to career transitions. Thus, research should adhere to longitudinal designs, capturing the athletes' responses to various change-events and transitions concurrently, as well as the athletes' adaptation and the effects on their career pathways. Also, it is important to capture the views of coaches and other stakeholders (see Henriksen et al., 2014).

2. Theoretical Question: How Are Athletes' Careers Shaped by Transitions and Change-Events?

To date, the JST received almost exclusive research attention. Research suggested, however, that additional change-events (e.g., *joining a training-abroad program, deselection, a dispute with a coach, participation in the Olympic Games [OGs]*) are perceived as highly significant in athletes' careers (Blakelock et al., 2016; Samuel & Tenenbaum, 2011b, Samuel et al., 2016; Samuel, Stambulova, et al., 2020). These change-events received limited empirical consideration, mostly using cross-sectional and retrospective designs. Two longitudinal studies of injured athletes (Samuel et al., 2015) and handball players who underwent a cultural transition (Samuel, Stambulova, et al., 2020) are unique in this context, as they provided an in-depth analysis of the athletes' experiences and how they influenced their career pathways. Still, it remains unclear whether additional, yet to be identified, transitions or change-events are meaningful in athletes' careers, and what are their unique characteristics. A good example would be the 2020 coronavirus pandemic and the associated global repercussions, such the postponement of the Tokyo OGs (Schinke et al., 2020). Preparing athletes and coaches for potential significant change-events, thereby assuming a proactive standpoint toward athletes' careers, would allow more efficient support during these situations.

To best address this question, it is vital that researchers expand the horizons beyond the normative transitions such as the JST. Moreover, while athletes can experience multiple types of change-events in their careers, certain ones might influence career trajectories more significantly. Considering the potential transitional experiences, researchers should be aware of the unique sportive as well as cultural contexts within which the athlete is engaged (Stambulova et al., 2020). For instance, student-athletes and professional athletes likely experience unique change-events and transition experiences, and tennis players and soccer players have idiosyncratic (e.g., sport-specific) challenges in their career pathways. Likewise, the change-events shaping Chinese athletes might not parallel those experienced by American or European athletes.

Researchers should be aware that athletes tend to experience several concurrent transitions. Existing measurements, such the change-event inventory (Samuel & Tenenbaum, 2011b), might capture only part of the full transitional experience. A need remains to develop measurements that allow an accurate evaluation of a broader range of the transition experience, as well as direct comparison among various types of transitions and change-events. In addition, advancement can be achieved by adopting a mixed-methods longitudinal approach, aimed at capturing a more comprehensive transitional experience, within a specified context (e.g., see Stambulova & Samuel, 2020). Rather than stating general arguments about "the way" athletes develop in their careers, this area calls for a specification of career pathways contextualized within sport discipline environments (see Drew et al., 2019; Henriksen et al., 2014), which are further contextualized within unique sociocultural environments (see Ryba et al., 2018).

3. Theoretical Question: How Do Athletes Adapt During Transitions and Change-Events?

According to the athletic career transition model (Stambulova, 2016), the transition process is defined as "coping with a set of transition demands/challenges using relevant coping strategies and taking into consideration internal (person-related) and external (environment-related) resources and barriers" (p. 257). This suggests that coping is an inherent aspect of athletes' transitional experiences. However, the model does not specify what coping essentially is, other than the application of coping strategies. It is also unclear whether coping occurs implicitly or with conscious intention. Furthermore, the term *coping* is used to explain both the predictor and the outcome of the transitional experience. In cultural transition research (e.g., Ryba et al., 2016), the term *coping* is not used, and the common terms are *psychological adjustment* and *adaptation*. Therefore, it seems that an important factor of the transitional experience has not been well defined, both conceptually and methodologically.

Identifying this shortcoming, the SCSPP (Samuel & Tenenbaum, 2011a, 2011b) was developed, in part to account for what actually constitutes an effective coping process, in terms of psychological change, when athletes are facing disruptions of their career status quo. Within the change process, a distinction is made between the *perceived effectiveness of coping*, the *perceived satisfaction of coping*, and the *perceived outcome* of the change process (Samuel & Tenenbaum, 2013; Samuel et al., 2016). It is further suggested that athletes make conscious decisions (i.e., an initial *strategic decision* and a secondary *decision to change*) in response to a change process, as part of their personal adaptation. These ideas received empirical support regarding various types of change-events (Knowles & Lorimer, 2014; McEwen et al., 2018; Samuel & Tenenbaum, 2013; Samuel et al., 2015, 2016; Samuel, Stambulova, et al., 2020). Samuel and Tenenbaum (2013) also acknowledged the role of *coping strategies usage* as part of athletes' change processes. Specifically, it was found that *acceptance* and *instrumental support* predicted athletes' likelihood of making a decision to change.

To best address this question, researchers should first conceptualize what coping is, acknowledging the separate effects of coping effectiveness and coping satisfaction on the transition outcome and athletes' motivation, respectively. Moreover, a range of coping strategies frameworks (e.g., problem focused and emotion focused, adaptive and maladaptive) and associated measurements are currently used. This diversity creates difficulty in systematically and theoretically comparing among studies in this area. It is important to assess both athletes' decision-making processes (e.g., Park et al., 2013; Samuel & Tenenbaum, 2011b) and transition-specific coping strategy usage (e.g., Stambulova et al.,2012). This would provide a more accurate account of the adaptation process.

4. Theoretical Question: How Do Social Media and Globalization Shape Generation Z Athletes' Careers?

Career researchers should acknowledge the unique characteristics of Generation Z (Gen Z) athletes (Gould et al., 2020). Born after 1996, these athletes are living in a world heavily influenced by social media and globalization processes. They do not necessarily hold the long-term focus required to develop as athletes because they tend to be more focused on short-term outcome goals rather than the training process (Gould et al., 2020). As a result, they might experience high rates of transitions between several sport disciplines at the early stages of their sport development. They also find it difficult to organize their schedules so might feel overwhelmed by the number of daily/weekly tasks. This, in turn, can affect their dual-career development and lead to overcentralizing the sport dimension of their lives. Thus, Gen Z athletes might experience intensified emotional reactions to various change-events (Samuel & Tenenbaum, 2011a) and when dealing with adversity (Gould et al., 2020). Furthermore, these young individuals tend to have high achievement expectations (Gould et al., 2020), thereby increasing the risk of being too outcome oriented and experiencing burnout.

Gen Z athletes are also preoccupied with social media, having a constant "fear of missing out" (Gould et al., 2020). It is unclear, however, how social media influence their career decision-making. For example, who are the social agents and what are the underlying mechanisms affecting their motivation, aspirations, and choices? Also, how do social media affect athletes' reactions to various change-events such as winning a gold medal, losing in the first round of a major championship, or getting injured?

Gen Z individuals are also considered less independent in terms of obtaining a driver's license and moving out of the home (Gould et al., 2020). This might influence their ability to make autonomic career decisions and implement them effectively. At the same time, athletes nowadays are expected to engage in transnational mobility (Ryba et al., 2018). Thus, researchers are encouraged to examine how Gen Z athletes feel about leaving home for short- and long-term periods.

Currently, only a few studies examine Gen Z characteristics, not necessarily from a career transition perspective (e.g., David et al., 2018; Gould et al., 2020). Here, focus groups and anthropological designs are effective, as many of these characteristics are apparent in social interactions and might not surface when an athlete is examined individually. Researchers should be aware that much of the "psychological world" of Gen Z athletes can be found in social media, yet it influences their behavior in the real world; for example, how do they respond to critical posts and tweets on social media? (e.g., David et al., 2018). Being technologically savvy and speaking "Gen Z language" are imperative to effectively communicate with today's young athletes and provide effective support.

5. Applied Question: Is Current Career Support Tailored to Sport Performers' Needs?

Stambulova (2016) proposed the assistance in career transitions (ACT) model as a set of guidelines on how to plan a career transition intervention, including (a) foundations, (b) client's characteristics and relevant contexts, (c) goals, (d) contexts to work in, (e) time frames, (f) basic methods, (g) perspectives and content, and (h) assessment. The *preventive/supportive perspective* covers interventions aimed at enhancing athletes' awareness of the forthcoming/current transition demands and aiding in timely development of all the necessary resources for effective coping. The *crisis/negative consequences coping perspective* covers interventions that help athletes assess their crisis/traumatic situations and find the best available ways to cope.

It is important to re-evaluate the relevance and effectiveness of present career support programs and interventions. Practitioners are encouraged to adopt a whole-person approach, considering the various levels of development (Wylleman et al., 2013). In addition, practitioners should be aware of the concurrent transitions or change-events the athlete is experiencing (e.g., a JST accompanied by the change of a coach; see Samuel, 2013). Cultural and sport subcultural contexts are central in accurately assessing athletes' situations. Furthermore, evaluating the athlete's perception is important, as two athletes might perceive similar career situations differently. Conceptually, it is important to assess the stage of the transition. Some transitions (e.g., injuries, OG participation) progress through distinct stages, and this might influence the athlete's decision-making and adaptation.

Most importantly, the focus of counseling athletes in transitions should be on their adaptation to change, potentially through an emphasis on decision-making and implementation, supported by coping strategies (e.g., Samuel, 2013; Samuel, Stambulova, et al., 2020). Practitioners should not assume that athletes automatically cope with transitions, or that coping is effective, and acknowledge the difference between coping (satisfaction and effectiveness) and perceived outcome. Furthermore, it is important to be aware of the unique Gen Z characteristics and how global processes such as social media usage and international migration affect their responses to transitions and change-events. Evaluating the specific transitional experiences and unique contexts of other sport performers, such as referees and coaches, is critical to be able to provide them with adequate career support.

There are only a few intervention studies or case studies related to supporting athletes during transitional experiences, especially within career and in crisis. Some of the work was published in the early 2000s and might be out of context for today's Gen Z athletes who operate in complex sport environments. Thus, applied practice research is much needed, integrating the new developments of this field, considering aspects such as concurrent transitions, dual careers, cultural contexts, and Gen Z characteristics. Longitudinal designs (e.g., Pummell & Lavallee, 2019) are important; however, it is imperative to evaluate the actual effects of such interventions on athletes' long-term adaptation and transition pathways (e.g., Samuel, Stambulova, et al., 2020).

Conclusion

This chapter critically reviewed the recent developments in the area of career transitions and change in sport. Although many of these developments are attuned to the global human developments we witness nowadays (e.g., globalization, dual careers), researchers still are challenged to identify the complex contexts within which athletes are developing their careers. Considerable conceptual and empirical efforts are required to portray the careers of athletes (and other sport performers) and how transitions and change-events play a significant role in shaping career pathways. Both researchers and practitioners should be more critical when evaluating adaptation and coping in the context of transitional experiences. Finally, it is critical to acknowledge that as this field moves forward, so do the lives of sport performers; they have unique characteristics and "psychological worlds" that need to be carefully considered to effectively support them in their career pathways.

References

Blakelock, D. J., Chen, M., & Prescott, T. (2016). Psychological distress in elite adolescent soccer players following deselection. *Journal of Clinical Sport Psychology, 10*, 59–77. doi:10.1123/jcsp.2015-0010

David, J. L., Powless, M. D., Hyman, J. E., Purnell, D. M., Steinfeldt, J. A., & Fisher, S. (2018). College student athletes and social media: The psychological impacts of Twitter use. *International Journal of Sport Communication, 11*, 163–186. doi:10.1123/ijsc.2018-0044

Drew, K., Morris, R., Tod, D., & Eubank, M. (2019). A meta-study of qualitative research on the junior-to-senior transition in sport. *Psychology of Sport and Exercise, 45*, Article 101556. doi:10.1016/j.psychsport.2019.101556

Gould, D., Nalepa, J., & Mignano, M. (2020). Coaching Generation Z athletes. *Journal of Applied Sport Psychology, 32*(1), 104–120. doi:10.1080/10413200.2019.1581856

Henriksen, K., Larsen, C. H., & Christensen, M. K. (2014). Looking at success from its opposite pole: The case of a talent development golf environment in Denmark. *International Journal of Sport and Exercise Psychology, 12*, 134–149. doi:10.1080/1612197X.2013.853473

Ivarsson, A., Stambulova, N., & Johnson, U. (2018). Injury as a career transition: Experiences of a Swedish elite handball player. *International Journal of Sport and Exercise Psychology, 16*, 365–381. doi:10.1080/1612197X.2016.1242149

Knight, C. J., Rodgers, W. M., Reade, I. L., Mrak, J. M., & Hall, C. R. (2015). Coach transitions: Influence of interpersonal and work environment factors. *Sport, Exercise, and Performance Psychology, 4*, 170–187. doi:10.1037/spy0000036

Knowles, A., & Lorimer, R. (2014). A case study of an athlete's experience of multiple change-events moving between team and individual sports. *Journal of Applied Sport Psychology, 26*, 197–210. doi:10.1080/10413200.2013.819393

McEwen, C. E., Hurd Clarke, L., Bennett, E. V., Dawson, K. A., & Crocker, P. R. E. (2018). "It's this thing of being an Olympian that you don't get from anything else": Changing experiences of Canadian individual-sport athletes with Olympic team selection. *Sport Psychologist, 32*, 81–92. doi:10.1123/tsp.2016-0152

Park, S., Lavallee, D., & Tod, D. (2013). Athletes' career transition out of sport: A systematic review. *International Review of Sport and Exercise Psychology, 6*, 22–53. doi:10.1080/ 1750984X.2012.687053

Pehrson, S., Stambulova, N., & Olsson K. (2017). Revisiting the empirical model "Phases in the Junior-to-Senior Transition of Swedish Ice Hockey Players": External validation through focus groups and interviews. *International Journal of Sport Science and Coaching, 12*, 747–761. doi:10.1177/1747954117738897

Poczwardowski, A., Diehl, B., O'Neil, A., Cote, T., & Haberl, P. (2014). Successful transitions to the Olympic Training Center, Colorado Springs: A mixed-method exploration with six resident-athletes. *Journal of Applied Sport Psychology, 26*, 33–51. doi:10.1080/10413200.2013.773950

Pummell, E. K. L., & Lavallee, D. (2019). Preparing UK tennis academy players for the junior-to-senior transition: Development, implementation, and evaluation of an intervention program. *Psychology of Sport & Exercise, 40*, 156–164. doi:10.1016/ j.psychsport.2018.07.007

Ryba, T. V., Schinke, R. J., Stambulova N., & Elbe, A-M. (2018). ISSP Position Stand: Transnationalism, mobility, and acculturation in and through sport. *International Journal of Sport and Exercise Psychology, 16*, 520–534. doi:10.1080/ 1612197X.2017.1280836

Ryba, T. V., Stambulova, N. B., & Ronkainen, N. J. (2016). The work of cultural transition: An emerging model. *Frontiers in Psychology, 7*, 427. doi:10.3389/fpsyg.2016.00427

Samuel, R. D. (2013). Counseling athletes in career change-events: Applying the Scheme of Change for Sport Psychology Practice. *Journal of Sport Psychology in Action, 4*, 152– 168. doi:10.1080/21520704.2013.804015

Samuel, R. D., Basevitch, I., Wildikan, L., Prosoli, R., & McDonald, K. (2020). Please stop changing the rules! The modifications of judo regulations as a change-event in judokas' and coaches' careers. *Sport in Society, 23*(4), 774–794. doi:10.1080/ 17430437.2019.1669911

Samuel, R. D., Galily, Y., & Tenenbaum, G. (2017). Who are you, ref? Defining the soccer referee's career using a change-based perspective. *International Journal of Sport & Exercise Psychology, 15*, 118–130. doi:10.1080/1612197X.2015.1079792

Samuel, R. D., Stambulova, N., & Ashkenazi, Y. (2020). Cultural transition of the Israeli men's U18 national handball team migrated to Germany: A case study. *Sport in Society, 23*(4), 697–716. doi:10.1080/17430437.2019.1565706

Samuel, R. D., & Tenenbaum, G. (2011a). The role of change in athletes' careers: A scheme of change for sport psychology practice. *Sport Psychologist, 25*, 233–252. doi:10.1123/ tsp.25.2.233

Samuel, R. D., & Tenenbaum, G. (2011b). How do athletes perceive and respond to change events: An exploratory measurement tool. *Psychology of Sport and Exercise, 12*, 392– 406. doi:10.1016/j.psychsport.2011.03.002

Samuel, R. D., & Tenenbaum, G. (2013). Athletes' decision-making in career change-events. *Sport Psychologist, 27*, 78–82. doi:10.1123/tsp.27.1.78

Samuel, R. D., Tenenbaum, G., & Gil Bar-Mecher, H. (2016). The Olympic Games as a career change-event: Israeli athletes' and coaches' perceptions of London 2012. *Psychology of Sport and Exercise, 24*, 38–47. doi:10.1016/j.psychsport.2016.01.003

Samuel, R. D., Tenenbaum, G., Mangel, E., Virshuvski, R., Chen, T., & Badir, A. (2015). Athletes' experiences of severe injuries as a career change-event. *Journal of Sport Psychology in Action, 6*, 99–120. doi:10.1080/21520704.2015.1012249

Schinke, R., Papaioannou, A., Henriksen, K., Gangyan, S., Zhang, L., & Haberl, P. (2020). Sport psychology services to high performance athletes during COVID-19. *International Journal of Sport and Exercise Psychology, 18*(3), 269–272.. doi:10.1080/1612197X.2020.1754616

Schinke, R. J., Stambulova, N. B., Trepanier, D., & Oghene, O. (2015). Psychological support for the Canadian Olympic Boxing Team in meta-transitions through the National Team Program. *International Journal of Sport and Exercise Psychology, 13*, 74–89. doi:10.1080/1612197X.2014.959982

Stambulova, N. (2016). Theoretical developments in career transition research: Contributions of European sport psychology. In M. Raab, P. Wylleman, R. Seiler, A-M. Elbe, & A. Hatzigeorgiadis (Eds.), *Sport and exercise psychology research: From theory to practice* (pp. 251–268) Elsevier.

Stambulova, N., Franck, A., & Weibull, F. (2012). Assessment of the transition from junior to-senior sports in Swedish athletes. *International Journal of Sport and Exercise Psychology, 10*, 79–95. doi:10.1080/1612197X.2012.645136

Stambulova, N. B., Ryba, T. V., & Henriksen, K. (2020). Career development and transitions of athletes: The International Society of Sport Psychology Position Stand revisited. *International Journal of Sport and Exercise Psychology.* Advance online publication. doi:10.1080/1612197X.2020.1737836

Stambulova, N., & Samuel, R. D. (2020). Career transitions. In D. Hackfort & R. Schinke (Eds.), *The Routledge international encyclopedia of sport and exercise psychology* (Vol. 2, pp. 119–133). Routledge.

Stambulova, N. B., & Wylleman, P. (2019). Psychology of athletes' dual careers: A state-of the-art critical review of the European discourse. *Psychology of Sport and Exercise, 42*, 74–88. doi:10.1016/j.psychsport.2018.11.013

Wylleman, P., Reints, A., & De Knop, P. (2013). A developmental and holistic perspective on athletic career development. In P. Sotiaradou & V. De Bosscher (Eds.), *Managing high performance sport* (pp. 159–182). Routledge.

20

Fatigue, Overtraining, and Burnout

Robert C. Eklund and J. D. DeFreese

State of the Art

Sport is an ideal environment for the study of human physiological and psychosocial responses to the physical, mental, and social demands of intensive training and competition. Fatigue, overtraining, and burnout are important biopsychosocial outcomes of intensive sport involvement sharing overlapping territory that are too frequently conflated. Nonetheless, these constructs also represent key areas of focus for theoretical and applied research and intervention. The goal of this chapter is to synthesize the current state of the literature as well as to provide a roadmap to inform future research and practice efforts of sport scientists.

In this chapter, a brief overview and synthesis of extant theories and supporting research is provided on fatigue, overtraining, and burnout. Various theoretical perspectives are alluded to on the development of athlete burnout, but Smith's (1986) psychosocial stress and coping model is primarily focused upon because of its encompassing nature. An emphasis is placed on critical historical research milestones by reference to five key readings that have advanced sport science knowledge on these topics. Five major questions are also overviewed, the answers to which will have great informative value for advancing the knowledge base. After a literature review, these questions frame the remainder of the chapter.

Athlete biopsychosocial responses to the demand of sport and sport training have long been an area of interest for sport scientists, coaches, sport psychology practitioners, and the athletes themselves. The network of variables mediating and/or moderating athlete training load responses is complex and ranges across matters relating to individual differences in fitness and strength training, skill development, psychosocial stress, emotional regulation, and so on. Fatigue is the most acute and transient issue of the three outcomes defining this chapter. It is a relatively acute response to

Robert C. Eklund and J. D. DeFreese, *Fatigue, Overtraining, and Burnout* In: *Sport, Exercise and Performance Psychology.* Edited by: Edson Filho and Itay Basevitch, Oxford University Press. © Oxford University Press 2021.
DOI: 10.1093/oso/9780197512494.003.0020

training load/demands that can be monitored via athlete self-perceptions, autonomic nervous system responses, physical performance, and biochemical/hormonal/immunological function (Thorpe et al., 2017; Van Cutsem et al., 2017). Fatigue is an expected normative response to training and competition, but exposure to those stresses also has the potential to result in more maladaptive responses such as overtrained states and/or burnout.

Overtraining, an imbalance between training and recovery, can involve maladaptive responses that can be exacerbated by the presence of psychosocial stressors. Athletes undergoing overreach training (i.e., knowing engagement in a training regime resulting in short-term reductions in training performance to spur adaptations resulting in improved performance after a tapering period) to an excessive degree can experience the overtraining syndrome (OTS, decrements in performance and feelings of exhaustion that can be resistant to attenuation even with training load reductions or the introduction of periods of rest). This chronic condition involves, at its core, systemic (e.g., neurologic, endocrinologic, and immunologic) maladaptive responses to chronic training stress. Prolonged periods of rest are often implicated in recovery elicitation (Meeusen et al., 2013).

Athletes can also experience burnout as a maladaptive response to the chronic exposure to psychosocial stress in training and competition (Eklund & DeFreese, 2020). Evidence suggests that burnout may be driven in some degree by training load, but it can occur in its absence. This occurrence represents a consequence of individualized cognitive and affective responses in the experience of chronic psychosocial stress in sport. Athlete burnout has been conceptualized as a cognitive-affective syndrome characterized by symptomatic dimensions of emotional and physical exhaustion, reduced accomplishment, and sport devaluation (Raedeke & Smith, 2009). This maladaptive experiential state has been associated with deleterious affective and motivational states in sport participation (Eklund & DeFreese, 2020; Goodger et al., 2007). Altogether, athlete responses to training and competition can be complex, and differentiation of fatigue from OTS and/or athlete burnout can be difficult for coaches and athletes—and sport scientists as well. The sport stress literature, with a focus on burnout, has differentiated among these concepts, as indicated in five key readings (see Table 20.1).

Answering a warranted call by sport scientists for definitional and conceptual clarity, Smith (1986) drew upon Lazarus and Folkman's (1984) theoretical contentions on the stress process to conceptualize athlete burnout as a chronic experiential state resulting from prolonged exposure to psychosocial stress. Specifically, burnout was posited to be a result of psychological stress arising from the physical and mental demands of sport training and/or competition. Athletes unable to cope with this stress successfully were posited to experience myriad potential outcomes including heightened perceptions of stress, maladaptive mood states, and, in some instances, athlete burnout. Factors posited to be relevant in Smith's model included individual differences in motivation, social perceptions (e.g., social support), and personality (e.g., perfectionism). It is certainly not the only prominent conceptualization of processes leading to athlete burnout, as issues relating to identity and control (Coakley, 1992) and fundamental psychological need satisfaction (Deci & Ryan, 1985) have also been posited—neither of which are meaningfully incompatible with Smith's perspective. Ultimately, this model has been important to the study of burnout to date and is well positioned to inform this chapter as its particular focus on psychosocial stress aids in the differentiation of athlete burnout from fatigue and OTS. Moreover, it represents a potential synergy with the emerging sport science area of recovery science (Kellmann et al., 2018). In the extant body of literature, athlete burnout has been positively associated with athlete perceptions of psychological stress and negatively associated with perceptions of social support (Goodger et al., 2007). Four seminal psychological stress-based studies are reviewed with a focus on athlete burnout, psychological stress, and how each adds to our discussion of these experiences relative to fatigue, overtraining, and (potentially) recovery.

Considering psychological stress and athlete motivation, both factors relevant to the psychosocial stress and coping model, DeFreese and Smith (2014) completed a prospective, longitudinal study of collegiate swimming/diving and track and field athletes ($N = 465$). They examined temporal associations of social support and negative social interactions with athlete burnout and life satisfaction across a competitive season after accounting for psychological stress, sport motivation, and dispositional factors. Social support was found to be an inverse predictor of athlete burnout, while negative social interactions were a positive predictor of athlete burnout over time. Importantly, the psychosocial stress and coping framework of burnout was expanded in this study to include social perceptions.

Personality factors such as perfectionism were also identified as potentially contributing to athlete burnout in the psychosocial stress and coping model—a matter considered by Madigan, Stoeber, and Passfield (2016) in a longitudinal investigation of motivation, perfectionism, and burnout.

Their study involved the collection of data from a sample of junior sport academy athletes ($N = 141$) at three time points over a 6-month period of active training. Autonomous motivation was found to mediate the negative relationship between perfectionistic strivings and burnout at both the between- and within-person levels of analysis. Controlled motivation, however, mediated the positive relationship between perfectionistic concerns and burnout only at the between-person level. This study highlighted the potential role of perfectionism in athlete burnout development.

Individual difference factors such as age and gender also have relevance to the development of athlete burnout within the stress and coping model—matters considered by Isoard-Gautheur et al. (2015) in their multilevel growth curve analysis examination of trajectories of development of individual burnout dimensions at the beginning, middle, and end of a 2-year period. They obtained data from an initial sample of 895 adolescent French handball athletes. Unique patterns in the development of burnout perceptions among adolescents were observed over time, with some trajectories differing across genders (see Table 20.1 for additional details), suggesting the need to consider gender and age when examining developmental patterns in burnout.

Meta-analyses have also been instrumental in synthesizing and benchmarking the current state of literature on athlete burnout. Pacewicz, Mellano, and Smith (2019), for example, conducted a recent meta-analysis of post-2000 quantitative studies focused on the association between social constructs and athlete burnout. Results provided indications that positive social perceptions may mitigate the experience of athlete burnout, while negative social perceptions (albeit based on relatively few studies, $n = 20$) may promote this aversive experiential state.

As may be inferred from the studies highlighted, few of the strongest historical studies of athlete burnout development have considered fatigue and/or overtraining variables. We posit three reasons for this empirical discrepancy: (a) problems of differentiating burnout from overtraining because of the shared implication of fatigue and similarities in some areas of symptomology, (b) a poor interface in scholarship across sport scientists focused on either physiological or psychological responses to training load and psychosocial stress, and (c) the lack of a unifying framework to guide such work. We posit that recovery science may represent a suitable unifying framework.

Recovery science is focused on an active, multifaceted (i.e., physiological and psychological) approach to athlete recovery in terms of restoring individual athlete biopsychosocial fitness. Recovery science provides a nuanced view of the process that extends beyond viewing recovery as merely a matter of rest or training load reduction/cessation (Kellmann et al., 2018). Athlete recovery is about far more than sleeping or taking time off from training. Both qualitative (Eccles & Kazmier, 2019) and quantitative (Balk et al., 2017) sport science data support the potential utility of this framework in guiding the assessment of athlete rest and recovery. We feel this framework has potential to unite the research areas on fatigue, overtraining, and burnout in sport.

Table 20.1 Five Key Readings in Fatigue, Overtraining, and Burnout

Authors	Methodological Design	Key Findings
DeFreese & Smith (2014)	Prospective, longitudinal	Social support (negative relationship) and negative social interactions (positive relationship) are significant predictors of athlete burnout over a competition season when stress, sport motivation, and personality factors are accounted for.
Isoard-Gautheur et al. (2015)	Prospective, longitudinal	Reduced accomplishment dimension of burnout decreases occurred over time, with the strongest effects for girls. A quadratic relationship for emotional and physical exhaustion occurred for age, with initial increases followed by decreases at older ages. Sport devaluation increased to a greater degree among girls than boys studied.
Madigan et al. (2016)	Prospective, longitudinal	Autonomous motivation mediated the negative relationship between perfectionistic strivings and burnout at both the between- and within-person levels. Controlled motivation mediated the positive relationship between perfectionistic concerns and burnout at the between-person level.
Pacewicz et al. (2019)	Meta-analysis	Positive social perceptions mitigate athlete burnout, while negative social perceptions promote it.
Smith (1986)	Conceptual review	Athlete burnout should be considered as one potential outcome of the psychosocial stress and coping model.

Questions to Move the Field Forward

In accordance with the theme of the book, the remainder of the chapter is guided by five major questions addressing important areas of applied intervention, theory, or methodology. We have sought to provide cogently stimulating answers to each of these major questions by addressing the what, why, and how of each. We begin with two applied questions, follow up with two theory questions, and conclude with one methodology question.

1. Applied Question: What Interventions Are Best Suited to Prevent and/or Ameliorate Maladaptive Responses to the Sport Experience Including (Unrelenting) Fatigue, Overtraining Syndrome, and Athlete Burnout?

What. One of the primary reasons for conducting prospective, longitudinal studies of athlete burnout (and overtraining) is so that a deeper understanding of variables potentially impacting development of these maladaptive states can inform intervention development. We propose, therefore, a detailed discussion of potential interventions. Answering this question, in our opinion, remains the biggest science-to-practice need in the athlete burnout literature because, at present, conjecture remains the primary contour of a course of action for intervention.

Why. Burnout has recently been characterized as an "occupational phenomenon" for workers (World Health Organization, 2019). Unsurprisingly, social scientists are much further ahead in the topic relative to the burnout of working professionals. Yet, the sport science knowledge base is well positioned to "catch up" relative to intervention development. Intervention research does not need to come at the expense of collecting additional data on burnout and overtraining predictors including fatigue. Specifically, interventions combined with monitoring provide an opportunity to collect additional data to further refine predictive algorithms while simultaneously promoting athlete health and well-being.

How. A variety of athlete burnout predictors have been well established in cross-sectional research and subsequently borne out in (limited) longitudinal research. Blending the psychosocial stress and coping perspective and recovery science, interventions educating training athletes on stress management and coping strategies as well as active recovery processes (i.e., nutrition, hydration, dynamic stretching, mindfulness) may represent reasonable target points. Moreover, the social dynamics of sport, including social support and negative social interactions/conflict with various sport-based social actors (i.e., teammates, coaches, parents), have been shown to be important predictors of burnout (Barcza-Renner et al., 2016; Cresswell & Eklund, 2006a) and may also represent key starting points for burnout prevention. The fit between workers and their organizational structures has been an area of interest in workplace burnout intervention efforts. Some preliminary evidence (albeit cross-sectional and descriptive in nature) presented by DeFreese and Smith (2013) suggests promise for this perspective in athlete populations. Variables within this "areas of worklife" framework (Leiter & Maslach, 2004) include workload, control, reward, community, fairness, and values. These variables represent targets for intervention that have potential utility for interfacing well with the recovery science framework. Properly construed for relevance to the sport setting (a task in need of future empirical efforts), they may well help athletes rebound from unrelenting fatigue while also helping to prevent overtraining. Finally, while there are no clinical diagnostic criteria for athlete burnout, interventions can be created to uniquely target athletes who are experiencing relatively severe burnout symptoms. There is certainly utility in exploring whether additional intervention foci and/or duration may be needed by this population as compared to athletes experiencing low to moderate symptom levels. All aforementioned work would be more effective if these interventions included a robust safety monitoring and evaluation plan.

2. Applied Question: How Will Novel Theory-Based Intervention Strategies Be Effectively Evaluated to Ensure Their Efficacy, Safety, and Effectiveness in Athlete Populations?

What. Successful intervention should be theory based, be well designed, adhere to American Psychological Association guidelines, and be carefully evaluated. The thorough evaluation of intervention impact requires that all topics are assessed so continued intervention development is properly informed.

Why. Interventions need to improve patient efficacy in a safe manner to be effective. Moreover, interventions must be feasible so as to promote athlete adherence. Finally, intervention outcomes of burnout, overtraining, and fatigue symptom counts are certainly necessary. Outcomes consistent with recovery science measures including heart rate variability, physical performance, neuromuscular function, and markers of inflammation also represent novel outcomes to target within specified interventions.

How. Psychometric assessment of athlete burnout, overtraining, and athlete fatigue exists in varying degrees of adequacy. These subjective, self-report assessments, however, should be triangulated with data from other observers of athlete psychosocial health including sports medicine providers (i.e., athletic trainers, team physicians), coaches, and parents. Additionally, the availability of neuro-bio-psycho-social marker data on fatigue may present a major opportunity for knowledge about burnout to be moved forward. These data may provide opportunities for insight on how this cognitive-affective syndrome links with athlete physiology and perhaps provide opportunities to positively impact athlete performance. Overall, the use of recovery science as a guide to merge psychological markers of burnout with physiological markers may provide innovative possibilities crucial to intervention assessment and a move toward better understanding of the physiological burden associated with this psychologically maladaptive state. Ultimately, a merging of psychosocial perspectives on burnout with recovery science, along with a blend of subjective and objective assessments, will be of utilitarian benefit to future research on fatigue, overtraining, and burnout in athlete populations.

3. Theoretical Question: Is There a Theoretical Conceptualization That Characterizes and Differentiates Fatigue, Overtraining, and Burnout?

What. Consideration of the extant literature makes apparent that conceptual understanding of the similarities and differences among the constructs of fatigue, overtraining syndrome, and burnout has been an issue from the beginning of the study of these constructs in sport (Eklund & DeFreese, 2015, 2020). The need for such a conceptualization represents an important conceptual step in future work aiming to understand athlete burnout development.

Why. The answer to this question is crucial to future basic and applied research efforts seeking to understand and/or intervene upon variables important to athlete performance and psychosocial health. For researchers to accomplish any of these important goals (and, moreover, to do so in the most effective ways possible), the constructs of fatigue, overtraining, and burnout must be clearly and distinguishably defined and accurately assessed to afford opportunities to pose meaningful research questions and design potentially meaningful intervention studies. Psychometric advancements in assessment and clear operational definition of constructs will be crucial for applied research efforts targeting these constructs individually or concomitantly.

How. Clear, theory-based methodological approaches are needed that examine the sequelae of training and competitive stress among competitive athletes relative to the constructs of fatigue, overtraining, and athlete burnout. Such approaches should afford the use of complex longitudinal analyses to predict these variables at both the between- and within-athlete levels using variables with discriminatory potential relative to their development. These may include variables relating to athlete perceptions of stress and fatigue, coping, sport motivation, training load, and demographic (e.g., gender) and personality (e.g., perfectionism) constructs as well as potential indicators of systemic maladaptive responses relating to neurologic, endocrinologic, and/or immunologic function. Such work may also provide grist for advanced factor analytic or discriminant function analytic strategies to advance clearer differentiation among the constructs and their predictors, as well as their shared territory. The Athlete Burnout Questionnaire (ABQ; Raedeke & Smith, 2009) has, historically, proven to be a valid and reliable psychometric instrument to this point, but the availability of similarly sound psychometric indices of fatigue and overtraining have yet to be employed in sport psychology at this point. The Recovery-Stress Questionnaire (RESTQ-Sport) represents one potential psychometric measure to aid in such important work (Kellmann & Kallus, 2016; Nicolas et al., 2019). Assessment of theoretically relevant markers of these psychobiological states (e.g., Cresswell & Eklund, 2007; Van Cutsem et al., 2017) will also be needed to afford advances in understanding of shared territory and key discriminators. Future prospective longitudinal studies of fatigue, overtraining, and burnout symptoms in athletes will require careful consideration of guiding theory as well as advances in and integration of psychometric and biomarker assessment.

4. Theoretical Question: Does Recovery Science Represent a Useful Conceptual Model to Guide the Next Decade of Topical Research on Fatigue, Overtraining, and Athlete Burnout?

What. Theoretical/conceptual frameworks in sport science that are germane to understanding and supporting athlete health and well-being exist. However, the extent to which they have been used to monitor and understand more distal physiological and psychological sequelae of training and competitive stress (i.e., overtraining syndrome, burnout) among athletes is limited. Based on our review of the literature and its utility to inform both research and practice, we propose recovery science as an informative framework to guide research to advance knowledge in this area. Recovery science is a burgeoning topic in sport science with clear links to fatigue and clear conceptual links to overtraining as a result of its focus on active strategies to optimize mental and physical recovery from training. The integration of athlete burnout into this perspective represents a logical potential next conceptual step forward.

Why. The efforts to focus on intervention relative to athlete burnout and overtraining in sport have been limited and largely without overarching and unifying conceptual grounding. Research examining burnout in the workplace has made greater strides toward this aim (Maslach & Leiter, 1997). An innovative focus on athlete recovery provides a needed opportunity to shift the focus on maladaptive sequelae to training and competitive stress among athletes further yet into the world of intervention under the guidance of a clear conceptual framework.

How. Recovery science involves an emphasis on measurement with a primary focus on monitoring fatigue relative to both external load (i.e., work completed by the athlete regardless of internal response characteristics) and internal load (i.e., physiological strain resulting from external demands; see Halson, 2014). This can involve athlete self-report measures as well as biomarkers of the autonomic nervous system (i.e., submaximal heart rate, heart rate variability, heart rate recovery), physical performance (i.e., neuromuscular function, joint range of motion/flexibility), and biochemical/hormonal/immunological function (i.e., creatine kinase, inflammation markers, cortisone, testosterone). Though some of these measures have been investigated in relation to athlete burnout in small pilot studies (e.g., Cresswell & Eklund, 2007), these common markers of recovery science have not been included in an overarching study of athlete burnout development. Many sport teams at various levels of competition have already begun to monitor external and internal training load; accordingly, adding consistent assessment of athlete burnout to such protocols would be fruitful. The creation of large-scale athlete data sets of markers of recovery, overtraining, and burnout symptoms would represent a major step in our understanding and effective monitoring of these markers with primary implications for the design of safe and effective interventions to optimize athlete mental and physical health. Specifically, algorithms could be created from such data sets that identify individual or combinations of recovery variables best suited for prevention of overtraining syndrome and/or burnout as well as promotion of athlete recovery.

5. Methodological Question: What Research Designs Represent Scientifically Efficacious and Ethical Ways to Concomitantly Investigate the Development of Fatigue, Overtraining, and/or Burnout in Athletes?

What. A need exists for well-designed research studies well suited to using theory to answer the aforementioned research questions. Cross-sectional research designs were frequently used in early studies of athlete burnout, but longitudinal studies aimed at understanding burnout development have increasingly emerged over the last decade. Going forward, longitudinal research design should continue to be prioritized to further advance knowledge about interrelationships among fatigue, overtraining, and burnout. Certainly, this question in and of itself suggests the need for multi-time-point designs because of the emphasis on development. However, myriad seasonal (or out-of-season) windows for the assessment points as well as developmental windows (i.e., linked to chronological or biological age) for assessment represent key considerations going forward.

Why. Research design is an extremely important, yet too often underrated, aspect of the conceptual brainstorming required to move knowledge forward on a topic. To date, the number of and duration between time points in longitudinal studies of overtraining and burnout, and recovery science-driven studies of fatigue and training load have varied wildly. Assessment windows have ranged from being across seasons and years of developing athletes' careers to multiple in-season time points ranging from weeks to months apart to even a subset of weeks within a training or competition period (e.g., Cresswell & Eklund, 2005, 2006b; Isoard-Gautheur et al., 2015). The use of more systematic designs for work in these areas to afford both comparability and efficient contrast of developmental time frames will represent a potentially important innovation for the advancement of the knowledge base.

How. Recovery science may again be helpful to the creation of more standardized windows for the assessment of the development of overtraining and burnout symptoms. Specifically, a focus on parameters for assessing daily and/or weekly internal and external training load could also be used to assess overtraining and burnout symptom development. Lemyre, Treasures, and Roberts (2006) conducted a study of burnout, motivation, and affect during collegiate swimming training that may represent a guide for continued development work in this area. At minimum, the assessment protocols of relevance for competitive seasons, off-seasons, and cross-training time points probably differ. Additionally, multiyear designs to look at athlete burnout over time should involve more than one assessment per year. Ultimately, a standardization of monitoring windows relative to training load (e.g., periodized training phases) and athlete outcomes will be useful for advancing knowledge about overtraining and burnout development as well as being informative for translation of resultant knowledge into interventions to prevent and treat overtraining and burnout among athletes. Importantly, the epidemiology of burnout and overtraining syndrome (i.e., prevalence as one marker) is still unknown in any meaningful way despite years of research (Eklund & DeFreese, 2015, 2020).

Conclusion

Overall, this chapter presents a synthesis and roadmap for the next decade of sport science research with the goal to advance the scope of knowledge on these three important sport psychology topics. The concepts of fatigue, overtraining, and burnout are conceptually complex, but that complexity provides sport science scholars with many exciting opportunities to be innovative on applied, theoretical, and methodological accounts. It will take interdisciplinary scholarship to continue to define and differentiate these constructs. The use of relevant theory and appropriate designs to understand the shared and unique components of their development should be revealing in ways that will allow successful intervention and meaningful evaluation to promote athlete health and well-being. We feel recovery science represents a conceptual framework that, along with relevant theory and extant athlete burnout research, could provide a valuable guide for the use of the prospective, longitudinal, and theoretically informed interventions best suited for answering these complex questions. Ultimately, we hope this chapter provides a useful guide to researchers who, like ourselves, are interested in furthering knowledge on these important topics of fatigue, overtraining, and burnout in sport.

Acknowledgments

We acknowledge and thank the members of the recently created Burnout in Sport Network for their gracious and thoughtful suggestions on topical ideas for this chapter.

References

Balk, Y. A., de Jonge, J., Oerlemans, W. G. M., & Geurts, S. A. E. (2017). Testing the triple-match principle among Dutch elite athletes: A day-level study on sport demands, detachment and recovery. *Psychology of Sport and Exercise, 33*, 1–17.

Barcza-Renner, K., Eklund, R. C., Morin, A., & Habeeb, C. (2016). Controlling coaching behaviors and athlete burnout: Investigating the mediating role of perfectionism and motivation. *Journal of Sport and Exercise Psychology, 38*, 30–44.

Coakley, J. (1992). Burnout among adolescent athletes: A personal failure or social problem? *Sociology of Sport Journal, 9*, 271–285.

Cresswell, S. L., & Eklund, R. C. (2005). Changes in athlete burnout over a 12-week league tournament. *Medicine and Science in Sports and Exercise, 37*, 1957–1966.

Cresswell, S. L., & Eklund, R. C. (2006a). Changes in athlete burnout over a 30-wk "rugby year." *Journal of Science and Medicine in Sport, 9*, 125–134.

Cresswell, S. L., & Eklund, R. C. (2006b). The nature of player burnout in rugby. *Journal of Applied Sport Psychology, 18*, 219–239.

Cresswell, S. L., & Eklund, R. C. (2007). Athlete burnout and immune function. *New Zealand Journal of Sports Medicine, 34*, 5–11.

Deci, E. L., & Ryan, R. M. (1985). *Intrinsic motivation and self-determined human behavior*. Plenum Press.

DeFreese, J. D., & Smith, A. L. (2013). Areas of worklife and the athlete burnout–engagement relationship. *Journal of Applied Sport Psychology, 25*, 180–196.

DeFreese, J. D., & Smith, A. L. (2014). Athlete social support, negative social interactions, and psychological health across a competitive sport season. *Journal of Sport and Exercise Psychology, 36*, 619–630.

Eccles, D. W., & Kazmier, A. W. (2019). The psychology of rest in athletes: An empirical study and initial model. *Psychology of Sport and Exercise, 44*, 90–98.

Eklund, R. C., & DeFreese, J. D. (2015). Athlete burnout: What we know, and what we should be finding out about. *International Journal of Applied Sports Sciences, 27*, 63–75.

Eklund, R. C., & DeFreese, J. D. (2020). Athlete burnout. In G. Tenenbaum & R. C. Eklund (Eds.), *Handbook of sport psychology* (4th ed.). Wiley.

Goodger, K., Gorely, T., Lavallee, D., & Harwood, C. (2007). Burnout in sport: A systematic review. *Sport Psychologist, 21*, 127–151.

Halson, S. L. (2014). Monitoring training load to understand fatigue in athletes. *Sports Medicine, 44*, S139–S147.

Isoard-Gautheur, S., Guillet-Descas, E., Gaudreau, P., & Chanal, J. (2015). Development of burnout perceptions during adolescence among high level athletes: A developmental and gendered perspective. *Journal of Sport and Exercise Psychology, 37*, 436–448.

Kellmann, M., Bertollo, M., Bosquet, L., Brink, M., Coutts, A.J., Duffield, R., Erlacher, D., Halson, S. L., Hecksteden, A., Heidari, J., Kallus, K. W., Meeusen, R., Mujika, I., Robazza, C., Skorski, S., Venter, R., &Breckman, J. (2018). Recovery and performance in sport: Consensus statement. *International Journal of Sports & Physiology and Performance, 13*, 240–245.

Kellmann, M., & Kallus, K. W. (2016). *The recovery-stress questionnaires: User manual.* Pearson Assessment.

Lazarus, R. S., & Folkman, S. (1984). *Stress, appraisal and coping.* Springer.

Leiter, M. P., & Maslach, C. (2004). Areas of worklife: A structured approach to organizational predictors of job burnout. In P. L. Perrewé & D. C. Ganster (Eds.), *Research in occupational stress and well-being* (pp. 91–134). Elsevier.

Lemyre, P.-N., Treasure, D. C., & Roberts, G. C. (2006). Influence of variability in motivation and affect on elite athlete burnout susceptibility. *Journal of Sport and Exercise Psychology, 28*, 32–48.

Madigan, D. J., Stoeber, J., & Passfield, L. (2016). Motivation mediates the perfectionism-burnout relationship: A three-wave longitudinal study with junior athletes. *Journal of Sport & Exercise Psychology, 38*, 341–354.

Maslach, C., & Leiter, M. P. (1997). *The truth about burnout: How organizations cause personal stress and what to do about it.* Josey-Bass.

Meeusen, R., Duclos, M., Foster, C., Fry, A., Gleeson, M., Nieman, D., . . . Urhausen, A. (2013). Prevention, diagnosis and treatment of the overtraining syndrome: Joint consensus statement of the European College of Sport Science (ECSS) and the American College of Sports Medicine (ACSM). *European Journal of Sport Science, 13*, 1–24.

Nicolas, M., Vacher, P., Martinent, G., & Mourot, L. (2019). Monitoring stress and recovery states: Structural and external stages of the short version of the RESTQ sport in elite swimmers before championships. *Journal of Sport and Health Science, 8*, 77–88.

Pacewicz, C. E., Mellano, K. T., & Smith, A. L. (2019). A meta-analytic review of the relationship between social constructs and athlete burnout. *Psychology of Sport & Exercise, 43*, 155–164.

Raedeke, T. D., & Smith, A. L. (2009). *The Athlete Burnout Questionnaire manual.* West Virginia University.

Smith, R. E. (1986). Toward a cognitive-affective model of athletic burnout. *Journal of Sport Psychology, 8*, 36–50.

Thorpe, R. T., Atkinson, G., Drust, B., & Gregson, W. (2017). Monitoring fatigue status in elite team-sport athletes: Implications for practice. *International Journal of Sport Physiology and Performance, 12*, S227–S235.

Van Cutsem, J., Marcora, S., De Pauw, K., Bailey, S., Meeusen, R., & Roelands, B. (2017). The effects of mental fatigue on physical performance: A systematic review. *Sports Medicine, 47*, 1569–1588.

World Health Organization. (2019). Burn-out an "occupational phenomenon": International Classification of Diseases. https://www.who.int/mental_health/evidence/burn-out/en/

21

Injury and Concussion

Leslie Podlog, Stefanie Podlog, and Jeffrey G. Caron

State of the Art

In the 1980s, scholars began paying increased attention to the psychological aspects of sport injury. Much of the research since that time has focused on intrapersonal (e.g., stress, motivation, self-efficacy beliefs) and interpersonal (e.g., patient-practitioner relationships, social support) factors associated with injury risk, rehabilitation, and return to sport (Brewer & Redmond, 2017). In summarizing the research, we briefly highlight conceptual models guiding inquiry in this area. Table 21.1 highlights five seminal studies on the psychosocial aspects of sport injury.

Factors Influencing Injury Risk

The majority of research on psychological risk factors for acute injury has been guided by Williams and Andersen's stress-injury model (1988; revised, 1998). The researchers suggest that athletes' cognitive appraisals of potentially threatening sport situations elicit a stress response—characterized by attentional deficits (i.e., peripheral narrowing and distraction) and deleterious physiologic implications (e.g., fatigue, reduced timing and coordination)—the strength of which increases or decreases the likelihood of injury risk. Further, although findings generally support the hypothesized contention that personality traits, history of stressors, and coping resources all moderate the stress response and subsequent injury risk, a meta-analysis (Ivarsson et al., 2017) indicated that relationships between personality traits ($r = .01$, 80% confidence interval [CI] [–.01, .03]), history of stressors ($r = .13$, 80% CI [.11, .15]), coping resources ($r = -.07$, 80% CI [–.10, –.03]), and injury were marginal to small at best. Some support has also been found for the proposed mediators, specifically, that athletes with high life event stress

Leslie Podlog, Stefanie Podlog, and Jeffrey G. Caron, *Injury and Concussion* In: *Sport, Exercise and Performance Psychology*. Edited by: Edson Filho and Itay Basevitch, Oxford University Press. © Oxford University Press 2021.
DOI: 10.1093/oso/9780197512494.003.0021

may be more susceptible to attentional disruptions and subsequent injury (Ivarsson et al., 2017). Although much has been learned about the psychological factors predictive of musculoskeletal injury, virtually no research exists examining psychosocial variables that predict concussion or chronic injury. A concussion is a type of traumatic brain injury that results from direct or indirect blows to the face, head, or elsewhere on the body (McCrory et al., 2017). The neurological impairment that accompanies a concussion is often transient (i.e., 2 weeks for adults and 30 days for children and adolescents younger than 18 years of age). A concussed individual may experience one or more of the following: symptoms (somatic, cognitive, emotional), physical signs, behavioral changes, balance and cognitive impairment, and sleep disturbance. In an effort to target injury risk factors, researchers have also examined the effects of multimodal, cognitive behavioral interventions. A recent meta-analysis demonstrated that interventions focused on stress management and relaxation techniques had a large effect on reducing the number of injuries among athletes (Ivarsson et al., 2017).

Rehabilitation

In examining factors influencing rehabilitation, scholars have consistently used Wiese-Bjornstal and colleagues' (1998) integrated model of response to sport injury. The central assumption of the model is that the same individual and situational variables that influence injury risk also influence athletes' postinjury responses. In particular, a host of personal (e.g., injury-specific, psychological, demographic, physical) and situational (e.g., sport types, social, environmental) factors are posited to influence cognitive (e.g., goals, self-perceptions, injury attributions), emotional (e.g., frustration, grief), and behavioral responses to injury (e.g., adherence to rehabilitation, malingering) in a cyclical fashion, all of which are suggested to influence recovery outcomes (i.e., physical and psychological). In support of the model, numerous personal (e.g., self-motivation, pain tolerance, self-efficacy) and situational variables (e.g., social support, patient-practitioner rapport) have been associated with athletes' cognitive, emotional, and behavioral responses throughout the rehabilitation time frame (Brewer & Redmond, 2017). For instance, Caron and colleagues (2013) described the deleterious implications of repeated concussion on former National Hockey League players' cognitive, emotional, and behavioral/interpersonal functioning.

Athletes articulated feelings of alarm and distress associated with the physical symptoms of concussion (e.g., vision impairments, headaches), experiences of isolation and withdrawal, profound emotional upheaval (e.g., anxiety and depression), and changing self-perceptions during their transition out of professional sport. The importance of situational factors, namely social support, in coping with concussion and retirement was also described (Caron et al., 2013).

Psychological interventions such as imagery, relaxation, goal setting, and written emotional disclosure have been shown to improve emotional response, rehabilitation adherence, pain, and functional ability (Brewer & Redmond, 2017). Recent interdisciplinary efforts focused on understanding the mechanisms of intervention effects demonstrate that interventions such as imagery or relaxation may expedite the recovery process through neurophysiological changes, such as increased motor-force generation in the cortex and improved programming and planning in the motor system (Clark et al., 2014). For example, in their experimental study, Clark et al. (2014) found that mental imagery training attenuated the loss of muscle strength and voluntary activation (the nervous systems ability to fully activate muscle) by ~50% (23.8 ± 5.6% and 12.9 ± 3.2% reductions, respectively). Scholars have also found that interpersonal interventions focused on social support and positive patient-practitioner rapport can improve athlete rehabilitation adherence and well-being (Brewer & Redmond, 2017). Additional well-powered, experimental studies are needed, however, to support efficacy claims for various interventions such as imagery (Zach et al., 2018), social support, and emotional disclosure.

Return to Sport

The return-to-sport time frame refers to the period when athletes transition from rehabilitation to sport-specific training and competition. Evidence suggests that intrinsic or personally valued reasons for returning to sport (e.g., a love of the game) predict a greater likelihood of return to sport, more positive return-to-sport outcomes (e.g., greater sport appreciation, increased mental toughness), and more positive appraisals and emotions regarding an upcoming return to sport (Ardern et al., 2013; Podlog & Eklund, 2010). Substantial research also highlights the fact that competence (e.g., reinjury anxieties, worries about postinjury performance), autonomy (e.g., pressures to return to sport, a lack of control over rehabilitation progress), and relatedness (e.g., feelings of isolation from one's teammates) issues are pertinent as athletes' re-enter the competitive arena (Ardern et al., 2013). For instance, a key competence-based concern—reinjury anxiety—has been shown to delay or prevent a return to sport, increase attentional distraction, and adversely impact athletes' postinjury performances (e.g., Ardern et al., 2013; Gray, 2015). Gray (2015) found experimental evidence that injured expert position baseball players ($n = 10$) who received medical clearance to return to sport but had not yet begun playing competitively performed significantly worse on a simulated batting task compared to noninjured experts ($n = 10$). Moreover, comparisons between injured and noninjured experts on a secondary judgment task involving perceptions of one's knee angle while swinging the bat revealed that injured experts were more aware of their knee angles while at bat compared to their noninjured counterparts. The latter finding indicated that injury induced an internal focus of attention, which may have in part accounted for performance decrements on the simulated batting task.

Although there is evidence of greater interdisciplinary collaboration, traditionally, research on the psychosocial aspects of sport injury has been siloed and/or limited in focus. We believe there are several explanations for this. First, pragmatic considerations such as the need to obtain a particular sample size for statistical analyses and the challenges inherent in objectively assessing performance across a variety of sports (e.g., effective postinjury performance in swimming may be different than in rugby) have typically led researchers to retrospectively examine whether one perception (e.g., motivations to return to sport) correlates with another perception (e.g., postinjury performance). In doing so, researchers have ultimately limited the types of postinjury outcomes (e.g., objective performance, movement patterns, reinjury rates) that have been examined and precluded the need for interdisciplinary collaboration. Limited and competitive funding for research focused on injured athlete populations has also restricted the likelihood that researchers examine the types of questions that necessitate interdisciplinary methods, for example, examining the influence of psychological factors (e.g., cognitive or emotional response to injury) on physiological (e.g., hormonal) or motor performance behaviors. A final explanation for siloed research in this area may pertain to interest in collaborating across disciplinary lines.

While caution is warranted in making broad generalizations, researchers in the physical sciences (e.g., physiology, biomechanics) have traditionally viewed nonexperimental approaches—such as qualitative and cross-sectional designs typically employed in the psychology of sport injury—as "soft science" and may, therefore, be less interested in working with psychology of sport injury researchers. Despite these challenges, theoretical, methodological, and practical advances in sport injury research may be gained through further interdisciplinary research. In the next section, we articulate five questions spanning the three phases—preinjury, rehabilitation, and return to sport—that are best addressed from an interdisciplinary perspective. An interdisciplinary approach is one in which the expertise of scholars from different disciplines is brought to bear on the research problem in question.

Table 21.1 Five Key Readings in Psychosocial Aspects of Sport Injury

Authors	Methodological Design	Key Findings
Caron et al. (2013)	Qualitative—a focus on the rehabilitation and retirement phases	National Hockey League players described how concussion symptoms adversely affected their professional careers, personal relationships, and quality of life.
Clark et al. (2014)	Experimental—a focus on the rehabilitation phase	Imagery can reduce muscle weakness and mitigate voluntary activation. The neocortex may have an important impact on muscle strength.
Gray (2015)	Experimental—a focus on the return-to-sport phase	Injury induces an internal focus and results in diminished motor performance.
Ivarsson et al. (2017)	Meta-analysis—a focus on the preinjury phase	Stress is a consistent predictor of increased injury risk. Psychosocial interventions can mitigate injury risk.
Podlog & Eklund (2010)	Experimental—a focus on the return-to-sport phase	Greater self-determination in the return to competition resulted in more positive appraisals (increased desirability, reduced threat, unfairness, ego damage) and enhanced positive affect (greater happiness and excitement).

Questions to Move the Field Forward

1. Applied and Theoretical Question: Which Biopsychosocial Risk Factors Predict Chronic Injury?

Why Is It Important to Address the Question?
The vast majority of research has focused on antecedents of acute sport injury. Acute injuries occur suddenly, typically following traumatic confrontation of the physical body. Conversely, overuse injuries result from repeated exposure to physical training (Heidari et al., 2017). Although psychological factors such as stress have been shown to increase pain or acute injury risk (Ivarsson et al., 2017), it seems likely that chronic injury may be more a by-product of an interaction between biological factors, psychological variables (e.g., personality traits, repetitive behaviors), and sociocultural factors (e.g., norms promoting pushing through pain) that encourage sport participation at the expense of health and well-being. While evidence highlights the role of physical and biomechanical factors (inadequate tissue repair, maladaptive movement patterns, anatomic misalignment) in chronic injury (Paterno et al., 2013), much less support has been garnered for the role of psychosocial factors in chronic injury. In one of the only studies examining psychological factors and chronic injury, Rip, Fortin, and Vallerand (2006) found that obsessive passion for dance (controlled engagement in an activity characterized by contingent feelings of self-worth) was associated with prolonged suffering from chronic injuries.

Research examining predictors of chronic injury is important for several reasons. First, mounting evidence suggests that chronic injuries are increasingly commonplace among athletes of all levels, including youth participants (Paterno et al., 2013). Such injuries may deny younger athletes the opportunity to reap the benefits of long-term sport involvement. Second, chronic injuries may take a particularly insidious toll on athlete well-being, given the uncertain nature of recovery progressions and the indeterminacy of symptom resolution. Third, an understanding of the biopsychosocial factors involved in injury risk can help maximize the quality of athletes' training environments through the development of optimal workout programs and motivationally healthy climates. Overall, research on this topic can lay the foundation for applied interventions aimed at reducing chronic injury occurrence. In so doing, athletes may avoid the debilitating experience of chronic injury and continue to pursue their athletic aspirations.

What Is the Best Way to Address the Question?

In examining chronic injury, we advocate examination of the interaction between biological, psychological, and social factors. For example, sociocultural factors such as sport norms encouraging athletes to deny or disrespect pain may influence athletes' psyches (e.g., beliefs about playing/training through pain) and behaviors (e.g., excessive or prolonged practice), as well as their biological functioning (e.g., tissue repair, immune functioning) or biomechanics (e.g., maladaptive movement patterns). Collectively, these factors may influence the development of chronic injuries. Toward this end, physiologists, biomechanists, sport psychologists, and sociologists may combine their expertise to consider relationships between potentially relevant injury risk factors. From an analytic standpoint, it may be that a conjunctive analysis of factors may provide a stronger prediction equation of chronic injury. In particular, person-centered analyses such as latent profile analysis (i.e., a model-based approach to identifying clusters of individuals by providing probability estimates of group membership and fit indices to differentiate between multiple possible cluster solutions) may be valuable in examining individual profiles of biopsychosocial risk factors of chronic injury.

2. Methodological and Applied Question: Does Use of Smartphone Apps Help Reduce Injury Risk and Facilitate Effective Rehabilitation or Return to Sport?

Why Is It Important to Address the Question?

As indicated previously, a variety of cognitive behavioral interventions have demonstrated efficacy in reducing injury occurrence (Ivarsson et al., 2017). Moreover, empirical evidence supports the value of several sport psychology interventions (e.g., goal setting, imagery, social support, communication training, role models) in facilitating sport injury rehabilitation (Brewer & Redmond, 2017). Such interventions, however, have generally been conducted by qualified researchers or psychologists in relatively controlled contexts. With the exception of well-funded collegiate or professional sport teams, many sport teams do not have access to sport psychology practitioners. Furthermore, training and practice time is often limited and coaches may be reluctant to "give away" their valuable training time for inclusion of psychological skill interventions or other work that may be perceived as peripheral to the physical training and preparation of athletes. Finally, training facilities may be crowded, or space issues may preclude opportunities to carry out face-to-face interventions. Given these circumstances, novel approaches in the delivery of psychological skill interventions for reducing injury and enhancing sport injury rehabilitation are needed.

What Is the Best Way to Address the Question?

One potentially valuable method for introducing psychological skill interventions that circumnavigate issues associated with traditional skill delivery is the use of smartphone applications—commonly termed apps. Smartphone apps may be valuable in the delivery of skills for several reasons. First, apps are commonly used among millions of individuals worldwide (Islam & Mazumder, 2010). Second, and related to point one, individuals spend substantial amounts of time on their phones (e.g., an average of 5 hours per day among college students; Lepp et al., 2013). Third, injured athletes may be reluctant to seek help as it may be perceived as a sign of weakness or vulnerability. Use of phones and apps helps avoid such stigma by allowing athletes to engage with content in a confidential manner and at a convenient time and location.

To examine the effectiveness of apps in reducing sport injury occurrence and facilitating recovery, several steps are required. First, the development of apps requires the knowledge and skills of an interdisciplinary team, namely app developers as well as content experts in the psychology of sport injury and rehabilitation providers (e.g., sport medicine professionals). Additionally, extramural funding to support the development of content (e.g., videos) is needed. The content should target known risk factors for injury and/or factors shown to influence the effectiveness of injury rehabilitation. Second, once the apps are developed, there is a need to beta-test their effectiveness with regard to accessibility across various devices/platforms and to ensure they are appealing, engaging, and user-friendly. Third, well-controlled randomized clinical trials are needed to test whether the apps are effective in reducing injury rates and enhancing injury recovery and return-to-sport outcomes. Researchers should also assess dose-response effects, that is, to examine how much app usage is required to reduce injury risk or elicit injury recovery benefits (e.g., expedited recovery times). Development and testing of apps have broad methodological implications for the effective delivery of psychological interventions aimed at reducing injury risk and facilitating effective injury rehabilitation.

3. Theoretical and Applied Question: How Can Concussion Education Make a More Meaningful Impact on Athletes' and Coaches' Concussion Attitudes and Reporting/Management Behaviors?

Why Is It Important to Address the Question?

Concussion education has been disseminated in the form of printed educational materials, web-based platforms (e.g., websites, social networking sites), and, to a lesser extent, targeted interventions. Despite these efforts, researchers have reported that athletes and coaches report a lack of knowledge regarding signs, symptoms, and management of the recovery process (Nanos et al., 2017). A further problem is that even when athletes and coaches are equipped with sufficient knowledge of concussions, such knowledge may—in and of itself—be insufficient in initiating concussion prevention measures or safer decision-making, such as reporting possible concussions (Delaney et al., 2018). For example, Delaney and colleagues (2018) found that of the 106 professional football players (23.4% of the 454 athletes surveyed) who believed they had suffered a concussion in the previous season, 82% (87/106) reported that they did not seek medical attention despite their awareness of the potential adverse short- and long-term health implications associated with the injury. Such findings suggest that educational interventions focused solely on improving knowledge of concussion symptoms and consequences are unlikely to result in meaningful changes in attitudes (i.e., about the severity of the concussions) and behaviors (e.g., reporting concussions, avoiding dangerous contact and collisions).

What Is the Best Way to Address the Question?

Psychological theories provide researchers with a roadmap for understanding behavior by hypothesizing relationships between a set of variables and behaviors of interest (Michie et al., 2014). To date, health behavior interventions have mostly been unsuccessful because they have traditionally focused on disseminating knowledge to participants, which assumes that individuals will act rationally once they are made aware of the negative implications of engaging in an unhealthy/problematic behavior (Kelly & Barker, 2016). Researchers have found that among the health behavior interventions that have purported to use theory, the majority have only been *inspired* by theory and not *grounded* in theory (Conner & Norman, 2017). For an intervention to be grounded in theory, each intervention component must be directly linked to each component of a psychological theory (Michie et al., 2014). As such, grounding concussion education interventions in theory appears to be a useful strategy for researchers to balance messaging about concussion knowledge with theory-driven strategies that will improve athletes' concussion-related attitudes and help them understand how to engage in safer on-field behaviors. Developing sound educational interventions should involve interdisciplinary collaboration. For example, public health researchers, communication scholars, and sport medicine providers should be involved in the development of concussion education interventions.

4. Theoretical and Methodological Question: What Are the Key Attributes of "Readiness" to Return to Sport and Can a Comprehensive Measure of Readiness to Return to Sport Predict Return-to-Sport Outcomes?

Why Is It Important to Address the Question?
Traditionally, athletes' clearance to return to sport following musculoskeletal injury has been based on assessment of physical function, or in the case of concussion, tests such as neurocognitive assessment, gait/balance testing, reaction time, and oculomotor screening (McCrory et al., 2017). The assumption underlining such tests is that athletes who pass them are ready to perform at or exceed previous performance levels and are less likely to incur reinjury or a new injury. Unfortunately, increasing evidence suggests that such assumptions may be unwarranted. A growing body of science indicates that an exclusive reliance on test batteries of physical or neurocognitive function alone may be insufficient for assessing athletes' readiness to resume sport participation following musculoskeletal and concussive injury (Webster & Hewett, 2019). For example, in their meta-analytic examination of the validity of return-to-sport tests after anterior cruciate ligament (ACL) surgery, Webster and Hewett (2019) found that only one out of 18 studies showed

that passing return-to-sport (RTS) test batteries led to greater RTS rates. Moreover, two studies revealed that passing RTS test batteries did not significantly reduce the risk of a further knee injury (risk ratio [RR] = .28 [95% CI .04–.94], p = .09), while five studies showed that passing RTS test batteries did not reduce the risk for all subsequent ACL injuries (RR = .80 [95% CI .27–2.30], p = .70). Counterintuitively, passing an RTS test battery actually increased the risk for a subsequent contralateral ACL injury (RR = 3.35 [95% CI 1.52–7.37], p = 0.003]. These findings suggest that commonly employed tests (e.g., agility, strength, muscle mass/size) designed to assess athletes' readiness to resume sport participation and avoid reinjury or new injury may be inadequate or incomplete. As such, more comprehensive and/or sensitive tools are needed to assess athletes' readiness to resume sport participation.

What Is the Best Way to Address the Question?
In an effort to address neglected dimensions of readiness to return, scholars have in recent years developed survey instruments focused on the psychological aspects of readiness. Perhaps the most widely used inventory to date is Glazer's (2009) Injury-Psychological Readiness to Return to Sport (I-PRRS) Scale. However, equating confidence with "readiness" to return to sport after musculoskeletal injury may be incomplete (Podlog et al., 2015). Furthermore, given the unique pathophysiology of concussions, its symptomology, and the uncertain timeline for symptom resolution, measures sensitive to addressing the unique nature of concussion may be needed to address readiness among concussed athletes. Consequently, we argue here that the development of a biopsychosocial approach is needed to fully capture the dimensions of readiness. Presumably, a more holistic measure of readiness would be composed of perceptions of one's biological healing, psychological (e.g., confidence, emotions), and social elements (e.g., perceptions of trust/value in the expertise of care providers, social support). Further work is also needed to better understand whether "readiness" is about the relative absence of negative states (e.g., reinjury anxiety) or about experiencing the presence of particular states of mind. The creation of a biopsychosocial assessment tool of readiness to return to sport should ideally be established based on interactions between sport science/sport medicine practitioners with a knowledge of the biological aspects of healing (e.g., physiatrists, physiotherapists) and the psychosocial aspects of injury (e.g., rehabilitation and sport psychologists) likely to influence readiness perceptions.

5. Applied Question: Does the Development and Implementation of a Standardized Return-to-Learn Protocol Impact the Reduction of Concussion Symptomology?

Why Is It Important to Address the Question?

Concussed learners are a major public health concern, since they are likely to miss more days of school than those with a musculoskeletal injury (Romm et al., 2018). Incidence data suggest that up to 1.9 million youth are affected by sports- and recreation-related concussions each year (Chrisman et al., 2019). Given the tendency of learners to underreport their symptoms, such figures may be conservative (Asken et al., 2016). Furthermore, it is estimated that 5% of students participating in contact sports such as football may sustain concussion each season (Chrisman et al., 2019).

To avoid exacerbation of symptoms following a concussion, cognitive rest for a period of 24 to 48 hours has been advocated before resuming symptom-limited scholarly activities (McCrory et al., 2017). Unfortunately, premature return to learning poses a number of potential problems for the learner. For example, attempts to keep pace with course requirements may exacerbate concussion symptoms such as insomnia, concentration, and memory. Additionally, athletes who return to learning environments too soon have reported a variety of complaints including headaches, an inability to keep up with homework requirements, poor performance, and fatigue (Iverson & Gioia, 2016). Given these issues, there is a need for intervention strategies to help concussed athletes resume cognitive and academic activities without aggravating symptoms.

What Is the Best Way to Address the Question?

One approach that has been proposed is a graduated four-step return-to-learn (RTL) strategy (McCrory et al., 2017). The RTL strategy emphasizes rest following concussion and a gradual resumption of activities. Stage 1 focuses on gradual resumption of typical activities at home (e.g., reading, screen time), while in stage 2, individuals attempt to increase tolerance of cognitive work. Stage 3 is characterized by an increase in academic activities and a return to school part time. If symptoms are not exacerbated, individuals can progress to stage 4, in which scholastic engagements can be gradually resumed until a full day is tolerated. Ideally, the RTL process would be individualized based on the concussed learner's needs and involve input and communication between health care providers, school personnel (e.g., teachers), and, if or when needed, parents. This process requires a constructive and interprofessional relationship between school and health care providers who manage the RTL process.

Conclusion

In this chapter, we have reviewed research focused on the psychosocial aspects of musculoskeletal injury and sport-related concussion. Our review synthesized scholarship spanning three phases of the injury experience, namely psychological antecedents, rehabilitation, and the return to sport following rehabilitation. In examining this body of work, we argued that research on the psychology of sport injury has traditionally been siloed from other disciplines. In articulating five questions pertaining to sport injury, our goal has been to inspire further interdisciplinary work. By utilizing interdisciplinary teams, researchers may better understand nuanced interactions and connections between mind and body that influence injury risk, recovery, and return to sport. Ultimately, such understanding can inform evidence-based practice and clinical intervention with injured athletes.

References

Ardern, C. L., Taylor, N. F., Feller, J. A., & Webster, K. E. (2013). A systematic review of the psychological factors associated with returning to sport following injury. *British Journal of Sports Medicine, 47*, 1120–1126. doi:10.1136/bjsports-2012-091203

Asken, B. M., McCrea, M. A., Clugston, J. R., Snyder, A. R., Houck, Z. M., & Bauer, R. M. (2016). "Playing through it": Delayed reporting and removal from athletic activity after concussion predicts prolonged recovery. *Journal of Athletic Training, 51*, 329–335. doi:10.4085/1062-6050-51.5.02

Brewer, B. W., & Redmond, C. (2017). *Psychology of sport injury*. Human Kinetics.

Caron, J. G., Bloom, G. A., Johnston, K. M., & Sabiston, C. M. (2013). Effects of multiple concussions on retired national hockey league players. *Journal of Sport and Exercise Psychology, 35*, 168–179.

Chrisman, S. P., Lowry, S., Herring, S. A., Kroshus, E., Hoopes, T. R., Higgins, S. K., & Rivara, F. P. (2019). Concussion incidence, duration, and return to school and sport in 5- to 14-year-old American football athletes. *Journal of Pediatrics, 207*, 176–184. doi:10.1016/j.jpeds.2018.11.003

Clark, B. C., Mahato, N. K., Nakazawa, M., Law, T. D., & Thomas, J. S. (2014). The power of the mind: The cortex as a critical determinant of muscle strength/weakness. *Journal of Neurophysiology, 112*, 3219–3226.

Conner, M., & Norman, P. (2017). Health behaviour: Current issues and challenges. *Psychology and Health, 32*, 895–906. doi:10.1080/08870446.2017.1336240

Delaney, J. S., Caron, J. G., Correa, J. A., & Bloom, G. A. (2018). Why professional football players chose not to reveal their concussion symptoms during a practice or game. *Clinical Journal of Sports Medicine, 28*, 1–12. doi:10.1097/JSM.0000000000000495

Glazer, D. D. (2009). Development and preliminary validation of the Injury-Psychological Readiness to Return to Sport (I-PRRS) Scale. *Journal of Athletic Training, 44*, 185–189.

Gray, R. (2015). Differences in attentional focus associated with recovery from sports injury: Does injury induce an internal focus? *Journal of Sport and Exercise Psychology, 37*, 607–616.

Heidari, J., Hasenbring, M., Kleinert, J., & Kellmann, M. (2017). Stress-related psychological factors for back pain among athletes: Important topic with scarce evidence. *European Journal of Sport Science, 17*, 351–359.

Islam, R., & Mazumder, T. (2010). Mobile application and its global impact. *International Journal of Engineering and Technology, 10*, 72–78.

Ivarsson, A., Johnson, U., Andersen, M. B., Tranaeus, U., Stenling, A., & Lindwall, M. (2017). Psychosocial factors and sport injuries: Meta-analyses for prediction and prevention. *Sports Medicine, 47*, 353–365.

Iverson, G. L., & Gioia, G. A. (2016). Returning to school following sport-related concussion. *Physical Medicine and Rehabilitation Clinics of North America, 27*, 429–436. doi:10.1016/j.pmr.2015.12.002

Kelly, M. P., & Barker, M. (2016). Why is changing health-related behaviour so difficult? *Public Health, 136*, 109–116. doi:10.1016/j.puhe.2016.03.030

Lepp, A., Barkley, J. E., Sanders, G. J., Rebold, M., & Gates, P. (2013). The relationship between cell phone use, physical and sedentary activity, and cardiorespiratory fitness in a sample of U.S. college students. *International Journal of Behavioral Nutrition and Physical Activity, 10*, 79.

McCrory, P., Meeuwisse, W., Dvorak, J., Aubry, M., Bailes, J., Broglio, S., . . . Vos, P. E. (2017). Consensus statement on concussion in sport—The 5th international conference on concussion in sport held in Berlin, October 2016. *British Journal of Sports Medicine, 51*(11), 838–847.

Michie, S., Atkins, L., & West, R. (2014). *The behaviour change wheel: A guide to designing interventions.* Silverback Publishing.

Nanos, K. N., Franco, J. M., Larson, D., Mara, K., & Laskowski, E. R. (2017, December). Youth sport-related concussions: Perceived and measured baseline knowledge of concussions among community coaches, athletes, and parents. *Mayo Clinic Proceedings, 92*, 1782–1790. doi:10.1016/j.mayocp.2017.10.003

Paterno, M. V., Taylor-Haas, J. A., Myer, G. D., & Hewett, T. E. (2013). Prevention of overuse sports injuries in the young athlete. *Orthopedic Clinics of North America, 44*, 553–564. doi:10.1016/j.ocl.2013.06.009

Podlog, L., Banham, S. M., Wadey, R., & Hannon, J. C. (2015). Psychological readiness to return to competitive sport following injury: A qualitative study. *Sport Psychologist, 29*, 1–14. http://dx.doi.org/10.1123/tsp.2014-0063

Podlog, L., & Eklund, R. C. (2010). Returning to competition following a serious injury: The role of self-determination. *Journal of Sports Sciences, 28*, 819–831. doi:10.1080/02640411003792729

Rip, B., Fortin, S., & Vallerand, R. J. (2006). The relationship between passion and injury in dance students. *Journal of Dance Medicine and Science, 10*, 14–20.

Romm, K. E., Ambegaonkar, J. P., Caswell, A. M., Parham, C., Cortes, N. E., Kerr, Z., . . . Caswell, S. V. (2018). Schoolteachers and administrators perceptions of concussion management and implementation of return-to-learn guideline. *Journal of School Health, 88*, 813–820. doi:10.1111/josh.12687

Webster, K. E., & Hewett, T. E. (2019). What is the evidence for and validity of return-to-sport testing after anterior cruciate ligament reconstruction surgery? A systematic review and meta-analysis. *Sports Medicine, 49*, 917–929.

Wiese-Bjornstal, D. M., Smith, A. M., Shaffer, S. M., & Morrey, M. A. (1998). An integrated model of response to sport injury: Psychological and sociological dynamics. *Journal of Applied Sport Psychology, 10*, 46–69. http://dx.doi.org/10.1080/10413209808406377

Williams, J. M., & Andersen, M. B. (1998). Psychosocial antecedents of sport injury: Review and critique of the stress and injury model. *Journal of Applied Sport Psychology, 10*, 5–25. doi.org/10.1080/10413209808406375

Zach, S., Dobersek, U., Filho, E., Inglis, V., & Tenenbaum, G. (2018). A meta-analysis of mental imagery effects on post-injury functional mobility, perceived pain, and self-efficacy. *Psychology of Sport and Exercise, 34*, 79–87. https://doi.org/10.1016/j.psychsport.2017.09.011

22

Moral Behavior and Doping

Vassilis Barkoukis and Anne-Marie Elbe

State of the Art

Doping, considered to be one of the greatest threats to modern sports, is defined as the occurrence of one or more antidoping rule violations set forth in the Code of the World Anti-Doping Agency (WADA, 2019). The most common anti-doping rule violations are the presence in an athlete's urine or blood sample or the use, attempted use, or possession of prohibited substances or methods as outlined in WADA's list of prohibited substances and methods. Doping is problematic because it endangers the health of athletes, goes against the integrity of sport, destroys the idea of a "level playing field," and does not set a good example for young athletes (Kayser et al., 2007). Moral and ethical factors have been identified as contributing to the understanding of why athletes involved in competitive sports dope.

Morality refers to personal principles or habits with respect to right or wrong conduct (Gert, 2005). These principles are defined individually and are determined by culture and society. Moral factors that have been investigated with regard to doping are sportspersonship orientations, moral atmosphere, moral identity, and moral disengagement. Sportspersonship orientations reflect the individual differences in the predisposition to act morally. Moral atmosphere refers to norms regarding moral action, that is, the type of behavior considered acceptable in a group by its members. Moral identity refers to the cognitive schema people hold about their moral character; moral disengagement refers to cognitive mechanisms that individuals use to justify their choices and minimize anticipated negative affect (e.g., guilt, shame) when engaging in transgressive behavior (Bandura, 2002).

Studies on the association between doping and moral constructs indicate that the factors listed previously have a strong association with doping intentions and behaviors (Ntoumanis et al., 2014). Sportspersonship

Vassilis Barkoukis and Anne-Marie Elbe, *Moral Behavior and Doping* In: *Sport, Exercise and Performance Psychology.* Edited by: Edson Filho and Itay Basevitch, Oxford University Press. © Oxford University Press 2021.
DOI: 10.1093/oso/9780197512494.003.0022

orientations have been found to be negatively associated with doping intentions. This association was mediated by negative anticipated emotions and was stronger for non-doping users, thus highlighting the strong protective role sportspersonship orientations can play. However, athletes with high or low levels of sportspersonship orientations did not differ in their doping behavior or intentions for doping in the future (Ntoumanis et al., 2014).

With respect to moral atmosphere, past evidence suggests that an environment favoring doping is associated with more positive beliefs toward this behavior. For instance, beliefs that the social environment (i.e., coaches, peers, support personnel, family) approves doping were positively related to higher doping intentions (Lazuras et al., 2015). Similarly, moral identity has been found to influence the doping related decision-making process through moral disengagement and anticipated negative emotions (Kavussanu, Yukhymenko-Lescroart, et al., 2019).

In past research, moral disengagement has been the most extensively studied moral variable. Qualitative data confirmed that moral disengagement mechanisms are evident in amateur and competitive athletes (Boardley et al., 2015). This evidence revealed that athletes tend to rationalize and justify their choice and circumvent the health and moral-related concerns about doping. With respect to the prediction of doping behavior, research evidence consistently suggests that moral disengagement is strongly associated with doping behavior and doping intentions. Its effect on intentions and behavior is typically exerted through doping-related cognition such as attitudes and anticipated negative emotions (Ring & Hurst, 2019). Furthermore, Ntoumanis et al. (2017) concluded that moral disengagement mediates the effect of motivational variables (i.e., controlling motivational climate and basic psychological needs frustration) on doping intentions and behavior.

There is markedly less research with regard to the ethical aspects of doping. Ethics refers to the rules of conduct recognized in a particular group or culture (Solomon, 1984) and they are determined externally (e.g., by WADA, 2019). Ethical decision-making refers to the process of evaluating and choosing among alternatives in a manner consistent with ethical principles, whereas ethical climate refers to the climate within an environment/organization that captures the individuals' perceptions of the ethical policies, practices, and procedures (Martin & Cullen, 2006). To this extent, Elbe and Brand (2015) investigated athletes' ethical decision-making skills with regard to doping and showed that ethical decision-making training was successful in breaking up athletes' stereotypical style of reasoning about doping.

Furthermore, Burton, Welty Peachey, and Wells (2017) outlined that ethical climate is relevant for understanding and investigating ethical issues and sport scandals related to doping.

In sum, morality has been extensively studied in the context of doping. Social-cognitive approaches have dominated research (e.g., sportspersonship orientations, moral atmosphere and identity, and moral disengagement). We provide a list of key readings on the topic of sport and moral behavior in Table 22.1. The evidence suggests that moral-related variables can predict doping behavior and doping intentions and therefore serve in the fight against doping. In contrast, there is less research related to ethical aspects and doping. Despite the large amount of research on morality and doping, many questions warrant further research, as discussed next.

Table 22.1 Five Key Readings in Moral Behavior and Doping

Authors	Methodological Design	Key Findings
Barkoukis et al. (2019)	Qualitative study	Coaches and peers develop a social environment that may influence an athlete's decision to dope.
Elbe & Brand (2015)	Longitudinal study	Ethical decision-making training was successful in breaking up athletes' stereotypical style of reasoning about doping.
Gucciardi et al. (2015)	Literature review	Provides an overview of social desirability research with regard to doping.
Hemphill (2009)	Theoretical	A critical examination of the ethical foundations and arguments against doping.
Ntoumanis et al. (2014)	Meta-analysis	Morality and self-efficacy to refrain from doping had the strongest negative association with doping intentions and behaviors.

Questions to Move the Field Forward

1. Theoretical Question: Is Doping an Immoral Behavior or an Ethical Issue?

One could argue that doping is a performance enhancement aid like many others (e.g., nutritional supplements, high-altitude training, hypobaric chambers), and using doping substances is simply a violation of rules and, thus, an ethical issue. Others argue that doping is against the essence of the so-called "Spirit of Sport" and, thus, constitutes a moral problem (Loland & McNamee, 2019). The official approach of anti-doping authorities (i.e., WADA) assumes that doping is a moral problem for sports, whereas Elbe and Brand (2015) have shown that athletes and coaches perceive doping as an ethical issue.

This ambiguity has resulted in scattered research, the development of modestly effective anti-doping education, uncertainty in the prevalence of doping use (a range from approximately 3% to 57%; Sagoe et al., 2014; Ulrich et al., 2018), and concerns about the legitimacy of the anti-doping system. Resolving this ambiguity and determining whether doping is an ethical and/ or moral problem is expected to impact research, the content and the type of anti-doping education, and policy making in the future. In terms of research, endorsing the notion that doping is a moral problem reflects the notion that those who dope hold low moral values and may have encountered problems in their moral development process. Therefore, research could focus on the core human values and their association with doping, aiming to enhance our understanding of whether people lacking strong morals are more susceptible to doping. This also entails investigating whether there are core human values and if they are determined by culture. It has been argued that the Spirit of Sport values are based on a Western culture of predominantly White males (Loland & McNamee, 2019).

Endorsing the notion that doping is an ethical problem assumes that sport and anti-doping authorities are legitimate in developing and implementing the anti-doping regulations. In this sense, future research could focus on the legitimacy of anti-doping authorities and procedures and the rights of the athletes. It would provide data that could be used to alter the anti-doping regulations and procedures. Importantly, this approach would allow (a) for a more thorough and unbiased discussion of a common rule of conduct for athletes (irrespective of moral issues) and (b) to establish whether legalization of doping could be appropriate and just, and thus resolve the related ethical concerns.

In terms of education, an approach endorsing doping as immoral behavior would result in the development of interventions targeting concepts such as the Spirit of Sport, values of sport, moral reasoning, and moral development. On the other hand, if doping is conceptualized as an ethical issue, anti-doping education could focus on teaching what the common rules of conduct among athletes are, and which sanctions should be expected when the rules are broken. Resolving the morality versus ethics problem would help anti-doping authorities establish more effective prevention programs and policies against doping (see Hemphill, 2009; Loland & Hoppeler, 2012).

2. Theoretical Question: Whether and How Are Moral Factors (e.g., Moral Development, Moral Judgment) and Doping Behaviors Intertwined?

Morality is among the cornerstones of the fight against doping; however, to date, the study of morality and doping has been restricted to a small number of moral constructs. Thus, in terms of theory development, the quest for a robust theoretical approach will allow us to effectively understand the link between moral factors and doping behavior. More specifically, so far the doping literature has been dominated by social-cognitive theory and the concept of moral disengagement (Bandura, 2002). Extensive literature has shown that moral disengagement is closely associated with maladaptive beliefs about doping, such as positive doping attitudes and intentions, as well as doping behavior (Kavussanu, 2015). This line of research advanced our understanding of how athletes' justifications influence their decision to engage in an otherwise irrational behavior. In addition, past evidence has revealed that sportspersonship may also influence doping-related beliefs and cognitions (Ntoumanis et al., 2014). However, this social-cognitive approach limits our understanding of moral judgment about one's decision to dope, as it describes such decision on a static level and investigates the decision-making process at a single point in time. Furthermore, social-cognitive studies are reduced to a narrow set of cognitive variables and determinants of the decision-making process underpinning a "moral" behavior. Accordingly, future research should involve a wider set of variables and a longer time frame of investigation. For example, Hauw (2013) showed that the decision to dope is not a spur-of-the-moment decision, but rather a long and dynamic process.

Additional constructs providing a comprehensive conceptual framework to understand such moral development processes include moral competence and basic human values. Moral competence has been defined by Kohlberg (1964, p. 425) as "the capacity to make decisions and judgments which are moral (i.e. based on internal principles) and to act in accordance with such judgments." He further argued that people develop their moral competence through six stages (i.e., obedience and punishment orientation, self-interest orientation, interpersonal accord and conformity, authority and social-order-maintaining orientation, social contract orientation, and universal ethical principles) that require a long period of time to establish. If this is the case, this reinforces the notion that longitudinal designs would be warranted to investigate how athletes develop this competence. Schwartz (1992) identified 10 basic values (i.e., self-direction, stimulation, hedonism, achievement, power, security, conformity, tradition, benevolence, and universalism) that serve as trans-situational goals with varying importance that largely guide the behaviors of a person or group. An investigation of these values as related to sport might also advance our understanding of the moral basis of doping (see Ring et al., 2020). However, even if these values are endorsed by most athletes at the abstract level, they can become challenged by concrete real-life situations that athletes encounter. The gap between these abstract values (e.g., fair play) and the daily quest of performing better poses challenges to athletes' values.

3. Theoretical Question: What Is the Role of the Athletes' Entourage in Defining Moral Atmosphere and Ethical Climate?

In the extensive doping literature, the individual athlete has been the focus of investigation and intervention. However, athletes are not alone in the sporting environment, and their decisions are largely influenced by other social agents, such as parents, coaches, and peers. Hence, the role of the athlete's entourage in defining the moral atmosphere and ethical climate that can be associated with the decision to dope needs to be determined. Existing evidence indicates that athletes' entourage can influence their beliefs and doping behaviors (see Barkoukis et al., 2019). However, there is scarce evidence about how this influence is exerted over athletes. That is, previous research has not identified social environment aspects that can trigger doping-related beliefs, as well as the underlying processes that can affect athletes' decisions to dope. Recently, Barkoukis et al. (2019) demonstrated that coaches and peers (teammates and opponents) can influence the decision-making process through their interpersonal communication and impact on the overall team atmosphere. In this respect, an autonomy-supportive motivational climate is expected to deter doping behavior (Ntoumanis et al., 2017). Yet, the aspects of a "safe" environment and the situations that may trigger the decision to dope have not been clearly identified. Furthermore, the role of other social agents, such as parents, support personnel (e.g., trainers, doctors, physiotherapists), and media, in influencing athletes has not been fully addressed in the literature so far.

As our knowledge of the role that athletes' entourage play on the established moral atmosphere and athletes' decision to dope is limited, anti-doping efforts (e.g., doping controls and prevention interventions) remain focused on the athletes and largely neglect their entourage. In other words, anti-doping efforts neglect a wide range of people that may influence an athlete and who should be educated about doping. Furthermore, the lack of understanding on how athletes' entourage influences their doping behaviors limits the content and reach of educational interventions targeting athletes' support personnel and social environment. WADA's ADeL (Anti-Doping e-Learning) and project CoachMADE are notable exceptions as they provide anti-doping education for support personnel and coaches. Still, their effectiveness has not been ascertained, and thus interventions should be developed, implemented, and tested for their effectiveness. Specifically, future studies investigating the role of support personnel and other social agents in the development of moral atmosphere and the athletes' decisions to dope would allow for the development of evidence-based interventions promoting healthy moral atmospheres. In turn, the education of athletes' support personnel is expected to better safeguard those who wish to "compete clean" and to deter those who contemplate doping.

4. Methodological Question: How to Best Measure Doping Prevalence and Variables (e.g., Morality/Ethics, Attitudes, and Susceptibility of Doping) Related to the Decision to Dope?

Official WADA reports show that the percentage of athletes who dope is less than 2%. However, self-report surveys with elite athletes revealed that the prevalence of doping among athletes ranges from 3% to 15% (Sagoe et al., 2014). In addition, studies using indirect approaches, such as randomized response technique (RRT), yield much higher prevalence rates. Ulrich et al. (2018) suggested that the doping use prevalence may be between 39.4% and 57.1%. Assuming that these indirect measures are reliable, there is a large proportion of athletes who deliberately cheat when responding to survey questions concerning either their past or current doping use or their beliefs related to future use. This "cheating" might relate not only to questions about actual doping behavior but also to attitudes toward doping, doping susceptibility, and doping-related moral variables. Possible reasons for this might be the development of stereotypes about doping users, the stigmatization of doping as an "immoral" behavior, the strict penalties for those who dope, and social desirability (Gucciardi et al., 2015). If this is indeed the case, scientific evidence about doping prevalence and related variables so far may have been biased. Consequently, evidence-based interventions might not have been based on the most appropriate constructs.

For scientific research on doping to provide valuable information to practitioners, reliable data must be gathered. A key action to resolve the lack of trustworthy data would be to deal with social desirability in survey research targeting doping-related variables. Gucciardi et al. (2015) suggested the use of both proactive and post hoc approaches. More specifically, developing new scales utilizing techniques to prevent social desirability bias during scale completion (e.g., ensuring anonymity and confidentiality, bogus pipeline technique) has been proposed as a useful proactive approach. Furthermore, utilizing statistical techniques (e.g., common shared variance, bogus items) can assist in identifying unreliable data. Also, Wolff, Schindler, and Brand (2015) suggested that indirect methods (e.g., the doping brief implicit association test) may be useful in measuring athletes' doping attitudes and in identifying fake answers to doping-related surveys.

Another aspect to consider to increase the reliability of research on doping in sports consists of applying sport-specific measurement instruments. There is a research call in sport psychology to measure sport phenomena with sport-specific rather than general psychological instruments to decrease measurement error in sport-related research (Kellmann & Beckmann, 2003). In terms of morality, so far, two scales measuring doping-related moral disengagement have been developed (Kavussanu et al., 2016; Mallia et al., 2016). The use of hypothetical scenarios, vignettes, implementation intentions, behavioral expectations, and doping willingness (e.g., susceptibility and likelihood) is expected to increase the variance in participants' responses, thus allowing for a better understanding of the decision-making process anteceding doping behavior. Overall, the measurement reliability of the prevalence of doping should be improved through the inclusion of social-desirability-reducing techniques in survey assessments and the development of novel measures to provide valuable information about participants' beliefs and behaviors toward doping. By using correctly developed and sport-specific measures, we can understand the exact magnitude of the problem and investigate the effectiveness of preventive interventions.

5. Applied Question: What Is the Most Effective Content, Delivery Mode, and Target Groups for Moral-Based and Ethical Intervention?

The most common approach to tackling doping use has been that of regular doping controls and punishments for positive tests, which can also be termed a *detection and deterrence approach* (Mazanov & McDermott, 2009). However, this approach has been deemed ineffective in lowering the prevalence of doping. Furthermore, a number of education campaigns, such as WADA's APLHA and ADeL, and SATURN (Student Athlete Testing Using Random Notification; Goldberg et al., 2007), have focused on increasing awareness of doping control procedures. This approach, however, does not assist in the prevention of doping. The deterrence approach therefore has been complemented by a *prevention approach*, and many respective education programs have been launched (Barkoukis, 2015). Past evidence has shown that education-based interventions were modestly effective in changing athletes' beliefs toward doping (Ntoumanis et al., 2014). The majority of these interventions (e.g., Laure's educational intervention, ATLAS, ATHENA, Doping e-Learning Tools [DELTS]) focused on the health consequences of doping, whereas morality was underdeveloped or ignored.

So far, there are only a few interventions targeting the moral and ethical aspects of doping. The ethical decision-making training composed of moral dilemmas is a notable exception. The training resulted in a small decrease in negative attitudes toward doping and was successful in breaking up athletes' stereotypical style of reasoning about doping (Elbe & Brand, 2015). Projects HEROES and VIRTUE consisted of an intervention targeting moral disengagement and were found to be modestly effective in changing doping-related beliefs and cognition (Hurst et al., 2019; Kavussanu, Hatzigeorgiadis, et al., 2019). Hence, at the present moment, although there is educational material to inform athletes about the negative health effects of doping and the doping control procedure (e.g., the WADA code), morality-related educational material is rather scarce. Therefore, athletes generally hold a negative stance toward doping, but they cannot support it effectively as they lack knowledge and arguments about the moral aspects and hazards of doping. This makes them vulnerable to unreliable information and maladaptive influences (Barkoukis et al., 2019). Regardless of whether doping is immoral or unethical, effective moral/ethical interventions should be developed in the future. In this respect, the content of the intervention, the targeted constructs, the delivery mode of the intervention, the target groups (e.g., athletes, support personnel, students), level of participation, gender, and cultural issues should be taken into account (Tsorbatzoudis et al., 2015).

Conclusion

In conclusion, our chapter illustrates that there are numerous unanswered research questions regarding moral behavior and doping that pertain to theoretical, methodological, and applied aspects. It is our hope that by researching these questions a contribution to a deeper understanding of the relationship between morality, ethics, and doping and an accurate assessment of doping prevalence can be made. This knowledge could then be applied when developing educational interventions aimed at tackling one of the greatest threats of modern sports.

References

Bandura, A. (2002). Selective moral disengagement in the exercise of moral agency. *Journal of Moral Education, 31*, 101–119. https://doi.org/10.1080/0305724022014322

Barkoukis, V. (2015). Moving away from penalization: The role of education-based campaigns. In V. Barkoukis, L. Lazuras, & V. Tsorbatzoudis (Eds.), *Psychology of doping in sport* (pp. 241–255). Routledge.

Barkoukis, V., Brooke, L., Ntoumanis, N., Smith, B., & Gucciardi, D. F. (2019). The role of the athletes' entourage on attitudes to doping. *Journal of Sports Sciences, 37*(21), 2483–2491. https://doi.org/10.1080/02640414.2019.1643648

Boardley, I. D., Grix, J., & Harkin, J. (2015). Doping in team and individual sports: A qualitative investigation of moral disengagement and associated processes. *Qualitative Research in Sport, Exercise and Health, 7*(5), 698–717. https://doi.org/10.1080/2159676X.2014.992039

Burton, L. J., Welty Peachey, J., & Wells, J. E. (2017). The role of servant leadership in developing an ethical climate in sport organizations. *Journal of Sport Management, 31*(3), 229–240. https://doi.org/10.1123/jsm.2016-0047

Elbe, A.-M., & Brand, R. (2015). Ethical dilemma training – A new approach to doping prevention. In V. Barkoukis, L. Lazuras, & V. Tsorbatzoudis (Eds.), *Psychology of doping in sport* (pp. 165–180). Routledge.

Gert, B. (2005). *Morality: Its nature and justification*. Oxford University Press.

Goldberg, L., Elliot, D. L., MacKinnon, D. P., Moe, E. L., Kuehl, K. S., Yoon, M., Taylor, A., & Williams, J. (2007). Outcomes of a prospective trial of student-athlete drug testing: The Student Athlete Testing Using Random Notification (SATURN) study. *Journal of Adolescent Health, 41*(5), 421–429.

Gucciardi, D., Jalleh, G., & Donovan, R. (2015). Substantive and methodological considerations of social desirability for doping in sport. In V. Barkoukis, L. Lazuras, & V. Tsorbatzoudis (Eds.), *Psychology of doping in sport* (pp. 78–92). Routledge.

Hauw, D. (2013). Toward a situated and dynamic understanding of doping behaviors. In J. Tolleneer, S. Sterckx, & P. Bonte (Eds.), *Athletic enhancement, human nature and ethics* (pp. 219–235). Springer.

Hemphill, D. (2009). Performance enhancement and drug control in sport: Ethical considerations. *Sport in Society, 12*(3), 313–326. https://doi.org/10.1080/17430430802673668

Hurst, P., Kavussanu, M., King., A., Barkoukis, V., Skoufa, L., & Ring, C. (2019). *Preventing doping in sport: The VIRTUES project*. Conference of the European Society of Sport and Exercise Psychology, Muenster, Germany.

Kavussanu, M. (2015). Moral disengagement and doping. In V. Barkoukis, L. Lazuras, & H. Tsorbatzoudis (Eds.), *Routledge research in sport and exercise science: The psychology of doping in sport* (pp. 151–164). Routledge/Taylor & Francis Group.

Kavussanu, M., Hatzigeorgiadis, A., Elbe, A.-M., & Ring, C. (2016). The moral disengagement in doping scale. *Psychology of Sport and Exercise, 24*, 188–198. https://doi.org/10.1016/j.psychsport.2016.02.003

Kavussanu, M., Hatzigeorgiadis, A., Hurst, P., Galanis, E., & Ring, C. (2019). *Preventing doping in sport: The HEROES project*. Conference of the European Society of Sport and Exercise Psychology, Muenster, Germany.

Kavussanu, M., Yukhymenko-Lescroart, A. M., Elbe, A.-M., & Hatzigeorgiadis, A. (2019). Integrating moral and achievement variables to predict doping likelihood in football: A cross-cultural investigation. *Psychology of Sport and Exercise, 47*, 101518. https://doi.org/10.1016/j.psychsport.2019.04.008

Kayser, B., Mauron A., & Miah A. (2007). Current anti-doping policy: A critical appraisal. *BMC Medical Ethics, 8*, 2. https://doi.org/10.1186/1472-6939-8-2

Kellmann, M., & Beckmann, J. (2003). Research and intervention in sport psychology: New perspectives on an inherent conflict. *International Journal of Sport and Exercise Psychology, 1*, 13–26. https://doi.org/ 10.1080/1612197X.2003.9671701

Kohlberg, L. (1964). Development of moral character and moral ideology. In M. L. Hoffman & L. W. Hoffman (Eds.), *Review of child development research* (Vol. 1, pp. 381–431). Russel Sage Foundation.

Lazuras, L., Barkoukis, V., & Tsorbatzoudis, H. (2015). Toward an integrative model of doping use: An empirical study with adolescent athletes. *Journal of Sport and Exercise Psychology, 37*, 37–50. https://doi.org/10.1123/jsep.2013-0232

Loland, S., & Hoppeler, H. (2012). Justifying anti-doping: The fair opportunity principle and the biology of performance enhancement. *European Journal of Sport Science, 12*(4), 347–353. https://doi.org/10.1080/17461391.2011.566374

Loland, S., & McNamee, M. J. (2019). The "spirit of sport," WADAs code review, and the search for an overlapping consensus. *International Journal of Sport Policy and Politics, 11*, 325–339. https://doi.org/10.1080/19406940.2019.1581646

Mallia, L., Lazuras, L., Barkoukis, V., Brand, R., Baumgarten, F., Tsorbatzoudis, H., Zelli, A., & Lucidi, F. (2016). Doping use in sport teams: The development and validation of measures of team-based efficacy beliefs and moral disengagement from a cross-national perspective. *Psychology of Sport and Exercise, 25*, 78–88. https://doi.org/10.1016/j.psychsport.2016.04.005

Martin, K. D., & Cullen, J. B. (2006). Continuities and extensions of ethical climate theory: A meta-analytic review. *Journal of Business Ethics, 69*(2), 175–194. https://doi.org/10.1007/ s10551-006-9084-7

Mazanov, J., & McDermott, V. (2009). The case for a social science of drugs in sport. *Sport in Society, 12*, 276–295.

Ntoumanis, N., Barkoukis, V., Gucciardi, D. F., & Chan, D. K. C. (2017). Linking coach interpersonal style with athlete doping intentions and doping use: A prospective study. *Journal of Sport and Exercise Psychology, 39*, 188–198. https://doi.org/10.1123/jsep.2016-0243

Ntoumanis, N., Ng, J. Y. Y., Barkoukis, V., & Backhouse, S. (2014). Personal and psychosocial predictors of doping use in physical activity settings: A meta-analysis. *Sports Medicine, 44*, 1603–1624. https://doi.org/10.1007/s40279-014-0240-4

Ring, C., & Hurst, P. (2019). The effects of moral disengagement mechanisms on doping likelihood are mediated by guilt and moderated by moral traits. *Psychology of Sport and Exercise, 40*, 33–41. https://doi.org/10.1016/j.psychsport.2018.09.001

Ring, C., Kavussanu, M., & Gürpınar, B. (2020). Basic values predict doping likelihood. *Journal of Sports Sciences, 38*(4), 357–365. https://doi.org/10.1080/02640414.2019.1700669

Sagoe, D., Molde, H., Andreassen, C. S., Torsheim, T., & Pallesen, S. (2014). The global epidemiology of anabolic-androgenic steroid use: A meta-analysis and meta-regression analysis. *Annals of Epidemiology, 24*(5), 383–398. https://doi.org/10.1016/j.annepidem.2014.01.009

Schwartz, S. H. (1992). Universals in the content and structure of values: Theoretical advances and empirical tests in 20 countries. In M. P. Zanna (Ed.), *Advances in experimental social psychology* (Vol. 25, pp. 1–65). Academic Press. https://doi.org/10.1016/S0065-2601(08)60281-6

Solomon, R. C. (1984). *Ethics: A brief introduction.* McGraw-Hill.Tsorbatzoudis, H., Lazuras, L., & Barkoukis, V. (2015). 16 Next steps in doping research and prevention. In V. Barkoukis, L. Lazuras, & H. Tsorbatzoudis (Eds.), *Psychology of doping in sport* (pp. 230–243). Routledge.

Ulrich, R., Pope, H. G., Cleret, L., Petroczi, A., Nepusz, T., Schaffer, J., Kanayama, G., Comstock, R. D., & Simon, P. (2018). Doping in two elite athletics competitions assessed by randomized-response surveys. *Sports Medicine, 48*, 211–219. https://doi.org/10.1007/s40279-017-0765-4

WADA. (2019). The World Anti Doping Code. https://www.wada-ama.org/sites/default/files/resources/files/wada_anti-doping_code_2019_english_final_revised_v1_linked.pdf

Wolff, W., Schindler, S., & Brand, R. (2015). The effect of implicitly incentivized faking on explicit and implicit measures of doping attitude: When athletes want to pretend an even more negative attitude to doping. *PLoS ONE, 10*(4), Article e0118507. https://doi.org/10.1371/journal.pone.0118507

SECTION 3

CULTURAL AND PROFESSIONAL ISSUES

23

Ethics

Jack C. Watson II, Brandonn S. Harris, and Megan Byrd

State of the Art

Ethics can be thought of as a moral philosophy or code that guides the behaviors of an individual or group, based upon the values and moral principles of that individual or group and society at large. Ethical codes outline regulatory guidelines for behavior and often deal with complex dilemmas faced by those individuals functioning within a specific professional domain. Ethical codes often consist of ethical principles that are aspirational and promote the highest level of professional behavior and ethical standards that are more regulatory and specify what is and is not appropriate behavior within the profession.

The study of ethics is essential to the promotion of any profession, as ethics guide the behaviors of those within the profession based upon the values of that profession and help to educate practitioners and users of those services about appropriate and inappropriate behaviors, setting the guidelines for how professional relationships are intended to be structured. As technology and a profession evolve, new challenging dilemmas emerge and must be considered if professionals are to remain true to the values and moral principles espoused by their profession. Rarely are ethical issues straightforward and easy to identify or adjudicate. In most situations, the ethical issues faced by practitioners are more subtle and impacted by many factors that influence the dynamics of the situation. Research pertaining to ethical issues and decision-making is necessary to help individuals identify potential ethical issues and resolve them effectively before they have a negative impact upon their professional responsibilities and relationships. The field of sport, exercise, and performance psychology (SEPP) is unique from general psychology and other helping professions in that the responsibilities and scope of work in itself create potential ethical issues, thus requiring ethical codes specific to the field.

Jack C. Watson II, Brandonn S. Harris, and Megan Byrd, *Ethics* In: *Sport, Exercise and Performance Psychology.* Edited by: Edson Filho and Itay Basevitch, Oxford University Press. © Oxford University Press 2021. DOI: 10.1093/oso/9780197512494.003.0023

In SEPP most ethical issues are associated with the three major domains of work in which professionals engage: teaching, research, and practice. Given the diverse activities that SEPP professionals are engaged in, several organizations have developed codes of ethics to help guide and support the work of their members. For example, the Association for Applied Sport Psychology (AASP) adopted a code of ethics in 1996 to outline the responsibilities of AASP members to the public. The ethics code was developed based on the American Psychological Association's Ethical Principles of Psychologists code (1992). This code has since been modified slightly to account for the ever-changing role of technology within professional practice. More recently, the International Society of Sport Psychology produced and disseminated their own code of ethics to support the work of members across the international communities of the field (Quartiroli et al., 2020). These codes of ethics are connected to professional organizations and are intended to provide guidance to their members for dealing with the difficult work-related behaviors often encountered by professionals working in the field of SEPP.

Although writings related to ethical practices within the field of SEPP existed prior to the 1990s (e.g., Nideffer, 1981; Rotella & Connelly, 1984; Zeigler, 1987), a more consistent focus upon this work began in the early 1990s with the development of presentations, books, and articles focused on ethics from research, best practices, and case study perspectives (e.g., Berger, 1993; Henschen, 1991; Heyman, 1990; Petitpas et al., 1994; Sachs, 1993; Singer, 1993). These titles often utilized more descriptive methodologies and provided reviews aiming to identify the type and frequency of ethical dilemmas professionals found themselves encountering in practice and provided suggestions for those working in these specific areas. Since the early 1990s, presentations, articles, and book chapters related to ethics, ethical behaviors, and ethical decision-making in SEPP have become much more common.

While reviews are still published in the related literature (e.g., Watson et al., in press), more recently, attention has been given to more *applied* ethics in which normative ethics (e.g., theories and associated codes) are applied to dilemmas seen across the teaching, research, and practice domains. Yet SEPP is still thought of as a unique profession (Aoyagi & Portenga, 2010) because practitioners often interact with clients outside of traditional psychology practice settings to conform with the constraints commonly placed upon athletes because of their complex travel, meeting, and practice schedules as well as other systemic demands associated with the athletic culture (Brown

& Cogan, 2006). Although the ethical principles guiding sport psychology practitioners and licensed "sport" psychologists intersect, there are unique situations outside of a traditional clinical setting that a licensed psychologist may find difficult to navigate due to the nature of their training, conflicting ethical codes and laws, and complex nature of the culture of sport. These nontraditional interactions often lead to an increased opportunity for practitioners to find themselves in unanticipated ethically challenging situations. The differences associated with practice between licensed and nonlicensed practitioners in the sport domain have made it essential for ethics codes to be written specifically for those working in applied SEPP, and for researchers to write articles specific to this domain. Further, to increase the chance of making ethically sound decisions under pressure, authors have developed and encouraged the utilization of ethical decision-making models within SEPP settings (see Harris et al., 2009).

With the origins of ethics research in the profession and its subsequent development over the past three decades, certain scholarly works have had important influences on the ethics of research and practice in SEPP. Further, while not exhaustive, these writings have also helped professionals answer important questions within the profession of SEPP as well as highlighting the areas that are in direct need of future attention. The authors highlight five of these works (see Table 23.1) as well as address the following areas: (a) the most common ethical challenges faced by SEPP practitioners, (b) how SEPP practitioners make decisions when faced with ethical dilemmas, (c) how competent SEPP practitioners are at recognizing ethical dilemmas and acting appropriately upon those judgments, (d) the methodologies needed to comprehensively examine ethics in SEPP, and (e) what structural issues within the field of SEPP commonly lead to the development of ethical issues for practitioners.

Table 23.1 Five Key Readings in Ethics in Sport, Exercise, and Performance Psychology (SEPP)

Authors	Methodological Design	Key Findings
Aoyagi & Portenga (2010)	Review of literature with practical suggestions	Identifies SEPP challenges associated with multiple relationships, confidentiality, and self-regulation. Supports a positive and virtue ethics approach to ethics education. Encourages constant evolution and introspection of personal values and beliefs.

Continued

Table 23.1 *Continued*

Authors	Methodological Design	Key Findings
Brown & Cogan (2006)	Review of literature and ethical codes to provide practical solutions	Focuses on ethical challenges for licensed psychologists working in sport. Highlights issues of confidentiality, ethical diagnosing and third-party billing, competence and marketing, and boundaries. Provides suggestions for maintaining ethics while working with athletes.
Etzel et al. (2004)	Descriptive survey of Association for Applied Sport Psychology members' ethical training and beliefs	Surveyed SEPP practitioners about ethical beliefs and behaviors. Ethical dilemmas reflected currently identified ethical dilemmas (i.e., multicultural issues and tele-mental health). When compared to previous studies, fewer behaviors were indicated as controversial.
Harris et al. (2009)	Review of literature with practical suggestions	Outlines the importance of ethics codes and ethical decision-making models within SEPP. Use of ethical decision-making models improves the chance of making ethically sound decisions under pressure. A decision-making model is presented for use in SEPP.
Watson et al. (in press)	Review of literature with practical suggestions	Review of the ethical issues associated with teaching, research, and practice. Attention given to areas often neglected in other writings. Includes examples and recommendations for addressing issues in each of these professional domains.

Questions to Move the Field Forward

1. Applied Question: What Are the Most Common Ethical Challenges Faced by SEPP Practitioners?

This question is very important for helping advance applied SEPP interventions. SEPP practitioners must understand the common ethical challenges faced by those working in the profession if they are going to be mindful of how, why, and in what situations ethical challenges often evolve, and be able to develop effective strategies for dealing proactively with difficult situations.

Although not always the case, SEPP is often viewed as a luxury service. We often hear about clients making snap judgments about the entire profession based upon interactions with one professional. For example, a bad interaction with a SEPP practitioner may be viewed as an indictment of the entire profession. To the contrary, a bad interaction with a dentist is often perceived as an indication that the dentist is not someone you want to work with but is not reason to reject the entire profession. SEPP is also often viewed as a boutique industry, making it essential that practitioners take every opportunity to meet the highest standards of professionalism. Taking a positive, virtue ethics approach to SEPP practice not only helps practitioners avoid problems with ethics committees and the law but also does so by promoting an approach whereby practitioners utilize ethical codes to improve upon their practice and reach their full potential as a practitioner by focusing on their own personal character and who they want to be as a practitioner (Aoyagi & Portenga, 2010). Therefore, it is essential that SEPP practitioners identify who they are and want to be, as well as their professional aspirations for practice. The answers to these questions will help them to develop proactive plans to deal effectively with common ethical challenges, as well as handle the unexpected challenges that they are faced with.

Although SEPP practitioners face many of the same challenges as more traditional mental health professionals, the unique nature of their consulting brings with it many situations and challenges that appear to be more exclusive to this profession (Aoyagi & Portenga, 2010). To better understand and identify the common ethical challenges facing SEPP practitioners, the two most sensible approaches to research would entail a survey of practitioners similar to those conducted to identify the ethical beliefs and behaviors of sport psychology practitioners (Etzel et al., 2004; Petitpas et al., 1994) and an inductive qualitative study designed to better understand the common ethical challenges facing SEPP practitioners and how they handle them.

Survey methods designed to answer this question should attempt to overcome common sampling concerns associated with previous studies such as low response rates, use of practitioners associated with one professional organization, lack of practitioners from different training backgrounds, and working in different settings (Etzel et al., 2004; Petitpas et al., 1994). At present, survey methods in SEPP have primarily utilized professional listservs that are highly subscribed to by students and rarely subscribed to by those working as applied practitioners. Response rates have been very low, and the surveys have often been completed more frequently by academics and students than full-time SEPP practitioners (Etzel et al., 2004; Petitpas et al., 1994). It is essential that such surveys use sampling methods that maximize their respondents' professional experiences by reaching full-time practitioners who have different training backgrounds (i.e., sport sciences and mental health), holding different certifications and licensures, and working across different settings (e.g., private practice, collegiate sport, professional sport, military). Such surveys also need to reach practitioners working in different countries and within different cultures. These same considerations for maximum variation sampling are also important for effective qualitative research methods.

2. Applied Question: How Do Practitioners Make Decisions When Faced With Ethical Dilemmas?

This question is very important for helping advance applied SEPP interventions, but also important for the development of an ethical decision-making model in SEPP. SEPP is different from other mental health professions because of the unique setting in which practitioners work. Within this setting, it is sometimes difficult to identify the client, performance can be difficult to define, and practitioners often interact with clients in public settings and at nontraditional hours (Aoyagi & Portenga, 2010). Therefore, understanding how practitioners make ethical decisions and identifying an appropriate ethical decision-making process would be beneficial.

To better understand how practitioners make ethical decisions, two sequential approaches should be considered. The first approach is intended to answer this question at face value. Although a survey technique could effectively answer this question, it would be best to use qualitative methods to interview practitioners and identify their ethical decision-making processes. However, it is important to go beyond figuring out how practitioners make ethical decisions and look to identify a decision-making approach that would be specific and appropriate for SEPP using a Delphi method to reach consensus among practitioners.

It is first important for SEPP practitioners to understand the ethical decision-making processes of others. An inductive, qualitative study is proposed. This qualitative study should bring together a diverse group of practitioners and ask them: "What do you consider to be common ethical dilemmas in the practice of applied SEPP?" and then "What factors and approach do you use when making decisions regarding ethical dilemmas faced in SEPP practice?" The results of this study will be helpful in identifying the factors that are most commonly considered by SEPP practitioners when faced with ethical dilemmas and help to identify appropriate decision-making models.

Although knowledge of the most important factors to consider when faced with an ethical dilemma is important, it would be more important to identify an actual ethical decision-making model that is appropriate for SEPP. To answer this question, use of the Delphi method is suggested. Using the Delphi method, a group of expert SEPP practitioners would be identified. These experts should be practitioners from a variety of backgrounds who have been identified as knowledgeable about ethics and have avoided ethical problems throughout their careers. Results of the previous studies on ethical decision-making would then be used to structure a questionnaire related to ethical decision-making considerations. Several rounds of questionnaires would be sent to this group with the goal of providing a summary of the group response from previous rounds of questionnaires to respondents, allowing them to interpret these responses and adjust their own responses with the goal of developing consensus on how ethical decisions should be made.

Once an ethical decision-making model has been developed, future research should examine decision-making of individuals who use the model and those who do not. To examine this question along with the impact of other factors such as mood, educational level, training background, and culture on ethical decision-making, experimental studies could be developed that utilize ethical scenarios with different groups to evaluate between group ethical decision-making.

3. Applied Question: How Competent Are SEPP Practitioners at Recognizing Ethical Dilemmas and Acting Appropriately Upon Those Judgments?

A critical area associated with ethics in sport psychology involves competence. Indeed, a great deal of attention has been given to the importance of competent professionals in the field within teaching, research, and applied practice settings (see Moore, 2003). Further, relevant ethics codes of governing bodies (i.e., AASP, 1996) include specific principles and standards pertaining to competent work in SEPP. Interestingly, competence as it pertains to the ability to recognize *and* appropriately address ethical dilemmas in the field remains an area that has yet to be examined in sport psychology, which would advance our knowledge of the areas of graduate training and intervention work among professionals in the field.

The ability to recognize and address ethical dilemmas as a competency in sport psychology represents an important area of attention given the various dilemmas that can surface in teaching, research, and applied practice settings. Further, while these dilemmas may mirror those of other related fields (e.g., military psychology, counseling psychology), Aoyagi and Portenga (2010) also suggest additional challenges may exist that are unique to sport psychology settings. Thus, the idea of competent practice within teaching, research, and service provision must also include the ability of professionals to accurately recognize and manage any number of ethical dilemmas that can surface within each of the primary domains of the sport psychology profession.

A number of methodologies could be employed to better assess and understand this particular area of ethics in sport psychology. From a quantitative standpoint, survey methods could be advantageous for facilitating a more comprehensive examination of how competent decision-making is addressed globally in the field across graduate programs and practitioners within and outside of academia using such resources as listservs, the Directory of Graduate Programs in Applied Sport Psychology (Burke et al., 2018), AASP's Certified Mental Performance Consultant finder, and the International Society for Sport Psychology's Practitioner Registry. Experimental designs that involve ethical decision-making education as an intervention could address the effectiveness of such training. Further, the use of case scenarios with forced-choice responses querying appropriate decision-making and/or action steps based on each case could be addressed. It should be noted that methodologies have been known to encounter common limitations. These can include low response rates, the inclusion of practitioners who are affiliated with only one professional organization, and the lack of generalizable findings due to sampling methods that may not include practitioners and academics who come from different training backgrounds, work in different settings, or reside in different regions of the world. Qualitative methodologies that involve semistructured interviews of graduate students and faculty/supervisors could also provide more detailed feedback regarding perceptions of what abilities and skill sets make up competent ethical decision-making and how/if ethical decision-making is taught in graduate training programs.

4. Methodological Question: What Methodologies Are Needed to Comprehensively Examine Ethics in SEPP?

Advancements in SEPP teaching and applied practice generally stem from sound scientific processes and research methodologies. Interestingly, many codes of ethics have relatively little information within their standards and principles that address measurement and assessment for research and/or applied practice (Watson et al., 2012). With a great deal of importance placed on assessment, measurement, and research in the field, conducting such scholarship in an ethical manner remains a significant challenge and endeavor for professionals. An interesting extension of this involves examining ethics in SEPP given little is known about what methodologies would be most effective for the study of this area in the profession. Thus, this represents an area in which methodological approaches in sport psychology could be advanced.

The selection of a research methodology represents an important decision for SEPP professionals. Indeed, different methods require variable resources to carry out, as well as contain varied strengths and limitations in terms of the type of data obtained and question(s) that can be answered as a result. For ethics-related research, selecting and implementing appropriate methodologies is of importance, as the results of this area of research can influence graduate training as well as the care and safety of clients in applied settings.

A number of methodologies including quantitative, qualitative, and mixed-method designs would be critical in advancing the study of ethics in SEPP. For example, quantitative designs can help address questions pertaining to student and professional perceptions related to ethical behavior and frequencies associated with encountering and managing ethical dilemmas, as well as assess interventions designed to increase one's competence or ability to make ethical decisions. Similar to previous research in ethics, quantitative designs can sometimes be limited by lower response rates and an inability to generalize findings given varying sampling methods. These methods often do not result in a comparable number of practitioners and academics who come from different training backgrounds and work settings. To help overcome these common response rate and sampling concerns, perhaps one solution might involve the development of a centralized research database within the profession. Such a database could allow for improved communication between professional organizations around the world by allowing individuals to list themselves on a research database that categorizes each person based upon several different demographic variables (e.g., age, gender, training background, and practice status).

It is also possible that depending on the aspect of ethics being examined, participants may not feel comfortable disclosing experiences navigating ethical dilemmas if such experiences would involve admitting to having engaged in unethical behavior. Thus, social desirability and accuracy of findings remain a challenging aspect associated with this body of research regardless of methodology utilized. Safeguards designed to maintain the anonymity of research participants are of importance, as it is essential to protect the identity of respondents to help encourage more honest and accurate responses. Qualitative designs would allow for case examples, anecdotes, and experiences from participants to be explored in more detail as well. Perhaps the most comprehensive approach would include both methodologies in which select participants from a quantitative study are asked to engage in follow-up interviews in which more detailed information can be gathered to better understand an ethics-related question in SEPP.

5. Applied Question: What Structural Issues Within the Field of SEPP Commonly Lead to the Development of Ethical Issues for Practitioners?

Organizational ethics codes are created and adopted to guide users to engage in ethical behaviors deemed appropriate by the values and welfare of society. Practitioners may interpret ethical dilemmas differently based on several external issues including organizational, legal, and sport governing body regulations. These structural issues may influence perception of ethical dilemmas as well as one's decision-making process. If a practitioner belongs to more than one organization and the ethical codes for a certain behavior conflict (e.g., appropriateness of multiple relationships, consulting in nontraditional settings), a potential dilemma is created for ethical decision-making in that area. Similarly, practitioners must navigate the legal requirements bestowed upon them by their certification or licensure (i.e., psychologist) in addition to ethical codes. Regarding sport governing bodies, practitioners may find themselves in situations in which their ethical duty to their client may conflict with the rules and regulations of the governing body or the laws in their jurisdiction (e.g., client confidentiality vs. a coach's desire to know what is impacting an athlete's performance). The AASP Ethics Code

Standard 24 addresses this conflict and states that "if the demands of an organization with which AASP members are affiliated conflict with the Ethics Code, members clarify the nature of the conflict, make known their commitment to the Ethics Code, and to the extent feasible, seek to resolve the conflict in a way that permits the fullest adherence to the Ethics Code" (AASP, 1996). After consulting this ethical standard, the practitioner would still need to decide on their course of action following a potential ethical issue or dilemma. The course of action the practitioner decides to take may be impacted by structural issues. Understanding the structural issues that can impact ethical decision-making will help with the development of ethical theories and influence applied interventions.

In addition to navigating ethics codes from organizations and laws, practitioners may also have internal structural issues that influence their own standards, such as cultural, bias, moral, and personal factors. A person's demographic profile, including influences from personal, situational, and significant others such as support or institutional values (Hadjistravropoulos & Malloy, 2000), may influence how one conceptualizes and understands an ethical decision, thus influencing how they work to resolve the issue. By considering the important structural issues impacting a situation or the interpretation of that situation, one can consider the complexities of people and situations, which are reflected in the complex nature of ethical issues.

To answer this question about the structural issues that may exist and lead to ethical issues, several methodologies may be employed to advance current understanding of structural issues. To further the knowledge of the role of internal and external issues surrounding ethical dilemmas, a qualitative approach may be best. Practitioners who operate under multiple ethical codes could be prefaced with a vignette describing a common ethical belief or behavior as identified by previous studies (i.e., Etzel et al., 2004) and asked to discuss the congruence or dissonance between their ethical requirements in resolving this conflict. Probing questions from the researcher would specifically address potential internal structures, such as culture and morality. For example, the researcher may ask, "What led you to determine an ethical issue existed in this scenario?" or "What role do you believe culture plays in conceptualizing this scenario?"

To address the external structures that may influence ethical dilemmas, it is first necessary to identify which sport governing body regulations and restrictions are incongruent with ethical codes of SEPP practitioners.

This knowledge could be acquired by asking practitioners to identify situations in which they have had to navigate this predicament, or through a document analysis of regulations to classify where potential discrepancies exist. It would be important to include decision-makers within sport organizations in this research to further understand why certain regulations exist.

Conclusion

A paucity of literature focused on the assessment of ethical issues in SEPP existed prior to the turn of the 21st century. More recently the literature written on this topic has focused primarily upon the provision of practical suggestions to help practitioners address ethical issues while working in the field, with very few empirically based studies focused on ethics. In most cases, the practical suggestions in the literature stemmed from reviews of SEPP ethical standards that have been derived from the parent field of psychology. As suggested by Aoyagi and Portenga (2010), a stronger focus upon positive and virtue ethics within the profession could have the added benefit of encouraging students and practitioners to strive to find the best practitioner versions of themselves.

Ethics research in SEPP has also suffered from several methodological- and sampling-related issues. For instance, consistently low response rates within research focused on ethical issues often limit the generalizability of the findings. Thus, the suggestions within this chapter focused on the development of a more empirically based study of ethics in the field and identified suggested modifications to the research methodologies used. There is also a need to empirically understand the internal and external structural issues within the field that are commonly associated with ethical concerns, the common ethical beliefs and behaviors of practitioners, and the methods used by practitioners to make ethical decisions from a variety of methodological designs. These research questions are essential to the development of a better understanding of the ethical issues impacting professional behavior in SEPP. With an improved understanding of important and common ethical issues and how experienced practitioners navigate these issues and the factors that impact their decisions, we will be in a much better position to educate future practitioners relative to their ethical practices and behaviors.

References

Aoyagi, M. W., & Portenga, S. T. (2010). The role of positive ethics and virtues in the context of sport and performance psychology service delivery. *Professional Psychology: Research and Practice, 41*, 253–259.

Association for Applied Sport Psychology. (1996). *AASP code of ethical principles and standards.* http://www.appliedsportpsych.org/ethics/code2002.html

Berger, B. (1993). Ethical issues in clinical setting: A reaction to ethics in teaching, advising, and clinical services. *Quest, 45*, 106–119.

Brown, J. L., & Cogan, K. D. (2006). Ethical clinical practice and sport psychology: When two worlds collide. *Ethics and Behavior, 16*(1), 15–23.

Burke, K. L., Sachs, M. L., & Tomlinson, R. (2018). *Directory of graduate programs in applied sport psychology.* Association for Applied Sport Psychology.

Etzel, E. F., Watson, J. C., & Zizzi, S. (2004). A web-based survey of AAASP members' ethical beliefs and behaviors in the new millennium. *Journal of Applied Sport Psychology, 16*, 236–250. https://doi.org/10.1080/10413200490485595

Hadjistravropoulos, T., & Malloy, D. C. (2000). Making ethical choices: A comprehensive decision-making model for Canadian psychologists. *Canadian Psychology, 41*(2), 104–115.

Harris, B. S., Visek, A. J., & Watson, J. C. (2009). Ethical decision-making in sport psychology: Issues and implications for professional practice. In R. Schinke (Ed.), *Contemporary sport psychology* (pp. 217–232). Nova Science Publishers.

Henschen, K. (1991). Critical issues involving male consultants and female athletes. *The Sport Psychologist, 5*(4), 313–321.

Heyman, S. (1990). Ethical issues in performance enhancement approaches with amateur boxers. *The Sport Psychologist, 4*, 48–54.

Moore, Z. (2003). Ethical dilemmas in sport psychology: Discussion and recommendations for practice. *Professional Psychology: Research and Practice, 34*, 601–610.

Nideffer, R (1981). *The ethics and practice of applied sport psychology.* Mouvement.

Petitpas, A., Brewer, B., Rivera, P., & Van Raalte, J. (1994). Ethical beliefs and behaviors in applied sport psychology: The AAASP ethics survey. *Journal of Applied Sport Psychology, 6*, 135–151.

Quartiroli, A., Harris, B. S., Brückner, S., Chow, G. M., Connole, I. J., Cropley, B., Fogaça, J., Gonzalez, S. P., Guicciardi, M., Hau, A., Kao, S., Kavanagh, E. J., Keegan, R. J., Li, H. Y., Martin, G., Moyle, G. M., Noce, F., Peterson, K., Roy, J., Rubio, V. J., Wagstaff, C. R. D., Wong, R., Yousuf, S., & Zito, M. (2020). The International Society of Sport Psychology Registry (ISSP-R) ethical code for sport psychology practice. *International Journaly of Sport and Exercise Psychology, 0*, 1–22. doi:10.1080/1612197X.2020.1789317

Rotella, R., & Connelly, D. (1984). Individual ethics in the application of cognitive sport psychology. In W. Straub & J. Williams (Eds.), *Cognitive sport psychology* (pp. 102–112). Sport Science Association.

Sachs, M. (1993). Professional ethics in sport psychology. In R. Singer, M. Murphey, & K. Tennant (Eds.), *Handbook on research in sport psychology* (pp. 921–932). Macmillan.

Singer, R. (1993). Ethical issues in clinical services. *Quest, 45*, 88–105.

Watson II, J. W., Etzel, E. F., & Vosloo, J. (2012). Assessment and measurement in sport and exercise psychology. In G. Tenenbaum, R. C. Eklund, & A. Kamata (Eds.), *Measurement in sport and exercise psychology* (pp. 169–176). Human Kinetics.

Watson II, J. W., Harris, B. S., & Baille, P. (in press). Ethics in sport psychology. In G. Tenenbaum & R. Eklund (Eds.), *Handbook of sport psychology.* Wiley.

Zeigler, E. F. (1987). Rationale and suggested dimensions for a code of ethics for sport psychologists. *Sport Psychologist, 1*(2), 138–150.

24

Cross-Cultural, Multi-Cultural, and Intercultural Issues

Thierry R. F. Middleton, Robert J. Schinke, Brennan Petersen,
and Cole E. Giffin

State of the Art

During the 1990s, some sport psychology researchers began to call for an examination of how knowledge was generated (e.g., Dewar & Horn, 1992). One issue brought to the fore was the lack of diversity present in much of the work being conducted by sport psychology researchers (Duda & Allison, 1990). The development of cultural sport psychology (CSP) as a genre of research within sport psychology has brought attention to issues such as identity, equity, and cultural diversity within sport (Roper, 2016; Schinke, Blodgett, et al., 2019). We have chosen to highlight the diverse modes through which research around cultural issues may be conducted by focusing on one issue that has recently gained attention from researchers: the role of sport as an integrative context for newcomers.

With the focus from various governments on sport as an integrative tool (e.g., Canadian sport policy: Provincial/Territorial Governments of Canada, 2012; the European Commission's white paper on sport: European Commission, 2007), researchers have begun to explore the mechanisms by which sport may facilitate the successful integration of newcomers (Hatzigeorgiadis et al., 2013). Integration, as conceptualized by psychological researchers, entails newcomers (i.e., asylum seekers, refugees, and immigrants; Canadian Council for Refugees [CCR], 2010) maintaining their ethnic (i.e., home culture) identity while at the same time engaging in cultural learning with members of the host culture. Multicultural receiving communities (i.e., those willing to engage in a shared learning process with newcomers) have been found to be the most conducive to fostering the integration of newcomers (Berry & Hou, 2016).

Cross-cultural studies providing evidence for the aforementioned positions have largely been conducted using Berry's (2005) two-factor model

Thierry R. F. Middleton, Robert J. Schinke, Brennan Petersen, and Cole E. Giffin, *Cross-Cultural, Multi-Cultural, and Intercultural Issues* In: *Sport, Exercise and Performance Psychology*. Edited by: Edson Filho and Itay Basevitch, Oxford University Press. © Oxford University Press 2021. DOI: 10.1093/oso/9780197512494.003.0024 of acculturation in which adaptation to a new society is measured through changes to newcomers' food preferences, language acquisition and proficiency, and the adoption of receiving communities' form of dress and social norms (Chirkov, 2009). Recently, sport researchers in Europe have come together on a research initiative using Berry's theoretical conceptualization of integration to examine factors that may help regulate the integrative power of sport for both host and newcomer communities (Hatzigeorgiadis et al., 2013). Using the 18-item 5-point Likert-scale Ethnic/Cultural Identity Salience Questionnaire, researchers found that being supportive of sport participants' autonomy, focusing on building a task-oriented motivational climate, and fostering team cohesion are important factors for sport to become an integrative context (Elbe et al., 2018). Further, using the 12-item 5-point Likert-scale Host Community Acculturation Scale to measure host individuals' attitudes and perceptions in relation to newcomers, European researchers also found that host community adolescents who participated in sport showed a more accepting attitude toward interacting with newcomers in their community (Morela et al., 2017).

While the European research team provided generalized insight into how sport may be an integrative context, scholars using various qualitative methodologies have argued that the process of acculturation is one that is dynamic, negotiated, and not always under the control of the individual, as it is embedded within sociopolitical and historical forces (e.g., Chirkov, 2009). Burrmann et al. (2017) provided an example of the idiographic nature of newcomers' identity development as they navigate two (or more) cultural divides. Their case studies of four newcomers' journeys in Germany provide insight into how sport can provide newcomer youth with an avenue to build connections with members of their new community. The potential for sport to be an integrative context is shown as dependent on newcomer youths' willingness to learn unfamiliar cultural norms, their connection to their home culture, and the context-specific presence of perceived discrimination and prejudice in their local sport environment. Through interviews conducted with 15 professional and semiprofessional athletes, Ryba, Stambulova, and Ronkainen (2016) proposed examining athletes' acculturative journeys as a series of transitions. Their cultural transition model proposes that the acculturation journey is composed of a pretransition phase, an acute cultural adaptation phase, and a sociocultural adaptation phase. While presented as a sequential process, Ryba and colleagues (2016) noted that they believe each transition is negotiated in a dynamic, subjective, and relational manner. The insights provided by athletes willing to share their stories have highlighted the need for newcomer athletes to be involved in the research process so that they may feel in control of sharing the stories they see as important. Schinke and colleagues (see Middleton et al., 2020; Schinke et al., 2016) have embraced a social constructionist approach to their research and aimed to become more reflexive in their consideration of how their subjective positions have contributed to either the empowerment or marginalization of the athletes they work with. Using arts-based and mobile methods of data collection, athletes have been encouraged to share the stories they feel are important to them. The stories shared through this work have brought to life the dynamic and perpetual nature of acculturation, which is the process of developing and maintaining a sense of connection to varying cultural backgrounds dependent on context, time, and others who are present. One aspect that has been found to emanate from newcomer athletes' stories is the presence of family members and their role in providing support. Family member support has been storied as particularly important during the early stages of the acculturation process (Ronkainen et al., 2019; Schinke et al., 2016). Although athletes have spoken about navigating a divergence between their priorities and those of their parents at varying times during their journey, they have also noted that sharing success with their family members was made more meaningful due to obstacles they had to overcome together (Middleton et al., 2020). Notably, a key factor from the stories shared by both Burmann and colleagues (2017) and Middleton and colleagues (2020) was newcomer athletes' level of athletic ability and talent, which brought recognition from their receiving community and family, leading to an increase of self-efficacy and confirmation of their athletic identity in their new community.

CSP researchers have provided insight into how we can derive lessons from different forms of research (see Table 24.1 for five key readings). Newcomers' acculturation journeys should be explored and understood throughout pre-migration, during migration, and postmigration (see Ryba et al., 2016). At different times during the acculturative process sport may serve different purposes dependent on where newcomer youth come from and the cultural context to which they are adapting (Elbe et al., 2018). What is clear is that sport provides individuals from different cultural backgrounds an opportunity to find a common interest through which to learn more about each other, potentially leading to a greater opportunity for cultural exchanges to occur (Agergaard, 2017; Morela et al., 2017). The onus is on those in positions of power to develop culturally integrative sport programs, rather than merely assume newcomers will be able to successfully "integrate" into existing sport structures (Jeanes et al., 2015).

Table 24.1 Five Key Readings in Cross-Cultural, Multicultural, and Intercultural Issues

Authors	Methodological Design	Key Findings
Burmann et al. (2017)	Case studies	Sport clubs may provide newcomer youth with a place to belong. Experience of efficacy is the main mechanism through which youth can develop a long-lasting identification with sport and formation of affective bonds with those they train/compete with. Experiences of belonging are tied to personal and social conditions.
Elbe et al. (2018)	Cross-sectional multivariate analysis	Societal context and team composition can impact integrative potential of sport. Prosocial, supportive environments can help newcomers feel comfortable in expressing their heritage and ethnic (i.e., home culture) identity. Autonomy support and a task-oriented motivational climate can help foster an integrative context.
Hatzigeorgiadis et al. (2013)	Review	Sport by itself may not foster integration, but participation in a team context where personal development is promoted, the needs of the individual are valued and appreciated, and socio-moral values are fostered can help integration and multiculturalism flourish. Researchers examining the topic of integration have primarily employed qualitative methodologies; more quantitative research work could increase our understanding. The nature and type of sport may play an influential role in the integrative power of sport.
Ryba et al. (2018)	Position stand	Regardless of form of migration, newcomers all face the challenge of maintaining their ethnic identity (i.e., home culture) and developing their cultural identity (i.e., host culture). Knowledge should be produced that benefits both newcomers and host society members. Qualitative and quantitative research methodologies are needed.
Schinke, Blodgett, et al. (2019)	Review	Cultural sport psychology is meant to be open, inclusive, and pliable, rather than restricted to certain topics and methodologies. Decolonizing approaches can be used in research and practice to allow for work to be grounded in emancipatory action(s) and provide opportunity for increased athlete mental health.

Questions to Move the Field Forward

There remains much to be understood about how newcomers and host community members may be supported through a shared learning process (i.e., integration). The move to qualitative methodologies has brought about new knowledge that can provide transferable lessons for researchers and nonresearchers to learn from (Smith, 2018). With our belief that research should strive to bring about change to problems that face our community (at any level), the following five *unknown questions* provide guidance that we propose further this aim.

1. Theoretical Question: How Have Diverse Identities Been Accounted for Within Emerging Scholarship and How Might These Theoretical Orientations Be Expanded?

Feminist scholars in the early 1990s (e.g., Oglesby, 1993) began to voice their concern over the aim of many sport psychology researchers to find universal and objective laws that determined what "normal" was. Similarly, Duda and Allison (1990) cited an increasingly diverse community as a reason for researchers to begin to consider race and ethnicity as variables within their research. While progress has been made in bringing attention to the limitations of searching for universal theories, scholars need to continue to strive to work within multicultural frameworks that recognize the presence of multiple, intersecting identities and how these are impacted by power relations so that we may move forward to a more socially just manner of conducting sport (Gill, 2017). For example, working from an intersectional lens allows athletes' identities to be explored and understood as multiple, fluid, ever-changing, and not limited to success as an athlete, helping to ensure their mental health and holistic development (Schinke et al., 2017).

One common way that researchers have worked to understand athletes' identities has been through listening to and analyzing athletes' lives through the stories that they tell (Douglas, 2009). Using qualitative data collection methods intended to empower athletes to tell stories that are meaningful to them (e.g., arts-based methods) allows researchers to remain sensitive to the uniqueness of each individual story. However, the next step is to explore how researchers wishing to use quantitative methodologies can move beyond merely including certain variables at a surface level. One manner may be through conducting multistage research projects where in-depth qualitative methods with a smaller sample of athletes inform the variables used in the quantitative methods employed with a larger group of athletes. However, how these research methodologies and their underlying assumptions come together to deepen our theoretical understanding of the unique identities of the athletes we work with remains largely unexplored.

2. Methodological Question: How Have Researchers Accounted for Their Subjective Positions Within the Research Process and How Might These Methods Be Expanded to Augment Research Through Properly Executed Reflective and Reflexive Practice?

Concurrent to the broadening of research to include athletes' diverse identities is the critique of researchers working under the assumption that they can deliver objective, valid, and reliable accounts of the research participants they work with (Denzin, 2017). Qualitative researchers, who have been at the forefront of acknowledging their subjective position in relation to work they conduct, have begun to generally choose to engage in either reflective or reflexive practice, two terms that are often conflated (D'Cruz et al., 2007). Reflective practice is when a researcher develops an awareness of their own position in relation to gender, age, sexual orientation, and past personal experiences (among others) but does not assume that these impact the knowledge generated through the research process, merely their interpretation of that knowledge (D'Cruz et al., 2007). Reflexivity moves beyond the development of reflective practice to recognizing one's role in the co-construction of knowledge through the choices one makes during the research process (Schinke et al., 2012).

Generally, researchers have begun to situate themselves within their manuscript by including a section in which they provide brief, relevant details about themselves in relation to the research that was conducted. More recently, some researchers have begun to expand on reflexive approaches by including themselves within the stories that they share to bring to light their role in the co-construction of knowledge (i.e., authorial presence; Seoane & Hundt, 2018). Both reflective and reflexive practice can enhance our ability to bring about cultural understanding within sport, but this is still a relatively new progression in research, as evidenced by the continuing conflation of terms. Researchers should be encouraged to continue developing their ability to understand the role they play throughout their research so that they may critically analyze the information that is shared with them.

3. Methodological Question: What Can We Learn From Indigenous Decolonizing Research Practices and How Can These Be Transferred to Research Conducted Within the Sport Context?

One way in which researchers can ensure that the knowledge produced by their research will be meaningful to those they work with is to engage in decolonizing research practices. Stemming from work by Indigenous researchers such as Linda Tuhiwai Smith, a prominent Maori scholar, decolonizing research practices aim to move knowledge production beyond academic boundaries (Smith, 2012). These research practices were developed in response to Indigenous people's mistrust of researchers, as historically they were White, male researchers who came into Indigenous communities, gathered information they deemed valuable, and then disappeared. One form of research methodology that has developed from this desire to decolonize the research process is community-based participatory action research (CBPAR). This methodology calls for the academic researchers to reflexively work to shift power to community members throughout the research process from beginning to end, with the aim of generating knowledge in a collaborative manner (Kral, 2014). Schinke, Middleton, and colleagues (2019) described a project conducted with a Canadian Indigenous tribe to explore how community sport programming on their reserve may become more culturally sensitive. By working to include community members throughout the research process, the project resulted in generating meaningful answers to community-generated research questions, in turn leading to successful sport programs that have continued on past academic involvement. While this research project provides insight into how research may be decolonized to become culturally relevant to those we work with, there remain questions as to how this approach may translate to work with newcomer populations. While certain lessons such as building community capacity through the inclusion of community members in the research team have been adopted, ensuring that the research process continues to centralize community members is an ongoing and dynamic process (Schinke, Middleton, et al., 2019). The dynamic nature of the process entails researchers continuously work to understand who they are, what their intentions are and develop their ability to work with the communities that they become immersed in (Smith et al., 2019). There remains much to be learned from Indigenous researchers and much left to be understood about how the research process can further become decolonized.

4. Applied Question: How Can We Ensure That Findings Are Relevant for Those Working in the Field With Newcomers and Relevant to Differing Communities? How Can We Make Our Findings Concrete Rather Than Vague and Inaccessible?

Chirkov (2009) contended that researchers' overarching aim of finding generalizable results related to the process of acculturation through the use of quantitative methods did not translate into the production of useful knowledge for culturally diverse populations navigating unique acculturative journeys. Some researchers have responded to such criticism by employing qualitative methodologies with the aim of understanding the unique and detailed life stories told by newcomers (e.g., life story approaches; Ryba et al., 2016). Schinke, Middleton, and colleagues (2019) advocated for qualitative methodologies to be used by those working with immigrant athletes, as they allowed researchers to develop and demonstrate a genuine interest in learning about the immigrant athletes' home cultures, helping to build trust and aid in the acculturation process. However, qualitative research approaches lack generalizability as understood by researchers who work within a realist, positivist standpoint and are more comfortable with an objective, statistical-probabilistic generalizability approach (Smith, 2018). Nonetheless, this does not mean that qualitative findings cannot be generalized. For example, some qualitative researchers have strived for naturalistic generalizability, where the aim is to help readers recognize similarities and/

or differences between the research and their lives. This can be done by using techniques such as creating short videos and songs (e.g., Douglas & Carless, 2017) and composite storying methods such as vignettes (e.g., Schinke et al., 2016) and moving stories (e.g., Middleton et al., 2020) to represent data in a way that resonates more with the reader (Smith, 2018).

We propose that researchers continue to strive to use different data representation techniques that resonate with the audiences they aim to interact with, as these may also enhance the inferential generalizability (i.e., transferability) of research findings. As Smith (2018) outlined, for researchers whose work is underpinned by epistemological assumptions that there are multiple realities that are constructed and subjective in nature, generalizability does not necessitate that contexts be congruent, but rather that those reading a report feel that what they have learned may transfer to their own situation. To further make research findings accessible, we propose that researchers look to create partnerships with local organizations and create social media platforms from which knowledge may be disseminated to a nonacademic audience, in particular those individuals working with newcomer athletes. For example, the authors of this chapter have collaborated with a community agency to create a Facebook page dedicated to their work with newcomer youth athletes in their community (https://www.facebook.com/Activitypageforforcedimmigrantyouth). However, just as with the development of knowledge in relation to acculturation, methods of data representation and dissemination continue to develop. We encourage researchers to continue to push the boundaries in relation to making research relevant and accessible to those they work with, while remaining committed to grounding their work in the stories told by their research participants and broader findings shared by the research community. Researchers should also strive to be transparent and clear in the strengths and limitations of conducting qualitative research.

5. Applied Question: How Can We Engage in Context-Driven Practice With Sport Participants From a Specific Cultural Background, and How Might Such Approaches Transfer Into Work With Sport Participants From Other Cultural Backgrounds?

Context-driven practice entails informing and developing one's practice through immersing oneself, and reflecting upon, "relevant cultural/

sub-cultural contexts when planning and implementing sport and exercise psychology interventions" (Stambulova & Schinke, 2017, p. 131). One way that researchers and practitioners may engage in context-driven practice is through self-reflexivity (further detailed earlier in question 2; Schinke et al., 2012). Employing reflexive strategies can help ensure that understanding the differences between one's own cultural background and that of the sport participants one works with come to the fore. Reflexivity, in contrast to re-flection, involves drawing attention to power issues within relationships and continuously examining these prior to, during, and following interactions with athletes (Schinke et al., 2012). The constant awareness and apprecia-tion of our differences relative to the athletes we work with can help reposi-tion athletes as coparticipants in a shared learning process. This may require researchers and practitioners to engage in practices that may be uncomfort-able for them. For Thierry, one such situation was relinquishing control over a planned individual interview process during his work with refugee youth sport participants (see Schinke, Middleton, et al., 2019). Recognizing that the refugee youth and their families were the experts of their own stories, Thierry readily accepted the families' invitations to conduct the interviews within their homes. Each interview was conducted with family members present and accompanied by coffee and a variety of food dishes, many of which he had not tasted before. Conducting interviews in this way allowed him to learn more about the cultural backgrounds of the youth he was working with than if the interviews had been conducted in an academic of-fice setting. This was particularly impactful on helping Thierry appreciate the importance that family played in the lives of refugee youth. Engaging in context-driven practices such as sharing a meal can be beneficial for both athletes and consultants, as it can help consultants make their interventions more efficient, reduce their work stress, and increase their job satisfaction, while acknowledging the complex identities of athletes (Stambulova & Schinke, 2017). Learning from athletes from one cultural background may not necessarily directly relate to the understanding of athletes from other cultural backgrounds; however, this learning process can help consultants develop their ability to engage in reflective/reflexive practices, become more open to different ways of thinking and more comfortable in being uncom-fortable by acknowledging that they do not always have an immediate right answer. Although developing a diverse cultural skill set may be challenging, it will allow consultants to better deliver context-relevant and effective interventions for the athletes they work with.

Conclusion

Our aim in this chapter has been to highlight five unknowns related to cultural, cross-cultural, and intercultural issues in sport. The first of these is the need for further theoretical frameworks that enable researchers to recognize and explore the impact of athletes' multiple, intersecting identities. One proposal is for an exploration of how quantitative and qualitative methods may provide complementary knowledge in research examining how appreciating and empowering of athletes' diverse identities may contribute to their holistic development. Second, recognizing that researchers and practitioners also have diverse life stories, we encourage them to undertake a reflective/reflexive approach to understanding their position in relation to the athletes they are working with so that cultural differences may be acknowledged and brought to the fore through discussion. Third, conducting research in a reflexive manner can aid researchers in ensuring that their work is meaningful to the athletes they work with, which, fourth, may require researchers to critically interrogate how they represent their findings in a manner that is relevant and accessible to the athletes they work with. Presenting these methods in a transparent manner will help qualitative sport and exercise psychology researchers continue to develop innovative representation methods. Finally, ensuring that our work is grounded in the needs and desires of the athlete requires engaging in context-driven practices. Developing the skills needed to work with athletes from diverse cultural backgrounds in a reflexive and contextually-driven manner can help reposition the athletes we work with as partners in the research process. This is important as it recognizes athletes as experts of their own needs and desires, which should be a key determinant of the foci and approaches to research. Following the theme of the book, we encourage researchers and practitioners to take the unknowns we have posed as a starting point as they transfer our suggestions to their own practice and research. We look forward to the development and sharing of new creative methods through which we may best learn from those we work with.

References

Agergaard, S. (2017). Learning in landscapes of professional sports: Transnational perspectives on talent development and migration into Danish women's handball around the time of the financial crisis, 2004–2012. *Sport in Society, 20*, 1457–1469. http://dx.doi.org/10.1080/17430437.2016.1221068

Berry, J. W. (2005). Acculturation: Living successfully in two cultures. *International Journal of Intercultural Relations, 29,* 697–712 http://dx.doi.org/10.1016/j.ijintrel.2005.07.013

Berry, J. W., & Hou, F. (2016). Immigrant acculturation and wellbeing in Canada. *Canadian Psychology, 57,* 254–264. http://dx.doi.org/10.1037/cap0000064

Burrman, U., Brandmann, K., Mutz, M., & Zender, U. (2017). Ethnic identities, sense of belonging and the significance of sport: Stories from immigrant youths in Germany. *European Journal for Sport and Society, 14,* 184–204. http://dx.doi.org/10.1080/16138171.2017.1349643

Canadian Council for Refugees (CCR). (2010). *Refugees and immigrants: A glossary.* https://ccrweb.ca/en/glossary

Chirkov, V. (2009). Critical psychology of acculturation: What do we study and how do we study it, when we investigate acculturation? *International Journal of Intercultural Relations, 33,* 94–105. http://dx.doi.org/10.1016/j.ijintrel.2008.12.004

D'Cruz, H., Gillingham, P., & Melendez, S. (2007). Reflexivity, its meanings and relevance for social work: A critical review of the literature. *British Journal of Social Work, 37,* 73–90. http://dx.doi.org/10.1093/bjsw/bc1001

Denzin, N. K. (2017). Critical qualitative inquiry. *Qualitative Inquiry, 23,* 8–16. http://dx.doi.org/10.1177/1077800416681864

Dewar, A., & Horn, T. S. (1992). A critical analysis of knowledge construction in sport psychology. In T. S. Horn (Ed.), *Advances in sport psychology* (pp. 12–22). Human Kinetics.

Douglas, K. (2009). Storying myself: Negotiating a relational identity in professional sport. *Qualitative Research in Sport and Exercise, 1*(2), 176–190. https://doi.org/1080/19398440902909033

Douglas, K., & Carless, D. (2017, August 1). *We crossed the Tamar* [Video]. YouTube. https://www.youtube.com/watch?v=R4EGRN_bIw8

Duda, J. L., & Allison, M. T. (1990). Cross-cultural analysis in exercise and sport psychology: A void in the field. *Journal of Sport and Exercise Psychology, 12,* 114–131. http://dx.doi.org/10.1123/jsep.12.2.114

Elbe, A-M., Hatzigeorgiadis, A., Morela, E., Ries, F., Kouli, O., & Sanchez, X. (2018). Acculturation through sport: Different contexts different meanings. *International Journal of Sport and Exercise Psychology, 2,* 178–190. http://dx.doi.org/10.1080/1612197X.2016.1187654

European Commission. (2007). *White paper on sport.* https://eur-lex.europa.eu/legal-content/EN/TXT/?uri=celex:52007DC0391

Gill, D. L. (2017). Gender and cultural diversity in sport, exercise, and performance psychology. *Oxford Research Encyclopedia of Psychology.* http://dx.doi.org/10.1093/acrefore/9780190236557.013.148

Hatzigeorgiadis, A., Morela, E., Elbe, M. A., Kouli, O., & Sanchez, X. (2013). The integrative role of sport in multicultural societies. *European Psychologist, 18,* 191–202. http://dx.doi.org/10.1027/1016-9040/a000155

Jeanes, R., O'Connor, J., & Alfrey, L. (2015). Sport and the resettlement of young people from refugee backgrounds in Australia. *Journal of Sport and Social Issues, 39,* 480–500. http://dx.doi.org/10.1177/0193723514558929

Kral, M. J. (2014). The relational motif in participatory qualitative research. *Qualitative Inquiry, 20,* 144–150. http://dx.doi/org/10.1177/1077800413510871

Middleton, T. R. F., Schinke, R. J., Oghene, O. P., McGannon, K. R., Petersen, B., & Kao, S. (2020). Navigating times of harmony and discord: The ever-changing role played by the families of elite immigrant athletes during their acculturation. *Sport, Exercise, and Performance Psychology*, 9(1), 58–72. http://dx.doi.org/10.1037/spy0000171

Morela, E., Hatzigeorgiadis, A., Sanchez, X., Papaioannou, A., & Elbe, A-M. (2017). Empowering youth sport and acculturation: Examining the hosts' perspective in Greek adolescents. *Psychology of Sport and Exercise, 30*, 226–235. http://dx.doi.org/10.1016/j.psychsport.2017.03.007

Oglesby, C. A. (1993). Changed or different times – what's happening with "women's ways" of sport? *Journal of Physical education, Recreation, & Dance, 64*, 60–62. http://dx.doi.org/10.1080/07303084.1993.10606732

Provincial/Territorial Governments of Canada. (2012). *Canadian sport policy 2012.* https://canadiansporttourism.com/sites/default/files/docs/csp2012_en_lr.pdf

Ronkainen, N. J., Khomutova, A., & Ryba, T. V. (2019). "If my family is okay, I'm okay": Exploring relational processes of cultural transition. *International Journal of Sport and Exercise Psychology, 17*, 493–508. http://dx.doi.org/10.1080/1612197X.2017.1390485

Roper, E. A. (2016). Cultural studies in sport and exercise psychology. In R. J. Schinke, K. R. McGannon, & B. Smith (Eds.), *Routledge international handbook of sport psychology* (pp. 272–285). Routledge.

Ryba, T. V., Schinke, R. J., Stambulova, N. B., & Elbe, A-M. (2018). ISSP position stand: Transnationalism, mobility, and acculturation in and through sport. *International Journal of Sport and Exercise Psychology, 5*, 520–534. http://dx.doi.org/10.1080/1612197X.2017.1280836

Ryba, T. V., Stambulova, N. B., & Ronkainen, N. J. (2016). The work of cultural transition: An emerging model. *Frontiers in Psychology, 7*, 1–13. http://dx.doi.org/10.3389/fpsyg.2016.00427

Schinke, R. J., Blodgett, A. T., McGannon, K. R., & Ge, Y. (2016). Finding one's footing on foreign soil: A composite vignette of elite athlete acculturation. *Psychology of Sport and Exercise, 25*, 36–43. http://dx.doi.org/10.1016/j.psychsport.2016.04.001

Schinke, R. J., Blodgett, A. T., Ryba, T. V., Kao, S. F., & Middleton, T. R. F. (2019). Cultural sport psychology as a pathway to advances in identity and settlement research to practice. *Psychology of Sport and Exercise, 42*, 58–65. http://dx.doi.org/10.1016/j.psychsport.2018.09.004

Schinke, R. J., McGannon, K. R., Parham, W. D., & Lane, A. M. (2012). Toward cultural praxis and cultural sensitivity: Strategies for self-reflexive sport psychology practice. *Quest, 64*, 34–46. http://dx.doi.org/10.1080/00336297.2012.653264

Schinke, R. J., Middleton, T., Petersen, B., Kao, S., Lefebvre, D., & Habra, B. (2019). Social justice in sport and exercise psychology: A position statement. *Quest, 71*, 163–174. http://dx.doi.org/10.1080/00336297.2018.1544572

Schinke, R. J., Stambulova, N. B., Si. G., & Moore, Z. (2017). International society of sport psychology position stand: Athletes' mental health, performance, and development. *International Journal of Sport and Exercise Psychology, 16*(6), 622–639. http://dx.doi.org/10.1080/1612197X.2017.1295557

Seoane, E., & Hundt, M. (2018). Voice alternation and authorial presence: Variation across disciplinary areas in academic English. *Journal of English Linguistics, 46*, 3–22. http://dx.doi.org/10.1177/0075424217740938

Smith, B. (2018). Generalizability in qualitative research: Misunderstandings, opportunities, and recommendations for the sport and exercise science. *Qualitative*

Research in Sport, Exercise, and Health, 10, 137–149. http://dx.doi.org/10.1080/2159676X.2017.1393221

Smith, L. T. (2012). *Decolonizing methodologies: Research and Indigenous peoples* (2nd ed.). Otago University Press.

Smith, L. T., Tuck, E., & Yang, K. W. (2019). Introduction. In L. T. Smith, E. Tuck, & K. W. Yang (Eds.), *Indigenous and decolonizing studies in education: Mapping the long view* (pp. 1–23). Routledge.

Stambulova, N. B., & Schinke, R. J. (2017). Experts focus on the context: Postulates derived from the authors' shared experiences and wisdom. *Journal of Sport Psychology in Action, 8,* 131–134. http://dx.doi.org/10.1080/21520704.2017.1208715

25

Supervision

David Tod, Martin Eubank, Hayley E. McEwan,
Charlotte Chandler, and Moira Lafferty

Trainee sport psychologists often display anxieties about their initial attempts to help clients. They appreciate support from their supervisors. Equally, supervisors sometimes question their abilities to help trainees, and they may search the literature, hoping to find direction from the discipline's bank of knowledge. Some supervisors realize, however, that they need to expand their search into related disciplines, such as counseling and clinical psychology. Although counseling and clinical psychologists have a long history of discussing supervision, their sporting brethren are still becoming familiar with the topic and still grappling with how to translate the knowledge into practice. The first sport-related articles on supervision appeared in the mid-1990s (e.g., Andersen, 1994; Andersen et al., 1994), but they did not trigger research programs on the topic. Additional research will help individuals learn to supervise practitioners stepping into service delivery.

Supervision involves an interpersonal relationship in which supervisors help supervisees examine their perceptions, thoughts, feelings, and behaviors about their client interactions to achieve desirable outcomes (Van Raalte & Andersen, 2000). Primary outcomes include safeguarding clients' welfare; ensuring athletes receive effective and ethical services; and helping supervisees develop as humane, skillful, informed, and self-aware practitioners. In this chapter, we review existing research and propose avenues to advance knowledge, allowing professionals in the discipline to address challenges within supervision.

State of the Art

The earliest discussion on supervision appears to be a presentation at the 1992 Association for Applied Sport Psychology conference (Carr et al.,

David Tod, Martin Eubank, Hayley E. McEwan, Charlotte Chandler, and Moira Lafferty, *Supervision* In: *Sport, Exercise and Performance Psychology.* Edited by: Edson Filho and Itay Basevitch, Oxford University Press. © Oxford University Press 2021. DOI: 10.1093/oso/9780197512494.003.0025

1992). Andersen and his colleagues published the initial empirical and theoretical articles on supervision in sport psychology (e.g., Andersen, 1994; Andersen et al., 1994). Since these seminal articles, researchers have seldom positioned supervision as the primary focus of their investigations. Instead, supervision is typically a side dish to the main meal and appears in studies focused on topics such as trainee learning experiences (Tod et al., 2007), ethics (Etzel et al., 2004), practitioner development (McEwan et al., 2019), and career outcomes (Fitzpatrick et al., 2016). Table 25.1 presents five studies in which supervision was the main meal, and these investigations represent the major topics researchers have focused on.

The studies in Table 25.1 illustrate the breadth of the area researchers have explored. They have provided data on the types and amount of supervision occurring in the field (e.g., Watson et al., 2004), although given the age of these studies, the information is now likely outdated. Investigators have explored trainees', practitioners', and supervisors' perceptions and experiences related to supervision (Fogaca et al., 2018; Foltz et al., 2015; Sharp et al., 2021). Also, researchers have identified what trainees wish to learn in supervision (Hutter et al., 2015). When reviewing these studies with a primary focus on supervision, several key observations emerge.

There are few studies on any one topic, knowledge is fragmented, and many gaps exist across the terrain. For example, prevailing studies typically focus on the supervision of trainee sport psychologists. Such dyads have an inherent power imbalance, because the supervisor is typically an experienced and qualified practitioner, who is evaluating the supervisee's competence and acting as a gatekeeper to practice. Different types of relationships exist in supervision. Peer consultation is another type of relationship, involving colleagues of equal standing. Meta-supervision is a relationship where an individual supervises another person supervising a practitioner (Barney & Andersen, 2014a). Investigations on peer consultation and meta-supervision are lacking, but if conducted they would help guide practice.

More broadly, there is much scope for explorers to open up the supervision territory and stake a claim. The existing discipline-specific knowledge often rests on single studies, limiting our confidence in the transferability, credibility, and robustness of what we believe we know. We lack answers to many descriptive questions, such as what supervision is happening? Who is supervising and who is supervised? Why do people engage with or avoid supervision? When is supervision most likely to happen? How do people learn to supervise? What occurs during effective and healthy supervision?

Without a clear picture of the supervision that happens in the field, professionals need to draw on literature and research external to the discipline to advance theory and practice. Some professionals have drawn on counselor supervision and development theory to inform their research and help them suggest applied implications (Fogaca et al., 2018; McEwan et al., 2019). To date, sport psychologists have drawn primarily on Rønnestad and Skovholt's (2013) and Stoltenberg's (Stoltenberg & McNeill, 2009) theories when researching and discussing practitioner development and supervision. Evidence supports parallels between these counselor supervision and development theories and the findings on how sport psychologists mature and evolve (e.g., McEwan et al., 2019; Tod et al., 2011). Counselor psychologist supervision and development theories (and those from other helping professions) can enlighten sport psychology research and literature but best serve as a starting point because they are not tailored towards understanding the journey of the sport psychologist. For example, they do not document the specific demands that sport psychologists face as trainees or autonomous practitioners. Discipline-specific studies will uncover the contexts and cultures shaping supervision in sport psychology and represent an avenue of work that can lead to concrete and specific applied implications.

Supervision has emerged, however, as a theme in research focused on other topics. The most visible body of related work in which the topic arises is practitioner development. Practitioners, for example, rate supervision as one of the most influential learning activities in their growth as sport psychologists (McEwan & Tod, 2015; Tod et al., 2007). Longitudinal studies reveal ways in which supervision contributes to consultants moving from being practitioner-led problem solvers to client-led collaborators (McEwan et al., 2019; Tod et al., 2011).

Despite the lack of research, professionals have not ignored supervision completely. Authors have written opinion pieces, reflective articles, review papers, and case studies addressing topics such as challenges, benefits, and logistics associated with supervision (Van Raalte & Andersen, 2000). In recent years, reflective articles have discussed the role of mindfulness in enhancing the supervision relationship (Andersen et al., 2016; Barney & Andersen, 2014b). Nevertheless, researchers need to answer many questions before a complete understanding of supervision emerges that is grounded in empirical data.

Table 25.1 Five Key Readings on Supervision in Sports

Authors	Methodological Design	Key Findings
Fogaca et al. (2018)	Mixed-method study of nine supervision dyads involving the Consulting Skills Inventory, semistructured interviews, and reflective journals	• Supervisees' growth occurred when supervision involved regular meetings, close relationships, feedback, opportunities for trainee self-reflection, and supervisors adapting their guidance to students' developmental levels. • Supervisee background (e.g., knowledge, education, and previous experience) and the placement context (e.g., client variety, number, and interactions, and intern structure) also influence supervisee growth.
Foltz et al. (2015)	Qualitative analysis of semistructured interviews with nine trainee sport psychologists about their supervision experiences	• Data clustered into domains on *program factors*, *supervision process*, and *supervision content*. • Program factors described elements shaping supervision experience such as structure of supervision, modalities of delivery, inclusion of multiple perspectives, and the lack of an articulated model of supervision. • Supervision process reflected aspects of the supervisory relationship contributing to a positive and effective experience, including desired supervisor qualities, development of trust, receiving guidance, and collaboration. • Supervision content reflected factors needing to be addressed in supervision and included boundaries and roles, ethical and clinical competency, operating within sport environments, performance and mental health issues, and multiculturally relevant supervision.
Hutter et al. (2015)	Content analysis of the central issue 14 trainee sport psychologists wished to address, as self-reported in written supervision preparation assessments	• The two higher themes were *know-how* and *professional development*. • Know-how focused on learning how to act, with lower order themes related to (a) intake, (b) treatment planning, and (c) execution of interventions, evaluation, and termination. • Professional development focused on trainees' growth as practitioners, with lower order themes related to self-reflections, working principles, and coping with dilemmas.

Continued

Table 25.1 *Continued*

Authors	Methodological Design	Key Findings
Sharp et al. (2021)	Qualitative analysis of semistructured interviews with 10 experienced sport psychologists about the ethical challenges they have experienced and their engagement with supervision	• Practitioners believed that supervision is essential. • Supervision enabled consultants to monitor boundaries. • Supervision helped practitioners feel supported. • Supervision helped consultants get to know and care for themselves.
Watson et al. (2004)	Quantitative survey of 171 professional and 142 student members of the Association for Applied Sport Psychology, using a self-generated inventory	• A greater proportion of students received supervision than professionals (and received weekly supervision). • A greater proportion of students received supervision about program design and delivery than professionals. • The majority of professional members were not providing supervision and had received no training in supervision. • A minority of professionals received supervision, with no licensed certified individuals being supervised. • No differences emerged between sport science-based and psychology-based participants on supervision amount, frequency, or content.

Questions to Move the Field Forward

1. Theoretical and Applied Question: What Are the Amounts and Types of Supervision Practitioners Receive?

Professional bodies, such as the Association for Applied Sport Psychology (AASP, in the United States), the British Psychological Society (BPS, in the United Kingdom), and the Australian Psychological Society (APS, in Australia), prescribe the minimum hours and types of applied work and supervision students must achieve for certification or registration. The community, however, does not know if these requirements are being achieved or the quality of the contact. Some investigators have examined these questions when exploring sport psychology graduates' early career plans and outcomes, but these studies are largely dated (Andersen et al., 1997; Fitzpatrick et al., 2016; Williams & Scherzer, 2003). Understanding current supervision practices and graduates' career outcomes will help researchers to build theories that provide an accurate picture of the current supervision landscape and will help professional bodies and educators design and deliver supervisor training effectively.

Investigators could use quantitative surveys to describe the amount and types of current supervision practices and compare results against prescribed standards. Reliable surveys will emerge if professional bodies and universities collaborate to avoid errors associated with surveys. For example, education providers could detail the number and types of individuals enrolling and completing postgraduate qualifications leading to registration or certification. These data will define the population of trainees to help eschew coverage, sampling, and nonresponse errors (Ponto, 2015). In countries where professional bodies accredit or oversee the quality of education programs, communities could standardize data collection methods to evade measurement errors that erode confidence when pooling data from different training providers.

To complement these surveys, investigators can examine participants' experiences of supervision. Both quantitative and qualitative studies are relevant. Qualitative work could examine how people perceive, interpret, and structure their supervision experiences. Quantitative studies could explore the frequency of participants' perceptions and interpretations, along with identifying correlates. For example, investigators could assess if a greater proportion of neophyte trainees prefer supervisors to provide direct guidance than their advanced comrades. Further, researchers could also check if preferences for supervisor behavior correlate or predict trainees' levels of anxiety and confidence. These specific suggestions speak to models of supervision, another area where research will advance knowledge.

2. Theoretical and Applied Question: What Are the Optimal Ways to Match Models of Supervision With Trainees' Development Needs?

Supervisors can draw from several models to tailor their assistance towards supervisees' needs (Van Raalte & Andersen, 2000). Examples include behavioral, cognitive behavioral, phenomenological, psychodynamic, and developmental models. Beginning trainees may benefit from behavioral models, because the focus is on skill development and supervisors offer direct answers to specific questions. Seasoned practitioners may profit from phenomenological or psychodynamic models where the emphasis is on inter- and intrapersonal dynamics and supervisors collaborate with supervisees to explore issues arising in client sessions (Van Raalte & Andersen, 2000). Researchers have not explored, however, these conjectures in sport and exercise psychology contexts or even if supervisors are aware of supervision models.

These conjectures assume that learning to help clients begins with mastering communication skills before gaining insights into relationships and human interactions. Skills and insights, however, are intertwined. For example, insights about human interaction inform decisions about how to apply particular communication skills. Numerous communication skills exist, and relationships involve an endless variety of interactions. Both trainees' and autonomous practitioners' competencies in these numerous communication skills vary considerably, along with their abilities to interpret interactions with clients. Rather than stating that behavioral models suit trainees or that psychodynamic theories suit seasoned practitioners, a helpful suggestion is for supervisors to recognize the trainees' current needs, strengths, and situations before tailoring any guidance to ensure it is effective. This suggestion assumes supervisors can tailor their assistance and they have developed the competence to do so. The sport psychology literature does not contain evidence to help people decide when to apply, or move among, specific supervision models. Researchers who examine the role of supervision models in sport and exercise psychology will help stimulate the development of theories tailored to the discipline and provide data to ensure that applied practice is based on a solid foundation of evidence.

Longitudinal qualitative case studies describing supervision will allow for evidence-based decision-making. Researchers conducting longitudinal case studies will explore how supervisor skills and attributes, such as flexibility, humility, and ability to manage power, enhance trainee growth. The contributions that longitudinal case studies yield will be proportional to the extent they provide rich description of the supervision dyads examined. Fogaca and colleagues' (2018) longitudinal mixed-method study of nine supervision dyads illustrates the type of investigation that can advance theory. They employed interviews, participant diaries, and a quantitative inventory, and they were able to propose a theoretical understanding of supervision grounded in data. Researchers who provide rich and evocative descriptions will enhance the transferability of knowledge in ways that allow readers to reflect on their circumstances and theorists to paint comprehensive landscapes. Detailed maps of supervision will serve well those mentors wishing to learn how to guide their protégés and those professional bodies wanting to design supervisor training curricula.

3. Applied Question: How Can Educators Train Supervisors Effectively?

Few countries have formal training pathways for sport psychology supervisors, and currently most trainee education rests on the implicit assumption that qualified practitioners make suitable supervisors. Just as elite athletes do not always make helpful coaches, effective sport psychologists may not be useful or constructive supervisors. Some practitioners will be outstanding supervisors, whereas others will need support and training to gain supervision skills and knowledge. Research focused on how to prepare supervisors optimally will contribute to applied psychoeducational interventions or training programs that enhance the quality and effectiveness of supervision.

Supervisor training will yield individuals capable of establishing, maintaining, repairing, and terminating relationships with trainees. Various challenges exist that individuals need to navigate to ensure trainees benefit from supervision. Examples of these challenges include determining the fit between trainee and supervisor; the handling of personal and ethical boundaries; the cost of the supervisor's time and help; the frequency, duration, mode, and content of supervision meetings; and the way supervisors and supervisees handle disagreements.

Although professionals have not examined sport psychology supervisor training, research exists in related fields, such as clinical psychology, counseling, teaching, and coaching. An initial port of call for sport psychology researchers may be to conduct systematic reviews of supervisor training in related fields. Systematic review methodology has diversified in recent years (Tod, 2019), and scope exists to examine the supervisor training literature from multiple perspectives. Reviews of the topic in other disciplines will help sport psychology investigators from digging ground others have already plowed (e.g., Wheeler & Richards, 2007). It may be possible to gather the fruit from seeds others have sown.

The yields from reviews of other disciplines will complement empirical studies of supervisor training. Action research designs (Coghlan & Brydon-Miller, 2014), for example, will advance knowledge but also assist practitioners, professional bodies, educators, and researchers in implementing and assessing principles, strategies, and programs associated with supervisor training. Participative action research designs allow for researchers, practitioners, and other stakeholders to collaborate, helping ensure that training programs fit well with local landscapes and that relevant people have faith in the interventions (e.g., that diversity is celebrated; Coghlan & Brydon-Miller, 2014).

4. Theoretical Question: What Are the Active Ingredients in Supervision?

Active ingredients are variables allowing people to benefit from helping relationships (Tod et al., 2019). Few researchers have examined factors ensuring trainees benefit from supervision (Fogaca et al., 2018). In light of the limited number of studies in the area, research on the active ingredients in supervision will fuel theory development. Also, professionals will profit in several ways from studies exploring the topic. Supervisors, for example, will gain insights into facilitating supervision relationships, so that trainees have opportunities to grow as practitioners. Professional bodies will be able to develop evidence-based policies, guidelines, and supervisor training pathways. The benefits practitioners and professional organizations accrue may foster high levels of supervision that underpin trainee and consultant growth, which may contribute to improved athlete-client outcomes and service delivery relationships.

Investigators can advance knowledge about the active ingredients in supervision by conducting quantitative experiments and qualitative studies underpinned by narrative analysis. Experiments, especially randomized controlled trials, will let researchers address the question "Which variables cause positive outcomes in supervision?" A dismantling study is a useful experiment to conduct. Dismantling studies help researchers assess which elements in a supervision package cause change (Behar & Borkovec, 2003). Investigators randomly assign some participants to receive all components in a supervision package, whereas other individuals receive only some components. A principal advantage is that researchers hold many variables constant across the conditions, and dismantling studies control threats to internal validity, such as maturation, repeated testing, and regression to the mean.

Investigations underpinned by narrative analysis will examine the stories people tell about supervision. Researchers will gather data about the content, structure, and performance of supervision stories. The data will document how participants interpret their supervision experiences and the influence of cultural and social scripts. Through narrative analysis, investigators will generate understanding about individuals' beliefs regarding the active ingredients in supervision and how their stories shape their future behaviors.

5. Applied Question: How Do Culture and Context Shape Supervision?

In the parlance of Bronfenbrenner's (1979) theory on ecological systems, the previous questions have focused on the microsystem in which trainees interact directly with their supervisors. The supervision relationship exists within a wider context (i.e., the macrosystem), which impinges on and colors the processes within it. Across the world, for example, in Australia, New Zealand, the United States, and the United Kingdom, there are different ways to achieving recognition as a psychologist (with or without an endorsement in sport psychology), certified mental performance consultant, or accredited sport and exercise scientist. Further, within some countries (e.g., the United Kingdom), there are multiple pathways to attaining professional recognition. These different pathways vary in their structure, content, delivery, supervision requirements, and minimum number of work-experience hours. While training pathways are designed to ensure that regulators' standards and competencies are met, researchers could examine if the variations across the pathways (e.g., supervised work-experience hours) are associated with the knowledge and skills graduates attain, their career outcomes, and client satisfaction. Research on this topic will lead to applied interventions or educational programs that prepare practitioners optimally for satisfying and meaningful careers.

Bronfenbrenner's (1979) macrosystem level indicates that social and cultural values influence a person's development. The cultures of the sports and education environments where trainees operate may shape their development and supervision experiences. Researchers who explore cultural and social variables associated with supervision will provide knowledge that contributes to supervisor training and helps trainees and supervisors manage any such influences. For example, by understanding their own ethical, ethnic, cultural, sexual, and gender biases and prejudices, both supervisors and supervisees can become aware of the lenses through which they experience supervision and client interactions.

Ethnographies can provide detailed knowledge about the contexts and cultures associated with supervision. Although ethnography is still an emerging research method in sport psychology, investigators have used it to explore practitioner development and identity (Champ et al., 2020). The long-term engagement associated with ethnography will likely contribute to the understanding of several of the aforementioned questions, and not just about the influence of culture and context. Equally, although we have tethered specific research methods to each of the five major questions included, our suggestions do not preclude investigators from matching study designs to questions in ways that suit their needs, circumstances, and philosophies (we do not wish to encourage methodolatry). The lion's share of the research on supervision has employed descriptive quantitative surveys and qualitative studies with a realist aroma. Investigators who adopted alternative methods, such as those presented earlier, will help build a broader and more detailed knowledge base than might otherwise result from reliance on just two designs.

Conclusion

The supervisor-supervisee relationship can be a rewarding vehicle to ride when running smoothly. Both parties can learn about themselves, about each other, and about how to help athletes. They can also find time to enjoy the scenery as they navigate the twists and turns in the road. If, however, the fan belt breaks, a tire blows out, or oil levels drop to critical, then the individuals can lose their way, their momentum, and their goodwill towards each other. When learning how to drive, maintain, or even restore a car, drivers can often locate help from a manual tailored to their vehicle. In comparison, few manuals on sport psychology supervision exist. Nevertheless, helpful studies have been published that shine their headlights on avenues of future research. We present some avenues that, if upgraded into highways, would allow trainees and their professional elders to access the larger supervision territory. Increased access to the territory would pave the way for a well-maintained supervision superhighway or autobahn. Sound running supervision will lead to trainees with the skills, insights, and competencies to assist clients and benefit the wider profession.

References

Andersen, M. B. (1994). Ethical considerations in the supervision of applied sport psychology graduate students. *Journal of Applied Sport Psychology, 6*, 152–167. doi:10.1080/10413209408406291

Andersen, M. B., Barney, S. T., & Waterson, A. K. (2016). Mindfully dynamic meta-supervision: The case of AW and M. In J. G. Cremades & L. S. Tashman (Eds.), *Global practices and training in applied sport, exercise, and performance psychology: A case study approach* (pp. 330–342). Routledge.

Andersen, M. B., Van Raalte, J. L., & Brewer, B. W. (1994). Assessing the skills of sport psychology supervisors. *The Sport Psychologist, 8*, 238–247. doi:10.1123/tsp.8.3.238

Andersen, M. B., Williams, J. M., Aldridge, T., & Taylor, J. (1997). Tracking the training and careers of graduates of advanced degree programs in sport psychology, 1989 to 1994. *The Sport Psychologist, 11*, 326–344. doi:10.1123/tsp.11.3.326

Barney, S. T., & Andersen, M. B. (2014a). Meta-supervision: Training practitioners to help others on their paths. In J. G. Cremades & L. S. Tashman (Eds.), *Becoming a sport, exercise, and performance psychology professional: A global perspective* (pp. 339–346). Psychology Press.

Barney, S. T., & Andersen, M. B. (2014b). Mindful supervision in sport and performance psychology: Building the quality of the supervisor-supervisee relationship. In Z. Knowles, D. Gilbourne, B. Cropley, & L. Dugdill (Eds.), *Reflective practice in sport and exercise sciences: Contemporary issues* (pp. 147–159). Routledge.

Behar, E. S., & Borkovec, T. D. (2003). Psychotherapy outcome research. In J. A. Schinka & W. F. Velicer (Eds.), *Handbook of psychology: Volume 2, Research methods in psychology* (pp. 213–240). Wiley.

Bronfenbrenner, U. (1979). *The ecology of human development: Experiments by nature and design.* Harvard University Press.

Carr, C. M., Murphy, S. M., & McCann, S. (1992, October). *Supervision issues in clinical sport psychology.* Paper presented at the annual conference of the Association for the Advancement of Sport Psychology, Colorado Springs, CO.

Champ, F., Ronkainen, N. J., Nesti, M. S., Tod, D., & Littlewood, M. A. (2020). "Through the lens of ethnography": Perceptions, challenges, and experiences of an early career practitioner-researcher in professional football. *Qualitative Research in Sport, Exercise and Health, 12*, 513–529. doi:10.1080/2159676X.2019.1638444

Coghlan, D., & Brydon-Miller, M. (2014). *The SAGE encyclopedia of action research.* Sage.

Etzel, E. F., Watson, J. C., II, & Zizzi, S. (2004). A web-based survey of AAASP members' ethical beliefs and behaviors in the new millennium. *Journal of Applied Sport Psychology, 16*, 236–250. doi:10.1080/10413200490485595

Fitzpatrick, S. J., Monda, S. J., & Wooding, C. B. (2016). Great expectations: Career planning and training experiences of graduate students in sport and exercise psychology. *Journal of Applied Sport Psychology, 28*, 14–27. doi:10.1080/10413200.2015.1052891

Fogaca, J. L., Zizzi, S. J., & Andersen, M. B. (2018). Walking multiple paths of supervision in American sport psychology: A qualitative tale of novice supervisees' development. *The Sport Psychologist, 32*, 156–165. doi:10.1123/tsp.2017-0048

Foltz, B. D., Fisher, A. R., Denton, L. K., Campbell, W. L., Speight, Q. L., Steinfeldt, J., & Latorre, C. (2015). Applied sport psychology supervision experience: A qualitative analysis. *Journal of Applied Sport Psychology, 27*, 449–463. doi:10.1080/10413200.2015.1043162

Hutter, R. I. V., Oldenhof-Veldman, T., & Oudejans, R. R. D. (2015). What trainee sport psychologists want to learn in supervision. *Psychology of Sport and Exercise, 16*, 101–109. doi:10.1016/j.psychsport.2014.08.003

McEwan, H. E., & Tod, D. (2015). Learning experiences contributing to service-delivery competence in applied psychologists: Lessons for sport psychologists. *Journal of Applied Sport Psychology, 27*, 79–93. doi:10.1080/10413200.2014.952460

McEwan, H. E., Tod, D., & Eubank, M. (2019). The rocky road to individuation: Sport psychologists' perspectives on professional development. *Psychology of Sport and Exercise, 45*, Article 101542. doi:10.1016/j.psychsport.2019.101542

Ponto, J. (2015). Understanding and evaluating survey research. *Journal of the Advanced Practitioner in Oncology, 6*, 168–171. doi:10.6004/jadpro.2015.6.2.9

Rønnestad, M. H., & Skovholt, T. M. (2013). *The developing practitioner: Growth and stagnation of therapists and counselors.* Routledge.

Sharp, L.-A., Hodge, K., & Danish, S. (2021). "I wouldn't want to operate without it": The ethical challenges faced by experienced sport psychology consultant's and their engagement with supervision. *Journal of Applied Sport Psychology, 33*, 259–279. doi:10.1080/10413200.2019.1646838

Stoltenberg, C. D., & McNeill, B. W. (2009). *IDM supervision: An integrative developmental model for supervising counselors and therapists* (3rd ed.). Routledge.

Tod, D. (2019). *Conducting systematic reviews in sport, exercise, and physical activity.* Palgrave Macmillan.

Tod, D., Andersen, M. B., & Marchant, D. B. (2011). Six years up: Applied sport psychologists surviving (and thriving) after graduation. *Journal of Applied Sport Psychology, 23*, 93–109. doi:10.1080/10413200.2010.534543

Tod, D., Hardy, J., Lavallee, D., Eubank, M., & Ronkainen, N. (2019). Practitioners' narratives regarding active ingredients in service delivery: Collaboration-based problem solving. *Psychology of Sport and Exercise, 43*, 350–358. doi:10.1016/j.psychsport.2019.04.009

Tod, D., Marchant, D., & Andersen, M. B. (2007). Learning experiences contributing to service-delivery competence. *The Sport Psychologist, 21*, 317–334. doi:10.1123/tsp.21.3.317

Van Raalte, J. L., & Andersen, M. B. (2000). Supervision I: From models to doing. In M. B. Andersen (Ed.), *Doing sport psychology* (pp. 153–165). Human Kinetics.

Watson, J. C., II, Zizzi, S. J., Etzel, E. F., & Lubker, J. R. (2004). Applied sport psychology supervision: A survey of students and professionals. *The Sport Psychologist, 18*, 415–429. doi:10.1123/tsp.18.4.415

Wheeler, S., & Richards, K. (2007). *The impact of clinical supervision on counsellors and therapists, their practice and their clients: A systematic review of the literature.* British Association for Counselling & Psychotherapy.

Williams, J. M., & Scherzer, C. B. (2003). Tracking the training and careers of graduates of advanced degree programs in sport psychology, 1994 to 1999. *Journal of Applied Sport Psychology, 15*, 335–353. doi:10.1080/10413200390238013

Afterword

Itay Basevitch and Edson Filho

Wow, what a process! We definitely enjoyed it—well, at least most of it! After more than 10 years from idea to conclusion, we finally made our dream a reality. We have gathered leading experts in various areas in the sport, exercise, and performance psychology domain to share their knowledge and thoughts about the most pressing questions that will help move the field forward and direct the interested readers to the state-of-the-art literature in the domain. One way to consider and use this book is as a database of the most important questions and literature outputs in the field. Essentially, this book is a primary source for scholars and researchers at various levels and an effective guide toward research endeavors.

First, a bit of statistics and numbers. There are 125 questions in the book. The largest number of questions are applied in nature, $N = 45$, followed by questions addressing theoretical underpinnings, $N = 34$, and questions focusing on measurement and methodological issues, $N = 21$. The additional questions have a dual focus, $N = 25$, combining two closely related research aspects (Figure A.1).

Furthermore, the book consists of 125 essential literature outputs, and the majority, 62%, have been published within the past 5 years (Figure A.2). The literature outputs are varied with 77 research articles and 48 review articles or book chapters (i.e., meta-analyses, systematic reviews, or narrative reviews), as illustrated in Figure A.3.

Similar to a dictionary being an encompassing source of words and their definitions (Hackfort et al., 2019), we view this book as a comprehensive source of topics with key questions and readings in the domain. This is the first edition and volume of the book, and although it includes some of the most important and researched areas in the domain, we recognize that there are many other areas that are missing such as imagery (Filgueiras et al., 2018) and motivation (Vasconcellos et al., 2020). We hope to edit future volumes that will include additional research topics. Additionally, because

Itay Basevitch and Edson Filho, *Afterword* In: *Sport, Exercise and Performance Psychology*. Edited by: Edson Filho and Itay Basevitch, Oxford University Press. © Oxford University Press 2021. DOI: 10.1093/oso/9780197512494.003.0026

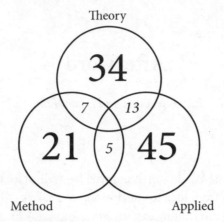

Figure A.1 Number of questions found in the book by question type (i.e., theory, applied, and/or method).

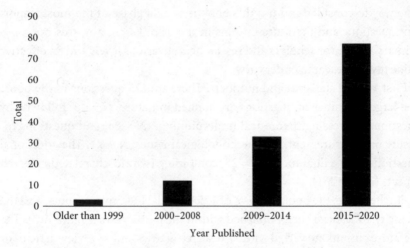

Figure A.2 Number of literature outputs found in the book by year published.

the domain is growing rapidly and new information is generated daily (Sly et al., 2020), revised editions of the topics will be updated periodically.

To do this we kindly ask you to keep us (and the chapter authors) updated with any new research findings and information related to each of the topics. It is our intention to have a parallel web-based platform (please visit http://bit.ly/SP-Book-Forumto access the online forum and start engaging with the community) that will enable communication among the authors, scholars, researchers, and readers on each topic for several purposes: (a) to ask the

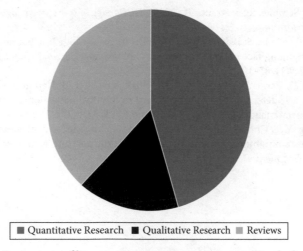

Figure A.3 Percentage of literature output types represented in the book.

authors questions about research in their expert topic area (e.g., what measurement tool should be used), (b) to discuss and share issues related to the topic area, (c) to update the authors when a research question has been addressed, and (d) to flag a research question that has yet to be addressed and is essential to move the field forward. We believe that there are many benefits of having both a book and a web-based platform, allowing readers to engage with the content of the chapters and with the authors as well, making the book a dynamic and interactive resource (Ye et al., 2015). We hope you take advantage of these features and we look forward to meeting you in the online forum.

Finally, whether you are a scholar, a researcher, an educator, a practitioner, or just a casual reader, we hope you enjoyed the structure and content of the book and found it beneficial for your purposes.

The important thing is not to stop questioning. Curiosity has its own reason for existing.

—Albert Einstein

References

Filgueiras, A., Conde, E. F. Q., & Hall, C. R. (2018). The neural basis of kinesthetic and visual imagery in sports: An ALE meta– analysis. *Brain Imaging and Behavior, 12*(5), 1513–1523.

Hackfort, D., Schinke, R., & Strauss, B. (2019). *Dictionary of sport psychology. Sport, exercise and performing arts*. Elsevier.

Sly, D., Mellalieu, S. D., & Wagstaff, C. R. (2020). "It's psychology Jim, but not as we know it!": The changing face of applied sport psychology. *Sport, Exercise, and Performance Psychology, 9*(1), 87–101.

Vasconcellos, D., Parker, P. D., Hilland, T., Cinelli, R., Owen, K. B., Kapsal, N., . . . Lonsdale, C. (2020). Self-determination theory applied to physical education: A systematic review and meta-analysis. *Journal of Educational Psychology, 112*(7), 1444.

Ye, H. J., Feng, Y., & Choi, B. C. (2015). Understanding knowledge contribution in online knowledge communities: A model of community support and forum leader support. *Electronic Commerce Research and Applications, 14*(1), 34–45.

Index

supervision
active ingredients in, 358–59
amounts of, 354–55
context and, 359–60
culture and, 359–60
key readings on, 353t
matching models to needs of
trainees, 355–57
outcomes of, 350
overview of, 350
state of the art on, 350–52
training of supervisors in, 357–58
types of, 351, 354–55
survey methods. *See also* Questionnaires
on doping, 314–15
sampling issues with, 327–28, 355
of SEPP practitioners, 327–28, 330
of youth, 259
Swann, C., 50t
synchronous communication, 171
SZOF (shared zones of optimal
functioning), 157

tai chi, 233–34
talent. *See also* Expert performance
athlete development and, 94–95
identification, ethics of, 99–100
nature *versus* nurture and, 92–93
predictions of, 94
Tanay, G., 224–25
targeting tasks, 23
task-specific knowledge, 105–6
team atmosphere, 313–14
team captains, 162
team cognition, 148, 153
team culture, 72–73, 166–67
teams. *See also* Group dynamics
attention in, 25–26, 28–29
characteristics of, 166–67
choking under pressure, 36, 40–41
cohesion in, 11, 151–53, 163
collective efficacy in, 6, 10–11
coordination in, 148, 155–56
decision-making in, 110–11
demographic factors, 110–11
diversity in, 151
gaze behavior in, 25–26

mental models in, 110–11, 148, 153
resilience of, 149, 154–55
roles within, 152
situational characteristics, 166–67
structure of, 152
teamwork
collective efficacy and, 11–12
meta-theoretical model, 148–49
promotion of, 162–63
technology
in communications, 171
exercise adherence and, 212–13
for mobile data collection, 27, 109–
10, 127
for neurophysiological measures, 27,
109–10, 127
smartphone apps and injuries, 299–301
use in studies of attention and
performance, 24, 27
Teixeira, P.J., 211t
Tenenbaum, G., 107t
tennis players, 81, 254
theory of implicit abilities, 258–59
theory of planned behavior, 244
"think aloud" technique, 41
Toner, J., 22t
TOPPS (Optimum Performance Program
in Sports), 180–81, 186–87
toughness, 82–83. *See also* Mental
toughness
training. *See also* Practice; Professional
training
adaptation, 136
evaluation, 64
genetic knowledge-based
personalization of, 139–40
individual responses to, 278–79
load, 278–79, 281–82, 287–88
maladaptive responses to, 278–79
overreach training (*see* Overtraining)
periodization, 139–40
recovery and, 281–82, 285, 287–88, 289
trait mindfulness, 223–26, 227–
30, 231–32
traits, 135, 136, 137
transactional leadership, 162–63, 165–66
transactive memory systems, 148